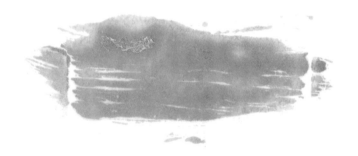

MANAGEMENT OF DISASTERS AND THEIR AFTERMATH

MANAGEMENT OF DISASTERS AND THEIR AFTERMATH

With experiences from

The M1 plane crash
The Manchester aircraft fire disaster
The Hillsborough football disaster
The Northern Ireland troubles
and other accidents

Edited by
W ANGUS WALLACE, FRCSEd FRCSEd(Orth)
Professor of Orthopaedic and Accident Surgery,
University Hospital, Queen's Medical Centre,
Nottingham, UK

JOHN M ROWLES, DM FRCS
NLDB Research Fellow,
Department of Orthopaedic and Accident Surgery,
University Hospital, Queen's Medical Centre,
Nottingham, UK

CHRISTOPHER L COLTON, FRCS FRCSEd(Orth)
Professor of Orthopaedic Surgery,
University Hospital, Queen's Medical Centre,
Nottingham, UK

BMJ
Publishing
Group

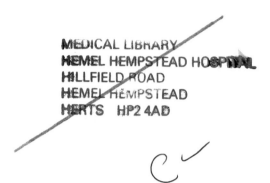
First published in 1994
by the BMJ Publishing Group, BMA House, Tavistock Square,
London WC1H 9JR

British Library Cataloguing in Publication Data

A catalogue record for this book is available
from the British Library

ISBN 0–7279–0841–3

Typeset, printed and bound in Great Britain by
Latimer Trend & Company Ltd., Estover, Plymouth

Contents

Preface

This book has been prepared following our experience in the East Midlands, and in particular in Nottingham, with dealing with the M1 aircraft accident in January 1989. Coping with the disaster was, for us, a new experience and we learned a number of lessons in the practical management of that major disaster which we felt many doctors, nurses, hospital managers, and health authority planners might benefit from learning about. Because the M1 aircraft accident focused on one particular type of accident we thought that a book devoted entirely to an aircraft accident was inappropriate, and we are very grateful to the authors of the other chapters for contributing their knowledge and their own experience from different incidents in the past.

By providing a rounded book that gives general experience of different accidents together with specific advice on the management of the patients, the hospital, and indeed the whole period of the disaster, both from the organisational and from the clinical point of view, we hope that readers will learn things that will place them in a much better position should they be unfortunate enough to experience a disaster in the future.

WA WALLACE
JM ROWLES
CL COLTON

Acknowledgements

We would like to acknowledge the following picture sources: figure 2.1, The Boeing Company; figures 2.3 and 2.4, Department of Transport; figures 4.1 and 4.2, Mr M Barnes; figure 4.3, Department of Medical Illustration, Leicester Royal Infirmary; figures 11.1 and 11.2, British Association of Social Workers (first appeared in *Order from Chaos*, Venture Press 1990); figures 12.1, 12.4, and 12.5, Photographic Services, US Air Base, Ramstein; figure 12.3, Dr C Carney; figure 15.1, *Dallas Morning News* and Juan Garcia; and figure 15.2, the *Guardian*.

Contributors

Michael J Allen, MB BS MRCP FRCS
Consultant, Accident and Emergency Department,
Leicester Royal Infirmary,
Leicester, UK

David Anton, MFOM DAvMed RAF
Biodynamics Division,
RAF Institute of Aviation Medicine,
Farnborough, UK

D Clive Bouch, MRCPath
Consultant Pathologist, Leicester Royal Infirmary,
Leicester, UK

Maureen A Bradford
Projects Manager, The Accident Research Unit,
in collaboration with Loughborough University of Technology,
Loughborough, UK

Peter Brownson, DM FRCSEd
NLDB Research Fellow, University Department of Orthopaedic and Accident
Surgery,
University Hospital, Queen's Medical Centre,
Nottingham, UK

Robert Carter, M Eng, C Eng, M RAeS
Senior Inspector of Aircraft Accidents (Engineering), Air Accidents
Investigation Branch, Department of Transport,
Farnborough, UK

Nigel Clifton, MA
Chief Executive, North Nottinghamshire Health Authority,
Ransom Hospital,
Mansfield, UK
(previously General Manager, University Hospital,
Queen's Medical Centre, Nottingham, UK)

Christopher Colton, FRCS FRCSEd(Orth)
Consultant Orthopaedic Surgeon, and Special Professor of Orthopaedic Surgery,
University Hospital, Queen's Medical Centre,
Nottingham, UK

William Curtin, MCh FRCSI(Orth)
Senior Registrar in Orthopaedic Surgery,
Beaumont Hospital,
Dublin, Eire

CONTRIBUTORS

Robert W Docherty, PhD
Assistant Firemaster (Operations), Strathclyde Fire Brigade,
Hamilton, UK

Andrew F Dove, MRCGP DObst
Consultant in Accident and Emergency Medicine,
University Hospital, Queen's Medical Centre,
Nottingham, UK

John L Firth, FRCSEd
Consultant Neurosurgeon, Department of Neurosurgery,
University Hospital, Queen's Medical Centre,
Nottingham, UK

JC Fitzpatrick, MD
Attending Surgeon, US Army Institute of Surgical Research,
Brooke Army Medical Center,
Fort Sam Houston, Texas, USA

Marion Gibson, MSSc, Dip SW, CQSW
Social Work Services Manager, South and East Belfast Community Unit,
Purdysburn Hospital,
Belfast, UK

Miles Irving, FRCS
Professor of Surgery, Department of Surgery,
University of Manchester, Hope Hospital,
Salford, UK

J Stephen Jones, FRCPath DMJ
Home Office and Consultant Pathologist, City Hospital,
and Special Professor of Forensic Medicine, University of Nottingham,
Nottingham, UK

Charles Malata, FRCS(Glas)
Research Fellow, Plastic Surgery and Burns Unit,
Bradford University, Bradford, UK,
and Honorary Registrar in Plastic Surgery,
Yorkshire Regional Health Authority, UK

Terence E Martin, DRCOG DAvMed MRAeS
Medical Officer, Biodynamics Section,
RAF Institute of Aviation Medicine,
Farnborough, UK

Raymon Moran, MCh(Orth) FRCSI
Consultant Orthopaedic Surgeon,
The Blackrock Clinic,
County Dublin, Eire
(previously Spinal Fellow, Queen's Medical Centre, Nottingham,
and Harlow Wood Orthopaedic Hospital, Nottinghamshire, UK)

BA Pruitt Jr, FACS
Commander and Director, US Army Institute of Surgical Research,
Brooke Army Medical Center,
Fort Sam Houston, Texas, USA

J Paul Robinson, CIS FBIM CDipAF DipMA
Deputy Chief Executive Officer, Mid-Western Health Board,
Limerick, Eire

John Rowles, DM FRCS
NLDB Research Fellow, Department of Orthopaedic and Accident Surgery,
University Hospital, Queen's Medical Centre,
Nottingham, UK

David T Sharpe, FRCS OBE
Director, Plastic Surgery and Burns Research Unit,
Bradford University,
and Consultant Plastic Surgeon, St Luke's Hospital,
Bradford, UK

Gavin R Tait, FRCS
Senior Orthopaedic Registrar,
Victoria Infirmary,
Glasgow, UK
(previously Orthopaedic Registrar to the Belfast Hospitals)

Peter D Thomas, BA(Physics)
Head, Accident Research Unit, ICE Ergonomics,
in collaboration with Loughborough University of Technology,
Loughborough, UK

W Angus Wallace, FRCSEd FRCSEd(Orth)
Professor of Orthopaedic and Accident Surgery,
University Hospital, Queen's Medical Centre,
Nottingham, UK

Jim Wardrope, FRCS
Consultant in Accident and Emergency Medicine,
Northern General Hospital,
Sheffield, UK

Barrie D White, FRCS
Neurosurgical Senior Registrar, Department of Neurosurgery,
University Hospital, Queen's Medical Centre,
Nottingham, UK

Nigel Williams, FRCS
Tutor in Surgery, Department of Surgery,
University of Manchester, Hope Hospital,
Salford, UK

1
It couldn't happen to us

W ANGUS WALLACE

Introduction

We all live in a world of our own surrounded by a protective cocoon that isolates us from most of the major problems that other people have. If you work in a hospital you acknowledge that major disasters are going to occur but it is unlikely that they will affect your hospital—you hope these things happen to others. You accept that disaster plans are made by people who prepare them as part of their job, but you hope they will never be put into action in a real "hot" situation, although you tolerate rehearsals "just in case." When the rehearsals occur you know you have many more important things to do; however, you do what is expected of you with a variable degree of enthusiasm. Like other orthopaedic surgeons, we have had some experiences of major incidents, particularly as a result of bad road traffic accidents, and I am sure these views were held by a number of my colleagues in Nottingham, Derby, and Leicester up until 8 January 1989—the date of the M1 Kegworth aircraft accident.

A major disaster is the classical "ambush" situation; we plan, prepare and exercise with great care and attention to detail and "out of the blue" the situation that presents is almost always a total surprise which does not quite "fit" the exercise pattern.

Jack A Costley, 1989[1]
Regional Health Emergency Planning Officer
Trent Regional Health Authority

The M1 plane crash: the first 24 hours[2]

Sunday 8 January 1989 was little different from any other Sunday. In the late afternoon I went into the office in the Queen's Medical Centre to clear some of the paperwork on my desk before another week of clinical work, teaching, research, and committees. My research fellow, Andrzej, was also at work in the department measuring cross sectional areas of bone—part of a Medical Research Council research project. At 8.55 pm Andrzej appeared at my door. "I've just been speaking to a doctor friend in Derby," he said. "The Derby Royal Infirmary switchboard says there has been a big plane crash at East Midlands Airport." My first reaction was disbelief but we both ran down to the accident department in case it was true and we could be of any help. Little did we realise the horrors of the night to come.

The first casualties from the M1 plane crash were already beginning to arrive. The major disaster arrangements had begun to swing into action with the accident department being quickly cleared of all non-urgent cases. At the door of the department triage of the patients into three groups was beginning to be carried out: the walking wounded in one area; the moderately injured but without life threatening problems in another area; and the severely injured in the resuscitation room. The initial problem was that the first batch of injured survivors all seemed to belong to the last category and although the resuscitation room was designed to take only four seriously injured patients on stretchers, we had eight seriously injured people in the first ten minutes. I met one of the consultants and he glanced up and said, "Angus, we've been training for this for years and I never believed it would ever happen." We both then concentrated on the injured. For the past three years I had taught the medical students how to manage patients with multiple injuries. I had warned them that in an emergency it was always difficult to remember what to do. Now I was the doctor not quite sure what to do. Every two minutes another severely injured patient at risk of dying arrived. Back to basics I said to myself. Then it all came back—the ABC of resuscitation—A for airway, B for breathing, and C for circulation—and then worry about the fractures. The troops then arrived— anaesthetists, general surgeons, and even physicians appeared in the department offering to help. The need during the first 30 minutes was for anaesthetists—many of the injured were not breathing well. Some needed simply to have their airways kept clear but three required immediate intubation. Several had pneumothoraces and I was impressed with one of my consultant orthopaedic colleagues (he had recently been on an acute trauma and life support—ATLS—course), who diagnosed and treated three collapsed lungs within the first half hour with the insertion of chest drains. There is a definite advantage in postgraduate courses on trauma.

Doctors and nurses were now in abundance—one nurse and at least one doctor per patient—and they were doing a superb job. Breathing was controlled, drips were going up fast, and injuries were receiving their first assessment. I spied a new admission requiring attention—a badly injured man whose leg was severely damaged and who also had head, chest, and abdominal injuries. There was no room for him in the resuscitation room and an initial assessment indicated that he was not about to die. "Take him to one of the cubicles," I said with authority (hiding the fact that I felt out of my depth) and went with him. Airway clear, breathing OK but laboured, circulation—blood pressure 80/60 mm Hg—not good—drip up, cross-match arranged, raise the legs. Oh no—the trolley was not designed to be raised with the foot elevated to the Trendelenberg position. Two chairs for the bottom wheels—that worked but one wheel fell off. The blood pressure came up to 110/70 mm Hg. Now fractures—there were broken bones—a possible skull fracture, clinically rib fractures, pelvic fractures, a right femur, and a compound left tibia—but in addition there was no blood supply to the left foot. This man was badly injured, might lose his foot, but was not going to die immediately. The leg was splinted. Now off to the x ray department with a nurse and junior doctor looking after him—verbal orders only—no time for me to write—a full x ray assessment of the injuries was now needed.

The consultant on call for trauma now called me. "Angus can you go up to the receiving ward and assess the injured." I did what I was told but took with me another medic—the professor of general practice no less—who with many other doctors had turned up spontaneously in the casualty department to help. Things were now under control. A 28 bedded ward had been cleared for the injured and the ward was now being filled with acutely injured patients. These patients had been sent here with moderate injuries which should not be life threatening. Our job was to assess them and make sure that there were no serious missed injuries. I took a six bedded bay and started to examine the patients—checking that their blood pressure was satisfactory and making sure that all bony injuries were identified and documented. This was the second assessment of injuries but this time I had time to carefully document all the injuries that I diagnosed and to decide whether any urgent investigations or treatment were required. There were several upper limb fractures—splintage was required and this was sent for. I looked round. I could not believe my eyes. This was the first occasion that I could recall when all ten orthopaedic consultants had been in the hospital at once—either in the casualty department or in the receiving ward. They were all there within one hour of the disaster and many without being formally called. I remembered the patient I had left in the x ray department. I found him with his full x ray assessment. Did we need an arteriogram as the foot was still white? No, let's take him to theatre and see what stabilising the fracture will do.

Theatre—here I come. At last I am in familiar surroundings and much more in control. I arrived in the theatre suite to find three operations in progress. A girl with a ruptured spleen was being treated with a laparotomy. A man with head and facial injuries was being treated for severe bleeding, and another lady with abdominal injuries and severe bilateral lower limb injuries was also having a laparotomy.

My senior registrar started to operate on the patient whom I had brought from the accident department. He treated the compound tibial fracture with toilet, debridement, and an external fixator and sutured the severe scalp laceration. There was a queue of patients for surgery so the closed femoral fracture would have to wait for definitive treatment. While this patient was receiving treatment I checked the other theatres. Four were now working and the theatre manager came up to me. "Prof," he said, "I can open another three or four more theatres. Have you got the orthopaedic staff?" Never have we been made an offer like that before. Usually it is the orthopaedic surgeon pleading with the theatre staff to open a theatre. We had the staff and we had many patients with compound fractures. Within an hour we had seven operating theatres working flat out from 11 pm to 5 am—what a team. I spent the next two hours fixing a nasty hip fracture in a 20 year old girl who had had two chest drains inserted and had required a splenectomy. My scrub nurse had worked the afternoon shift, was on her way home when the plane crash was announced, and had told the taxi driver to take her straight back to the hospital. Although she usually worked in the gynaecological theatre, she had done some orthopaedics in the past and acted superbly as scrub nurse and sole assistant to "the Prof."

By 4.00 am things were under control. I had cancelled my morning committee meeting for a regional health authority working party and had booked an operating list of accident victims for the morning. A few hours' sleep was probably wise. I went home but could not sleep. After such drama the memories are always difficult to subdue. I think I slept for one hour. Up at 7.00 am and back into the hospital. The ward round was important—each consultant had been allocated his own patients and I had to recheck that none of my patients had any missed injuries before going to theatre at 9.00 am. I spent most of the rest of the day in the operating theatre looking after the injured from the accident.

At the end of Monday the position was clearly under control and we could relax a little and review what had happened. What became clear was that this was one of the few "survivable plane crashes" that had occurred in recent years. This had been due primarily to superb emergency services—particularly the airport fire service who had the plane covered in foam within minutes of the accident. Perhaps there were lessons to be learnt from the accident? Should we be studying the injured and were there any ways in which the injuries could be reduced in future plane crashes? A research project was born.

The overriding feeling I was left with, however, was a deep pride in our hospital and our staff and the wonderful response of everyone to an emergency that, despite all the plans, was bigger than any disaster we could ever have foreseen. It was also clear that the hospitals in Leicester and Derby—although presented with smaller numbers—had also coped extremely well. We can all be proud of our National Health Service which provides in an emergency a response which is second to none.

Learning from the disaster

The lessons that can be learned from a disaster are often unexpected and far reaching but it is also surprising how frequently the same lessons are learned again and again with different disasters. Following the M1 aircraft accident on January 1989 there was intensive hospital activity for three weeks, as you will read in later chapters. However by four weeks the situation had begun to settle down, and at this stage it was time to reassess the events that had taken place and whether the emergency services and the hospitals had performed as well as they should have. A debriefing meeting was held on 7 February—four weeks after the disaster—at the Regional Ambulance Centre at Markfield in Leicestershie, which was attended by representatives of all three hospitals—Queen's Medical Centre, Derbyshire Royal Infirmary, and Leicester Royal Infirmary, as well as the police, ambulance, and fire and rescue services. Reports were prepared by all three hospitals, which had honestly reviewed the management of the disaster from their own hospital's point of view. Shortcomings were highlighted and recommendations for the future were made. These reports with additional information were collated by Mr Jack Costley the Trent regional health emergency planning officer and a full report of the accident was prepared and published.[1]

As a number of the experiences from the M1 aircraft accident are likely to apply to other major disasters, a selection of the conclusions and recommendations have been reproduced here for the guidance of others.

Some conclusions from the M1 plane crash

- Staff and services at all of the hospitals coped extremely well with the immediate and longer term effects of the accident

- Personnel of all disciplines responded rapidly and effectively—many who were off duty came in and worked throughout the night, and then completed their rostered shifts the following day. Staff from other hospitals and community services also volunteered their assistance

- Hospitals remained under pressure for at least 48 hours after the incident. However, the size of the hospitals involved, with the range of skills and facilities available under one roof, was a positive advantage enabling them to absorb the patients who were admitted without adversely affecting the care provided for those patients already in the hospital

- The longer term effects on the hospitals were significant. The range of work normally undertaken already placed considerable demands on operating theatres and intensive therapy units. In the case of Queen's Medical Centre both areas functioned at their maximum capacity for more than a week after the incident, and the number of ventilated patients in the intensive therapy unit severely restricted the hospital's ability to cope with further emergencies, and those patients undergoing planned major surgery

- The response to the incident demonstrated that some aspects of the major incident plan should be revised. In particular, the arrangement for calling out the Derbyshire Royal Infirmary flying squad, and communication systems both within and external to the hospitals, needed to be improved to cope with the intensity of activity and volume of information being handled. Police casualty bureau arrangements at hospital level could have been improved, and systems for recording and identifying casualties could have been more effective through shared police/NHS training

- The media response, and the simultaneous arrival of many of the relatives, demonstrated the importance of assigning senior staff to manage both functions. The prolonged aftermath, which affected a range of services, as well as producing unique managerial problems, was not anticipated and complicated the process of settling the hospitals back into a routine

- This incident emphasised the importance and the need to have well developed plans to help relatives in many practical ways—accommodation, clothing, currency exchange, transport, etc. On this occasion, British Midland Airways provided this assistance and expertise, and its staff are to be congratulated on the quality of their response.

Some recommendations arising from the M1 plane crash[1]

Ambulance communications: the Leicestershire ambulance mobile control and communications vehicle suffered technical failure on the way to the incident. Thereafter the ambulance incident officer used his car radio as mobile control. The use of a designated mobile communications vehicle has been reviewed.

Flying Squad communications: the Derbyshire Royal Infirmary (DRI) flying squad has a special role in the East Midlands Airport major disaster plan. The message received by the DRI from the Leicestershire police was unclear and led to delay in mobilising the flying squad. In future, Leicestershire ambulance service will alert the DRI flying squad.

Direct telephone contact between the hospital accident and emergency departments and the on-site flying squads is essential in order to:

- Regularly update the hospital on numbers and type of casualties they can expect

- Request further staff and equipment to support the scene

- Monitor the status of the hospital to continue to receive casualties.

The provision of miners' style head lamps: this should be considered in order to improve lighting for medical teams at the site.

Telephone communications: there was a major telephone communication problem between hospitals, medical staff, and with relatives because the police and telephone switchboards became jammed almost immediately. Methods of overcoming these difficulties have been discussed with British Telecom and advice received.

Alerting procedure and call out sequence: it was found that this needs to be simplified and made clear to everyone. Each hospital department should designate one person to maintain "cascade" call out lists which are updated regularly.

Triage: the designation of specific hospitals to receive certain classifications of casualties should be a routine part of 'triage' on site—for example, neurosurgery, spinal injuries, and burns should normally be transferred to regional specialty centres.

Site medical officer: there were difficulties of coordination on site particularly associated with the presence of three flying squads. The nomination and identification of *the* site medical officer early in the rescue operation is essential.

Documentation and identification of casualties: there was no standard procedure in use for the documentation and diagrammatic notation of triage nor for recording vital signs and treatment given. Subsequent to the accident it has been agreed that the METTAG II casualty label should be adopted until a national agreed label was identified. Two survivors who were transferred to a fourth hospital (Mansfield General Hospital), were overlooked and temporarily appeared on the mortality lists! This should be avoided by more careful on-site documentation in future.

The aftermath: hospital departments should include plans for coping with the aftermath, with particular emphasis on:

- The continuing demands on staff with special expertise

- The requirements for specialised equipment and consumables

- The ability to maintain urgent services—for example, by postponing routine operating lists, some clinics and other planned activity

- The counselling of staff, patients, and relatives.

7

The media: intense and sustained media interest must be anticipated. Senior personnel must be assigned to this function, preferably reporting to one central control point within the hospital. The press room *must* be kept separate from the accommodation areas for relatives to maintain privacy. Additional payphone facilities should be provided for the media.

Personal recommendations (by WAW) following the M1 plane crash

- Experience showed that the major disaster plans for both the accident site and for the hospitals were too complex. They should be kept simple in future.

- As a doctor, I felt untrained and not as competent as I would have liked when looking after the severely injured in the accident and emergency department on the night of the accident. I have since attended an advanced trauma and life support (ATLS) course and obtained a certificate from the Royal College of Surgeons of England. I recommend that all doctors who are likely to look after multiply injured patients in future should also do so.

- The first ambulances on the scene in this accident adopted a "scoop and run" policy for the first 30–45 minutes. Later this changed to an "initial on-site resuscitation of the injured and then transfer" policy. On reviewing the patient management this decision by the ambulance staff was felt to be correct and appropriate, with quick and early transfer of the first very sick patients to the well equipped accident departments where intensive resuscitation was possible. It is recommended that those designing major disaster plans should build into the plan a recommendation for an early "scoop and run" phase, as long as hospitals are near at hand and there are sufficient ambulances available.

- In the receiving accident and emergency departments an "attendant" or "scribe" should have been appointed to each injured patient, to act as a note taker and to remain with the patient at all times. There were plenty of available members of staff—nurses, medical students, and other volunteers. If we had used these attendants properly, we would have documented each patient's vital signs and injuries promptly and more accurately.

Conclusions

Involvement in a major disaster is a very humbling experience. First aid skills for medical staff have not been taught properly in the past but this is now being addressed. Communication problems remain the biggest challenge for those producing a major disaster plan and should not be underestimated. In nearly every major disaster communications have been cited as being a problem. Fortunately, common sense usually resolves difficulties experienced at this time of stress and common sense management prevailed at the scene of this accident. All those staff and voluntary helpers who took part in the early rescue procedures and later hospital management were totally committed to helping and giving their time and skills freely, and I am sure all the survivors remain grateful to this day for this help.

References

1 Trent Regional Health Authority. *Report on the Aircraft Accident BD 092, M1 Motorway, East Midlands Airport, Sunday 8th January 1989.* Available from Trent Health, Fulwood House, Old Fulwood Road, Sheffield S10 3TH. Ref Emergency Planning JAC/C17/24.
2 Wallace WA. Personal view—The M1 plane crash: the first 24 hours. *BMJ* 1989; **298**: 330–1.

2

A major disaster—the M1 plane crash—how it occurred

ROBERT CARTER

EDITORS' INTRODUCTION

Although sections of this chapter are somewhat technical, this summary of the Air Accident Investigation Branch (AAIB) report, AAR 4/90, "Report on the accident to Boeing 737–400 G–OBME near Kegworth, Leicestershire, on 8 January 1989", gives the reader insight into the depth of investigation, particularly on the engineering side, that is carried out as a routine by the AAIB.[1]

The aircraft design

The aircraft involved in the accident at Kegworth in January 1989 was a model 737-400 aircraft (figure 2.1) built by Boeing Commercial Airplanes in 1988. At the time of the accident this particular aircraft, carrying the British registration G-OBME, had accumulated just over 520 flying hours. Most of this time had been spent in carrying farepaying passengers for its operator, British Midland Airways Ltd.

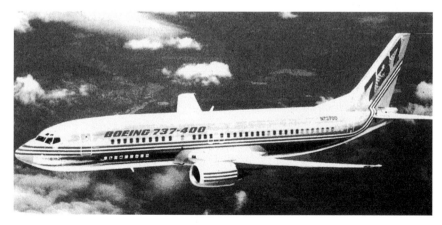

Figure 2.1—A Boeing 737-400.

At the time of the accident the 737-400 model was still a very new member of the family of Boeing 737 airliners and G-OBME was one of the first "-400" series to be delivered. Boeing had announced the new -400 series in June 1986, the first aircraft was "rolled-out" at Boeing's Renton plant near Seattle on 26th January 1988 and this version of the aircraft received its Federal Aviation Administration (FAA) "type certification" on 2 September 1988, with deliveries to airlines starting soon afterwards.

Despite the newness of the -400 variant, in general and G-OBME in particular, Boeing had started the 737 family in the 1960s with the development of the smaller 737-100, which first flew in April 1967 and entered airline service at the beginning of 1968. The "-100" series used Pratt & Whitney JT8D engines, as did the 737-200, which followed soon afterwards and was very similar. The major change in the programme came in 1980 when work began on the "-300" series, with the airlines receiving their first aircraft in November 1984. Changes incorporated in the -300 included a "stretch" of the fuselage by 104 inches, by means of two fuselage "plugs", and, more significantly, the powerplants were changed to the more powerful and more efficient CFM International CFM56-3B high bypass turbofan engines, built jointly by the SNECMA (France) and General Electric (USA) engine companies. For the 737-300 this engine was initially rated at 20 000 lbs of static thrust at sea level and later at 22 000 lbs.

The change to the 737-400 series from the -300 represented less of a step than between the -200 and -300 series. The fuselage was "stretched" by a further 120 inches, representing four rows of passenger seats, and the engine was a new version of the CFM56-3 engine, this time rated at 23 500 lbs. As with any new variant of an established basic design, Boeing took the opportunity to incorporate a number of other developments into the -400. One of these changes was the introduction of the electronic Engine Instrument System (EIS) solid state display, which replaced the electro-mechanical engine instruments found in earlier 737s and instead showed engine parameters (such as speeds, temperatures and vibrations) by means of light-emitting diodes (LEDs). Both the changes in the engines and the introduction of the EIS display were significant factors in the accident to G-OBME.

Seating configuration in G-OBME

At the time of the accident, G-OBME was configured with 156 passenger seats in a single class cabin with a total of 26 rows of pairs of triple seats (see figure 2.2). The seat pitch ranged from a maximum of 38 inches, for seat rows 12 and 14, adjacent to the overwing emergency exits, to a minimum of 30 inches for row 27L. The remaining seat pitches were either 31 or 32 inches.

The seat type was the Model 4001 tourist seat, manufactured by Weber

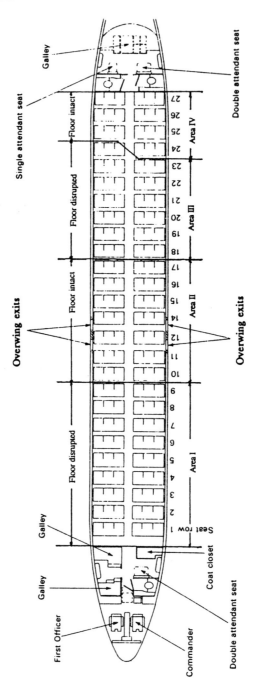

Figure 2.2—Plan showing seating in G-OBME.

Aircraft Inc. This design of seat had its origins in the work undertaken by the FAA in the 1980s concerning the upgrading of the Federal Aviation Requirements (FARs) dealing with seat strength and performance in crashes. This work led to the FAA issuing an Amendment ("25–64") in May 1988 requiring, for new aircraft type certifications in the "Transport Category" (that is, airliners), higher static load factors and two dynamic tests for the seats, one involving a velocity change of 35 ft/s up to a peak of 14 G and the other a velocity change of 44 ft/s up to a peak of 16 G. As the 737-400 was considered a "derivative" by the FAA and the Civil Aviation Authority (CAA), its seats were not required to meet these new standards, although the Weber 4001 seats had in fact been subjected to some dynamic testing on the FAA's Civil Aeromedical Institute (CAMI) track, with a view to meeting the requirements of a "16 G"seat.

For crew seating (see figure 2.2), the aircraft had conventional pilots' seats, positioned on floor-mounted tracks and equipped with 5-point harnesses. The aircraft had seating for five cabin attendants, arranged as two double seats and one single seat, all of which were rear facing. Both double seats were mounted on the left hand side of the aircraft, one just forward of the forward left passenger door and the other just forward of the rear left passenger door. The single attendant seat was mounted just forward of the rear right passenger door.

The aircraft was equipped with a total of 30 overhead stowage bins in the passenger compartment. Of these, 26 were of 60 inches in length and fully available for passenger hand baggage. The remaining two end pairs were shorter and partly used for cabin safety equipment.

History of the flight

The aircraft was on a "shuttle" flight between London Heathrow Airport and Belfast Aldergrove Airport. It took off for Belfast at 1952, with the first officer handling the aircraft. After take off the aircraft climbed initially to 6000 feet where it levelled off before receiving clearance to climb to flight level 120. Soon afterwards clearance was passed to climb to flight level 350 on a direct track to the VOR radio beacon at Trent.

At 2005.05, as the aircraft was climbing through flight level 283 (about 28 300 feet), the crew experienced moderate to severe vibration and a smell of fire. There was no fire warning or any other visual or aural warning on the flight deck. The commander stated afterwards that he saw and smelt air conditioning smoke. The first officer later remembered only a strong smell of burning. Later replay of the flight data recorder (FDR) showed that severe vibration had occurred in the No 1 (left) engine at this point, accompanied by marked fluctuations in fan speed, a rise in exhaust gas temperature, and low and fluctuating fuel flow.

The commander took control of the aircraft and disengaged the autopilot. He later stated that he looked at the engine instruments but did not gain from them any clear indication of the source of the problem. He also stated that he thought that the smoke and fumes were coming forward from the passenger cabin which, from his appreciation of the aircraft air conditioning system, led him to suspect the No. 2 (right) engine. The first officer also said that he monitored the engine instruments, and when asked by the commander which engine was causing the trouble he said, "It's the Le ... it's the right one", to which the commander responded by saying, "Okay, throttle it back." The autothrottle was then disengaged and the No 2 engine was throttled back. The first officer later had no recollection of what it was he saw on the engine instruments that led him to make his assessment. The commander later stated that the action of closing the No 2 engine throttle reduced the smell and the visual signs of smoke and that he remembered no continuation of the vibration after the No 2 throttle was closed.

Immediately after throttling back the No 2 engine, the first officer advised London Air Traffic Control Centre (LATCC) that they had an emergency situation which looked like an engine fire. The commander then ordered the first officer, "Shut it down." This order was given 43 seconds after the onset of the vibration but its execution was delayed when the commander said, "Seems to be running alright now. Let's just see if it comes in." The shutdown was further delayed as the first officer responded to radio messages from LATCC which advised the crew of the aircraft's position and asked which alternate airfield they wished to use. The first officer said that it looked as if they would take it to Castle Donington (East Midlands Airport) but LATCC were to stand by. At about this time a flight attendant used the cabin address system to advise the passengers to fasten their seat belts. The first officer then told the commander that he was about to start the "Engine Failure and Shutdown" checklist, saying at the same time, "Seems we have stabilised. We've still got the smoke". Again, action on the pilots' checklist was suspended as the commander called British Midland Airways Operations at East Midlands Airport to advise his company of the situation. At 2 minutes 7 seconds after the start of the vibration the fuel cock (start lever) of the No 2 engine was closed, thus shutting down that engine, and the auxiliary power unit (APU) was started.

The commander later recollected that, as soon as the No 2 engine had been shut down, all evidence of smell and smoke cleared from the flight deck, and this finally convinced him that the action he had taken was correct. Shortly afterwards power was further reduced on the No 1 engine, which continued to operate at reduced power with no symptoms of unserviceability other than a higher than normal level of indicated vibration and increased fuel flow. This high level of vibration continued for a further 3 minutes and then fell progressively until it reached a level of 2 units on the cockpit indicator, still a little higher than normal. After the accident, the commander stated that, during the remainder of the flight, the information that he had from the engine instruments, or any other source, were such as to indicate that the emergency had been successfully concluded and that the No 1 engine was operating normally.

In the cabin, the passengers and the cabin attendants had heard an unusual noise accompanied by moderate to severe vibration. Some passengers were also aware of what they described as smoke and some saw signs of fire from the left engine, which they described variously as "fire", "torching", or "sparks". Several of the cabin attendants described the noise as a low repetitive thudding, "like a car backfiring", and one described how the shuddering shook the walls of the forward galley. The three flight attendants in the rear of the cabin saw evidence of fire from the No 1 engine, and two of them briefly saw light coloured smoke in the cabin. Soon after the No 2 engine was shut down the commander called the flight service manager (FSM) to the flight deck and asked him "Did you get smoke in the cabin back there?", to which the FSM replied "We did, yes." The commander then instructed the FSM to clear up the cabin and pack everything away. About one minute later the FSM returned to the flight deck and said "Sorry to trouble you . . . the passengers are very very panicky." The commander then broadcast to the passengers on the cabin address system that there was trouble with the right engine which had produced some smoke in the cabin, that the engine was now shut down and that they could expect to land at East Midlands Airport in about 10 minutes. The flight attendants who saw signs of fire on the left engine later stated that they had not heard the commander's reference to the right engine. However, many of the passengers who saw fire from the No 1 engine heard and were puzzled by the commander's reference to the right engine but none brought the discrepancy to the attention of the cabin crew, even though several were aware of continuing vibration.

Approaching East Midlands Airport, the aircraft joined the runway centreline at 2000 feet above ground level. The commander called for the landing gear to be lowered and, as he passed the outer marker at 4.3 nautical miles from touchdown, called for 15° flap. One minute later, at 2023.49, when the aircraft was 2.4 nautical miles from touchdown at a height of 900 feet above ground level, there was an abrupt decrease in power from the No 1 engine. The commander called immediately for the first officer to relight (that is, restart) the other engine and the first officer attempted to comply. The commander then raised the nose of the aircaft in an effort to reach the runway. At 17 seconds after the power loss the fire warning system operated on the No 1 engine and 7 seconds later the ground proximity warning system glideslope warning sounded and continued with increasing repetitive frequency as the aircraft descended below the glidepath. At 2024.33 the commander broadcast a crash warning on the cabin address system using the words "Prepare for crash landing." Two seconds later, as the airspeed fell below 125 knots, the stall warning stick shaker operated, and continued to operate until the aircraft struck the ground at 2024.43. The last airspeed recorded on the flight data recorder was 115 knots. No power became available from the No 2 engine before the aircraft struck the ground.

The initial ground impact was in a nose high attitude on level ground just to the east of the M1 motorway. The aircraft then passed through trees and suffered its second and major impact 70 metres to the west and 10 metres lower, on the western (northbound) carriageway of the M1 motorway and the lower part of the western embankment (figures 2.3 and 2.4). The fuselage was extensively disrupted and the aircraft came to rest entirely on the wooded western embankment approximately 900 metres from the threshold of runway 27 and displaced 50 metres to the north of the extended runway centreline. At impact there was fire around the No 1 engine but, without a major release of fuel in the impact, this fire did not have time to develop further before it was extinguished by the airport fire service.

Thirty nine passengers died at the scene of the accident and a further eight passengers died later from their injuries. Of the 79 medium term survivors, 74 suffered serious injury.

The investigation by the Air Accidents Investigation Branch

In the United Kingdom the responsibility for the investigation of accidents to civil aircraft rests with the Air Accidents Investigation Branch (AAIB), part of the Department of Transport. This responsibility includes the production of a written report to the Secretary of State for Transport and this report should include any safety recommendations coming from the investigation. The AAIB was notified of the accident to G-OBME that evening and the on site investigation was commenced at 0040 on 9 January 1989.

The principal areas of the AAIB investigation were the Operations, Powerplants, Systems, Structures and Survivability aspects of the accident. In the Survivability portion of the AAIB investigation, a close link was established with the NLDB study group (the Nottingham, Leicester, Derby, Belfast crash study group), which had been established independently.

A study group of industry and government specialists from the USA also participated in the AAIB Structures and Survivability investigations. The interest of this group, who were involved in the development of certification requirements for aircraft seats, was largely generated by the fact that this was one of the first accidents to have occurred to a jet transport equipped with seats designed around the requirements of Federal Aviation Requirements Amendment 25–64—commonly called "16 G" seats.

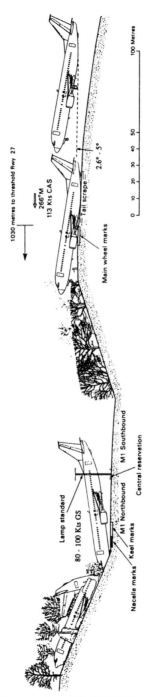

Figure 2.3—Cross-section of G-OBME impact sequence.

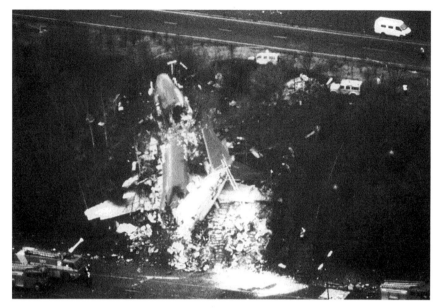

Figure 2.4—The final position of the aircraft at Kegworth.

The AAIB final report was published on 18 October 1990 and ran to 152 pages of text and a further six appendices[1]. It contained a total of 31 safety recommendations, addressed to the CAA. These recommendations covered all the areas of the AAIB investigation and included 11 concerning the Structures and Survivability investigations.

As to the cause of the accident, the conclusions of the AAIB report were as follows:

The cause of the accident was that the operating crew shut down the No 2 engine after a fan blade had fractured in the No 1 engine. This engine subsequently suffered a major thrust loss due to secondary fan damage after power had been increased during the final approach to land.

The following factors contributed to the incorrect response of the flight crew:

1. The combination of heavy engine vibration, noise, shuddering and an associated smell of fire were outside their training and experience.
2. They reacted to the initial engine problem prematurely and in a way that was contrary to their training.
3. They did not assimilate the indications on the engine instrument display before they throttled back the No 2 engine.
4. As the No 2 engine was throttled back, the noise and shuddering associated with the surging of the No 1 engine ceased, persuading them that they had correctly identified the defective engine.
5. They were not informed of the flames which had emanated from the No 1 engine and which had been observed by many on board, including 3 cabin attendants in the aft cabin.

The aircraft impact with the ground

As part of the Structures and Survivability portions of the investigation it was important to define the impact sequence and deceleration levels.

The first ground contact was made just before the eastern embankment of the M1 by the tail skid and aft fuselage, and started 29 metres east of the embankment boundary fence (figure 2.2). The ground marks showed that the main landing gears touched almost simultaneously with the tail and that, at first impact, the aircraft's atitude was approximately 13° nose up, with about 4° of right roll and 4.5° of left yaw.

The impact velocities had to be extrapolated from the final flight data recorder readings, giving a ground speed of between 104 knots (calibrated airspeed, corrected for wind) and 111 knots (from the aircraft inertial reference unit). The rate of descent was between 8.5 ft/s (barometric rate of descent) and 16 ft/s (radar altimeter rate corrected for terrain). These velocities combined to give an aircraft final flight path angle of between 2.5° and 5°.

The first impact detached the tail skid and auxiliary power unit door and the drag loads on the two main landing gears caused both legs to fail rearwards: the airframe remained otherwise intact. The aircraft then cut a swathe through the trees on the eastern embankment and, as it descended across the motorway, the left wing struck a central lamp standard, fracturing the standard at its base and removing the outboard 6 feet of the wing.

The second, and major impact occurred when the nose contacted the base of the western embankment. The first contact was made by the nose wheel on the road surface followed by the nose radome striking the embankment and the engine nacelles striking the road surface. The nose landing gear failed rearwards, the nose crushed against the embankment and both engine support structures failed upwards.

There was no indication of the velocity at the second impact from either the flight data recorder or the aircraft instrumentation. It became evident during the investigation that the major factor in determining the magnitude of the deceleration pulse in the second impact was the resultant (horizontal and vertical combined) velocity at this impact. Estimates covered the range of 77 knots (from a simple first order aerodynamic calculation) to 99 knots (from an impact analysis provided by the airframe manufacturer): AAIB concluded that the highest probability was in the range of 85–95 knots.

For determining the deceleration pulse transmitted to the cabin floor in the second impact AAIB considered four sources of information:

- The results of a KRASH computer simulation performed by the Cranfield Impact Centre[2]

- Calculation of the basic kinematics

- The damage to the passenger and pilot seating related to previous dynamic testing

- Comparison of airframe damage with previous calibrated tests.

All these sources of evidence indicated deceleration levels in the second impact in excess of the pulses defined in Amendment 25-64 and the balance of evidence indicated a resultant deceleration, within the centre section, with a peak value of between 22 and 28 G. The geometry of the impact showed that the initial pulse was primarily longitudinal, followed by a lower vertical pulse when the nacelles and centre section contacted the carriageway. The lack of damage in the tail section indicated a value there closer to but still above 14 G. Previous controlled impacts have indicated that the peak deceleration levels in the forward nose section would probably have been slightly higher than in the centre section.

Structural aspects

The structure of the cabin floor in the Boeing 737-400 is typical of this class of aircraft. It consists principally of a series of transverse floor beams that are mechanically attached, at each end, to the circumferential fuselage frames. The floor beams are, in general, placed at 20 inch spacing. The cabin flooring panels and longitudinal seat track members are secured on top of these beams.

Two major structural failures of the fuselage occurred in the impact, one slightly forward of the wing leading edge and one aft of the trailing edge. These failures left the structure in three principal sections (figure 2.3). In addition, all three landing gear legs and both engine supports failed, without rupturing the fuel tanks. In the case of the two main landing gear legs, the separations were clean and were as designed, failure occurring at the system of calibrated "fuse pin" bolts which attach the main landing gears to the wing structure. The engines were also designed to separate cleanly from the wing at the junction between the engine pylon and the wing leading edge. Although both engines did separate without rupturing the wing fuel tanks, all the "fuse pin" bolts were found intact and the structural failure had occurred within the pylon itself, approximately in the vertical plane of the forward wing spar.

The nose section sustained considerable crushing in the lower flight deck area and the belly skin disintegrated along the length of the forward passenger cabin. The floor of the forward passenger cabin was entirely disrupted and the stubs of the floor beams indicated that the failures aft of seat row one were in a forward and downward sense. The centre section remained intact and the wings remained attached, although the leading edges of both wings were extensively damaged by contact with the trees on both embankments. The tail section was almost inverted but had sustained less damage than the other fuselage sections.

So, of the total cabin floor, two areas survived the impact well, with the seats still attached, and two areas suffered substantial or total disruption of the floor structure. In the forward section, the floor was totally disrupted between row 1 and the front of the centre section (row 10). In the section of fuselage behind the wing and forward of the aft fuselage, the floor structure was disrupted but to a lesser degree than that forward of the wing. In some places, such as row 17, the seats had been retained by the floor beams which had remained intact, although separated from the fuselage wall.

The two surviving areas of floor were the overwing area and the aft fuselage section. In the overwing area there was evidence of high deceleration loads but the floor structure in this area is built on the wing centre section and is thus more robust than the areas immediately forward and aft. In the tail section there was less evidence of high deceleration, although the floor structure had sustained some damage from the seat inertial loads before the tail unit had rotated forwards into its final inverted position.

A distinctive pattern of failure emerged from the examination of the disrupted floor structure. The initial failure was of the longitudinal seat tracks under the inertial loading of the passenger triple seats. The resulting displacement of the seat track members from the floor panels prevented those floor panels from transmitting longitudinal crash loads and the transverse floor beams then failed under the longitudinal and torsional crash loads, for which they were not designed, as well as from the vertical loads.

The distribution of injuries with respect to the pattern of damage to the aircraft is discussed in chapter 3.

Seating

The seating plan is shown in figure 2.4.

Both pilots' seats were found still on their tracks and, despite the heavy impact damage to the flight deck area, both seats remained attached to the floor and the restraint systems were only slightly damaged. On both seats, the seat pans were found at the bottom of their vertical travel and this had caused additional seat damage. Similarly, all five attendant's seats suffered some damage but remained basically intact and attached to their respective toilet modules.

The greatest interest centred around the passenger seating. A total of 21 of the 52 triple seats remained fully attached to the cabin floor: 14 of these were in the overwing area and seven in the aft fuselage. During the rescue operations a total of 35 triple seats were removed from the aircraft, either intact or, in most cases, after being cut to allow the release of injured passengers. A further three were removed during the salvage operation.

After delivery of the wreckge to AAIB Farnborough, the cabin seating arrangement was reconstructed. Although there was variation in the damage to individual seats some distinctive patterns emerged.

In the forward area (rows 1–9) all the seats were totally separate from any floor structure. The rescue personnel who entered the forward section early in the rescue operation found that the seats and occupants had, in general, remained upright or tipped forward and had compressed together at the front of this section, with the occupants' heads at approximately the level at which the cabin floor had been before it collapsed. On most of the seats the rear attachments remained attached to segments of the seat track and in no instance did the seat structure fail at the rear track attachment. Where the rear attachments were found detached from the seat track, it was due either to a secondary failure or as a result of cutting by rescue personnel.

The centre (overwing) section corresponded to rows 10–17 (a total of 14 triple seats), and these triple seats remained attached to the cabin floor in the centre section with the exception of two individual outboard seats, which suffered complete bending failures of their horizontal front spars. Although these were the only seats where the front spar had separated, deformation occurred in several other seats.

The area immediately aft of the wing corresponded to rows 18 to 23/24, a total of 13 triple seats. In this area the seats had suffered varying degrees of disruption. Some seats (such as 18L) were almost intact, whereas others (such as 22R) were very extensively damaged. The damage generally related closely to that in the forward fuselage, with the additional damage apparently being caused by the buckling of the fuselage and the rescue operation.

The tail section corresponded to rows 24L to 27L and 25R to 27R, a total of seven triple seats. The seats in this area showed less damage and disruption than in any other part of the cabin and the seats were intact when the aircraft came to rest. All the rear track attachments remained properly engaged with the seat track and the front leg attachment to the front horizontal spar of the seat pan appeared undamaged on all 14 legs.

Overhead stowage bins

All the overhead stowage bins were recovered from the wreckage and their cabin positions determined. Photographs taken during the rescue operation and interview evidence from rescuers indicated that all the bins had become detached in the accident, apart from the forward bin on the right side (1R), which was partially detached. Almost all the bin doors were found detached from their bins.

The pattern of damage to the bins themselves reflected the cabin damage, with the least damaged bins in the overwing and tail sections and the most damaged being those creased and crushed in the buckled area aft of the wing.

On all the detached bins, the initial failure appeared to have occurred when the diagonal tie fitting pulled out of the bin upper surface. The lateral and vertical tie rods then failed when they were subjected to a longitudinal inertial load for which they were not designed. The failure sequence was consistent in all the bins that had detached and appeared to have been caused by a combination of the inertial loading of the bins themselves and the distortion of the fuselage attachments induced by the second impact.

The KRASH computer analysis of the impact

As part of the Structures and Survivability aspects of the investigation, it was decided to attempt a computer based modelling of the ground impact dynamics of G-OBME. The primary objective was to refine the deceleration levels at the cabin floor throughout the impact sequence. Secondary objectives were to determine the efficacy of such a computer based model and whether such a study could achieve useful results within the time scale of the overall accident investigation.

The two broad groups of computer programs available for impact dynamics may be classified as:

- Full "finite element" programs, which model a vehicle structure in detail using only geometric and material properties input data

- "Hybrid" programs, which use a simpler library of structural elements for the model and incorporate some test derived data for the collapse properties of key members within the structure.

KRASH is a hybrid program and has been developed specifically for the analysis of aircraft impact problems. Because of its simpler modelling and the availability of full scale test data from previous FAA full scale impact tests, Cranfield Impact Centre Limited was commissioned to perform the impact study, using the KRASH program.[2]

As the three main sections of fuselage (forward, centre, and tail) remained essentially complete, the wings, fuselage, and empennage were modelled as three lumped masses, divided by the two fuselage break points. The two engines, two main landing gears, and nose landing gear were individually represented by mass points, resulting in an eight-mass model. The effective masses and moments of inertia of the occupants, fuel, and luggage were added at the appropriate mass-points.

A key assumption made in this approach was that the deformation of the aircraft had been limited to localised areas of structure, that is, the fuselage break points and the lower fuselage. "Contact springs" were thus attached to the mass points to represent the force/deflection properties of those parts of the structure which would make contact with the ground and a simple beam model represented the bending behaviour of the fuselage.

Following the creation of the KRASH model, the impact sequence was run three times. Run 2 best represented the second impact after an assumed ballistic flight from the first impact, giving horizontal and vertical velocities of 48.9 m/s and 14.4 m/s respectively. Peak deceleration values for the centre section were 26.5 G (longitudinal axis) and 23 G (vertical axis): the peak resultant coincided with the 26.5 G longitudinal peak.

In run 2 the longitudinal deceleration signals were composed of a vibratory component of about 60 Hz, superimposed on a fundamental signal of approximately sine curve shape. The 60 Hz signal represented the low amplitude elastic deformations, whereas the fundamental wave represented the actual plastic deformation. The maximum value of this fundamental signal was 19.5 G for run 2.

The AAIB safety recommendations

The AAIB final report contained 11 safety recommendations to the CAA concerning Structures (crashworthiness) and Survivability issues.

Engine separation from the wings

One of these recommendations concerned the engine separations from the wings. Although the engine separations were benign, in that the wing fuel tanks were not ruptured, the structural failures occurred within the pylons themselves, leaving the "fuse pin" bolts in place. Thus AAIB recommended that:

The CAA should review the existing Joint Airworthiness Requirements concerning fuel tank protection from the effects of main landing gear and engine detachment during ground impact and include specific design requirements to protect the fuel tank integrity of those designs of aircraft with wing-mounted engines.

Seating

Four of the recommendations concerned aircraft seating. From the analysis of the major deceleration impulse it was clear that the forces encountered in the second impact were considerably greater than those for which the airframe and the furnishings were designed and certificated. It is in this context that the discussion around the seats' performance in G-OBME took place.

Both pilots' seats and the forward (rear facing) attendant seat suffered some structural damage in the accident and the aft (rear facing) double attendant seat moved with the bulkhead to which it was attached. But in general the crew seating performed well and, by remaining in position, limited the crew injuries resulting from secondary impacts with the cabin interior.

Of the passenger seating, it was true to say that "where the floor survived, so did the seats". The examination of previous accidents, the early dynamic testing of seats designed to the previous "9 G" static criteria and the dynamic testing of this model of passenger seat together indicated that fewer injuries occurred in this accident than would probably have been the case if the standard "9 G" seats had been fitted in the aircraft. However, some structural failures of the seats did occur, such as the front spar failures in the seats in the overwing section of the fuselage, and the AAIB recommended that:

The CAA should actively seek further improvement in the standards of JAR [Joint Airworthiness Requirements] 25.561/.562 and the level of such standards should not be constrained by the current FAA requirements.

Allied to this recommendation was one concerning seat detail design:

In addition to the dynamic test requirements, the CAA should seek to modify the JARs associated with detailed seat design to ensure that such seats are safety-engineered to minimise occupant injury in an impact.

It is worth noting that the fitting of the improved seats into G-OBME was not a legal requirement. The investigators considered that the performance of the passenger seats in G-OBME, however, strongly supported the case for fitting the improved seats into all newly manufactured aircraft coming onto the register and also refitting existing aircraft, at least on a seat replacement basis. The AAIB thus recommended that:

The CAA should require that, for aircraft passenger seats, the current loading and dynamic testing requirements of JAR 25.561 and .562 be applied to newly manufactured aircraft coming onto the UK register and, with the minimum of delay, to aircraft already on the UK register.

As for alternative seat designs, the investigators considered whether there was a case for recommending mandatory rear facing seats or upper torso restraints. Common to all the alternative seating configurations proposed was that implementation would have to be founded on a firm basis of research and development, including such questions as compatibility with the rest of the cabin, the level of passenger acceptance and the ability to provide protection in a wide range of impact conditions. The AAIB considered that little of this research had taken place in recent years and the limited use of rear facing seats in military transport aircraft had not answered these questions. The AAIB recommended, therefore, that:

The CAA should initiate and expedite a structured programme of research, in conjunction with the European airworthiness authorities, into passenger seat design, with particular emphasis on:
(i) Effective upper torso restraint
(ii) Aft-facing [rear facing] passenger seats.

Aircraft floors

Two of the recommendations concerned aircraft floors. The performance of the cabin floor in this accident was paradoxical in that, although large areas of the cabin floor failed, the full-scale dynamic tests performed in the USA indicated that the floor strength was, in fact, considerably higher than the "static 9 G" certification requirement. The answer to this paradox, which applied both to the cabin floor and to other furnishings in the aircraft, appeared to be in the geometric deformation that is inherent in any impact causing these high deceleration levels. The overall pattern of failure in G-OBME showed that relatively minor engineering changes could significantly improve the resilience and toughness of cabin floors in this category of aircraft and take fuller advantage of the improved passenger seats. In particular, AAIB believed there would be benefit in improved tolerance to out-of-plane loading and in providing multiple load paths.

Although questionable whether the cost would justify modification of existing airframes, the AAIB considered that future designs of cabin floor should certainly have to take account of dynamic loading criteria to ensure that the seats, and other floor mounted furnishings, remain in place in realistic impact cases. It was also considered reasonable that, at some point in the future, this should also apply to future production of existing designs. The AAIB recommendation thus read:

The certification requirements for cabin floors of new aircraft types should be modified to require that dynamic impulse and distortion be taken into account and these criteria should be applied to future production of existing designs.

The investigators also believed there to be scope for research into the feasibility of a significant increase in cabin floor toughness beyond the level of the current Joint Airworthiness Requirements/Federal Aviation Requirements (JAR/FAR) for seats. A further recommendation covered this area:

The CAA should initiate research, in conjunction with the European airworthiness authorities, into the feasibility of a significant increase in cabin floor toughness beyond the level of the current JAR/FAR seat requirements.

Infant and child restraints

Two of the recommendations concerned infant and child restraints. The AAIB report stated that the argument for child seats in motor cars had been well established for over a decade. It could be argued that the supplementary loop type belt provides some advantages over simple lap holding of infants but that it could provide an equivalent level of survivability to that provided for the adult passenger. The AAIB recommendations were that:

The CAA implement a programme to require that all infants and young children, who would not be safely restrained by supplementary or standard lap belts, be placed in child-seats for take-off, landing and flight in turbulence.

and

The CAA expedite the publication of a specification for child seat designs.

Stowage bins

Two of the recommendations concerned overhead stowage bins. All but one of the overhead stowage bins became detached in the impact and they did so in a very similar manner. Initially, the diagonal tie fitting separated from the upper surface of the stowage bin under the influence of the predominantly longitudinal inertial loads in the second impact; this was followed by the failure of the lateral and vertical ties when the bins moved forward.

Although it was not possible to determine the actual mass or distribution of passengers' belongings in the overhead bins, the results of the 1981–82 CAA survey indicated that the manufacturer's design and certification figure (3 lb/inch of bin length) was generously conservative and that the actual loading on G-OBME was about 33% of the placarded mass. It appears, therefore, that it was the dynamic nature of the loading, coupled with the general geometric distortion and disruption of the airframe, which caused the failure of the attachments.

This was clearly a serious matter for those injured by the bins and would have been very serious indeed had a major post-impact fire broken out. The accidents to G-OBME and other accidents to modern narrow body jet transports indicated great benefit in retaining cabin "items of mass" in position despite the deformation of the fuselage attachment structure and even after some disruption of the fuselage. Thus the AAIB recommended:

The certification requirements for cabin stowage bins, and other cabin items of mass, should be modified to ensure the retention of these items to fuselage structure when subjected to dynamic crash pulses substantially beyond the static load factors currently required.

There was also evidence that some of the bin doors opened during the last moments of flight, before the first impact. The inadvertent opening of overhead stowage bins has long been a problem, especially in turbulence, and some airlines now fit bins that incorporate secondary latching. The AAIB recommended that:

The CAA consider improving the airworthiness requirements for public transport aircraft to require some form of improved latching to be fitted to overhead stowage bins and this should also apply to new stowage bins fitted to existing aircraft.

A large number of people contributed to this investigation. They included: representatives of the National Transportation Safety Board, the Federal Aviation Administration, the Civil Aviation Authority and the airframe and equipment manufacturers. The author would like to thank them for their invaluable assistance and to compliment them on their steady professionalism. In particular, the independent work of the NLDB study group should be particularly commended.

1 Air Accidents Investigation Branch, DTp. *Aircraft accident report 4/90—report on the accident to Boeing 737-400 G-OBME near Kegworth, Leicestershire, on 8 January 1989.* HMSO, London; 1990.
2 *A computer-simulation of the G-OBME accident at Kegworth on January 8, 1989.* Cranfield Impact Centre Ltd, Cranfield. (CIC 14 November 1989.)
3 *Follow-up action on accident reports: accident to Boeing 737-400 G-OBME near Kegworth on 8 January 1989.* Civil Aviation Authority, Gatwick; 23 Oct 1990.

3

The injuries sustained in the M1 plane crash

JOHN M ROWLES, D CLIVE BOUCH

Introduction

This chapter reviews the injuries sustained by the occupants of the Boeing 737-400 involved in the aircrash on the M1 at Kegworth and analyses the causes of death. Although it is convenient to describe separately the injuries sustained by the survivors and the non-survivors, it is necessary to compare the injuries sustained by all the occupants of the aircraft if accurate and meaningful comparisons are to be made. Injury scoring techniques will be used to demonstrate such differences.

Of the 118 passengers (including a baby) and eight crew members on board the aircraft, 47 people, all passengers, died. Thirty nine bodies were removed from the scene of the accident, four initial survivors died in accident departments within a few hours, and a further four died some days later in hospital. Three of the late deaths were as a result of well recognised complications of major trauma.

Figure 3.1 demonstrates the age distribution of those on board the aircraft. Sixty three per cent (79) of the occupants were male.

A survivable aircraft accident is defined as:[1]

An accident in which the forces transmitted to the occupant through the seat and restraint system do not exceed the limits of human tolerance to abrupt accelerations, and in which the structure in the occupant's immediate environment remains substantially intact to the extent that a liveable volume is provided for the occupant throughout the crash sequence.

Thus essential to the analysis of the injuries sustained by occupants involved in an aircraft accident is an accurate seating plan of those on board. Using the original "boarding" seating plan (which is known to be inaccurate because passengers move seats) and statements from survivors,

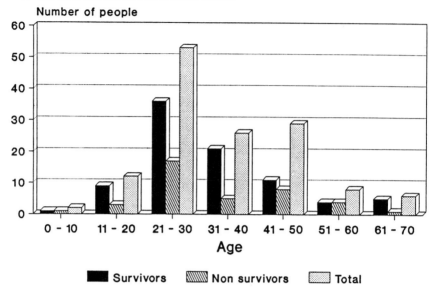

Figure 3.1—Age distribution of all passengers and crew.

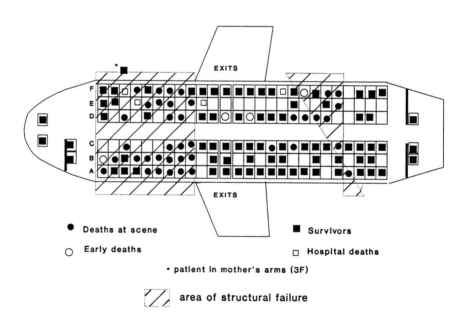

Figure 3.2—Seat plan showing the location and survival of the passengers.

an accurate seat plan was constructed (figure 3.2). The seat plan illustrates the locations of the occupants and their survivability in this accident. In

Box 3.1
Major injuries in the 87 survivors of the
M1 aircrash

Injury	No
Head	43
Thoracic	23
Abdominal (operated)	2
Spinal fractures	24
Pelvic/lower limb	142
open fractures	34
Upper limb	59
open fractures	6

this accident, the baby (3F) was seated in its mother's lap, restrained by an auxiliary lap belt. Twenty nine of the non-survivors were seated in the front section, five were seated in the central section and nine were seated in the rear section of the aircraft. Thus 88% of all early deaths occurred in those parts of the aircraft where there was greatest structural damage. Reference will be made to the seat plan to demonstrate the distribution of injuries on board the aircraft.

Injuries in survivors

Box 3.1 demonstrates the range of injuries seen in the 87 passengers and crew removed from the scene of the accident. The majority of the survivors were seated in regions of the aircraft that remained relatively intact and therefore, in most of these cases, a "liveable volume" was maintained.

Head injuries[2]

Seventy seven patients had evidence of head and facial injury including lacerations and bruising; of these, 43 had periods of amnesia surrounding the crash. Six of the initial adult survivors rescued from the aircraft demonstrated severe head injuries (box 3.2) including one patient with an extradural haematoma and one with a traumatic partial craniectomy (figure 3.3). Three died as a consequence of their head injuries and a fourth has survived with permanent severe neurological disability.

Examination of the patterns of head injury indicates that 21 patients (24%) had injuries to the backs of their heads, including five with severe head injury. This suggests that the victims may have been struck from behind. Three of these patients were seated in the middle of the aircraft,

---

Box 3.2
Severe head injuries sustained by six initial survivors of the crash

Patient injury	Outcome
1. Isolated posterior head injury: GCS 4 on arrival Lambdoid diastasis	Death from cerebral swelling
2. Isolated posterior head injury: GCS 5 on arrival Skull intact	Death from cerebral swelling
3. Posterior head injury, widened mediastinum: GCS 7 on arrival Skull intact	Death from cerebral swelling
4. Isolated posterior head injury: GCS 5 on arrival Parietal craniectomy with dural tear and brain herniation	Survived, tetraparetic in flexion
5. Isolated posterior head injury: Delayed deterioration to GCS 10 Posterior parietal fracture Acute extradural haematoma	Survived, no deficit
6. Head injury, atlantoaxial subluxation, Le fort III: GCS 7 on arrival Temporal contusion, C6 cord contusion Bilateral lower limb fractures	Survived, C6 tetraparesis

†GCS, Glasgow coma scale; MRC, Medical Research Council Muscle Strength Grading.

---

which remained structurally intact (apart from the overhead bins, which all failed).

Chest injuries[3]

Twenty three passengers sustained major chest trauma and all of these had injuries to other parts of the body. Five of these patients died within 12 hours of transfer to hospital. Fifteen patients sustained rib fractures, 11 patients had a haemothorax or pneumothorax, and 15 patients sustained lung contusions. In the six patients who demonstrated a widened mediastinum, investigations failed to identify a major vascular injury. Three survivors had electrocardiographic changes consistent with myocardial contusion, one of a severe nature.

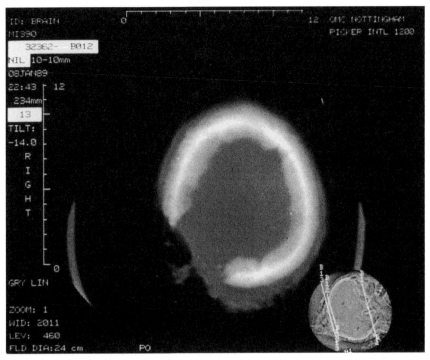

Figure 3.3—CT scan of traumatic craniotomy sustained by a survivor.

Box 3.3
Other injuries in 23 initial survivors
with chest trauma

Injury	No
Spinal fractures	9
Major head trauma	3
Limb fractures	19
Abdomen	2

Box 3.3 lists the range of associated injuries in those individuals with chest injuries. As can be seen, nearly all of them had limb fractures; however, only three had major head trauma. Most of the non-survivors demonstrated severe head and chest injuries occurring together.

Eight of the patients with chest trauma required ventilation. All had significant chest injuries, but spinal injury and head injury was the indication for ventilation in three patients. A significant correlation

Box 3.4
General surgery for abdominal injuries

Age (years)	Sex	ISS	TOA-OP† (min)	Injuries	Operation	Indication for laparotomy	Findings	Outcome
67	M	26	5	Multiple fractures Head	Laparotomy	Falling BP	None significant Mild bleeding from portahepatis	Deceased
61	M	27	25	Multiple fractures Head	Laparotomy	Falling BP	None significant	Deceased
					Fracture fixation	Tenderness	Mesenteric bruising	
				Chest Spinal fractures	Chest drain	Bruising		
52	F	45	30	Multiple fractures Head	Laparotomy	Falling BP	None significant	Survived
					Fracture fixation	Rigid abdomen	Liver haematoma	
				Chest	Chest drains			
32	F	27	55	Multiple fractures Chest	Splenectomy	Falling BP	Ruptured spleen	Survived
					Fracture fixation	Tense abdomen	Perinepheric haematoma	
23	M	19	95	Right limb fractures	Laparotomy	Tenderness	Ruptured bladder	Survived
				Diastasis of symphisis pubis	Wound toilet	Positive lavage	Tear of sigmoid colon	

†TOA-OP, time from arrival to operation.

between the age of patient and the number of rib fractures was evident such that with increasing age a greater number of rib fractures were seen. Younger patients had few or no rib fractures but still had a high incidence of lung contusion. Examination of the contusions in this group revealed a striking upper zone pattern.

Abdominal injuries[4]

Considering the apparent vulnerability of the abdomen to injury, only two patients sustained major intra-abdominal pathology; a further three patients required exploratory laparotomies but no major visceral injuries were identified (box 3.4). Both patients who sustained major intra-abdominal injuries were severely injured, with head, chest and limb injuries. One had a ruptured bladder, the other a ruptured spleen. All patients requiring

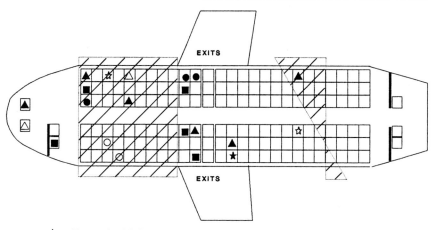

★   Two spinal injuries

▲   Lumbar spine fractures   ●   Cervical spine fractures

■   Thoracic spine fractures/disc prolapse   no fill ▪ neurology

Figure 3.4—Distribution of spinal injuries in the survivors.

laparotomies were operated on within 95 minutes of arrival at hospital, which suggests that their condition was of concern.

Thirty patients (34% of the initial survivors) demonstrated lower abdominal bruising associated with the wearing of lap type safety belts. Evidence of such bruising following an automobile accident suggests significant trauma has occurred and that intra-abdominal injury should be expected.[5,6]

Thirteen patients had haematuria, 11 microscopic and two macroscopic. Haematuria was recorded in seven patients with significant seat belt bruising, in one patient with a pelvic fracture, and in one patient with a lumbar spinal fracture. All cases were managed conservatively.

Spinal injuries

Twenty one survivors sustained a total of 24 spinal injuries, six cervical fracture or dislocations, six thoracic fracture or dislocations, and 12 lumbar fracture or dislocations. Figure 3.4 demonstrates the distribution within the aircraft of survivors with spinal injuries. Spinal injuries were more common towards the front of the aircraft where transmission of impact forces may have been higher.

Six patients sustained neurological injuries: three patients with a tetraparesis sustained by a translational type of injury to the cervical spine, one patient with an extension/distraction type injury to her thoracic spine, and two patients with burst fractures of the lumbar spine (figure 3.5).

35

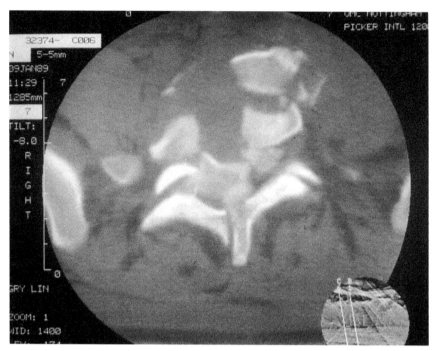

Figure 3.5—CT scan of a severe burst fracture of the lumbar spine.

In addition, of the 39 who died at the scene of the accident, 13 had spinal fractures (see later).

Pelvic and lower limb injuries

Pelvic and lower limb injuries were the commonest injuries sustained by the survivors, with 142 fractures or ligamentous injuries identified in 57 occupants (an average 2.5 injuries per patient). These included 23 pelvic injuries, 22 femoral fractures, 18 knee injuries, 31 fractured tibias, 26 ankle fractures, and 22 foot injuries. Thirty four (42%) of these lower limb injuries were open (compound) fractures.

Figures 3.6–3.9 demonstrate the distribution of pelvic and lower limb injuries for survivors and non-survivors. Many of the survivors who had pelvic fractures were in the intact centre region of the aircraft, whereas those with femoral fractures were distributed throughout the aircraft. Fractures of the tibia tended to occur in those regions of the aircraft that sustained the severest damage. However, a significant number of ankle fractures occurred in areas of the aircraft in which the floor remained intact.

A number of uncommon foot injuries were seen, namely eight compound talar fractures, the "aviator's astragalus" (figure 3.10) first described by

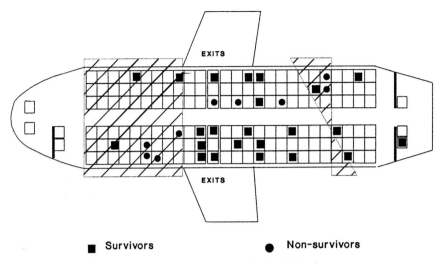

■ Survivors   ● Non-survivors

Figure 3.6—Distribution of pelvic injuries.

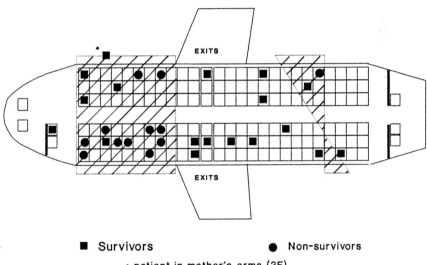

■ Survivors   ● Non-survivors

• patient in mother's arms (3F)

Figure 3.7—Distribution of femoral injuries.

Anderson in 1919 as being frequently sustained by pilots,[7,8] and six tarsometatarsal (Lisfranc) fracture/dislocations.

Upper limb injuries

Fifty nine upper limb and shoulder girdle fractures and/or dislocations were identified in 36 passengers. These included 19 fracture and/or

37

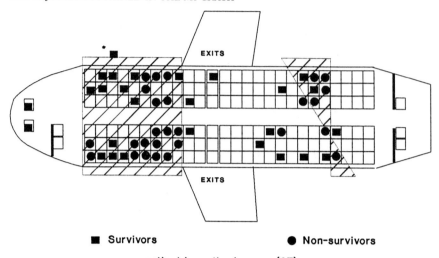

■ Survivors   **● Non-survivors**

• patient in mother's arms (3F)

Figure 3.8—Distribution of tibial fractures.

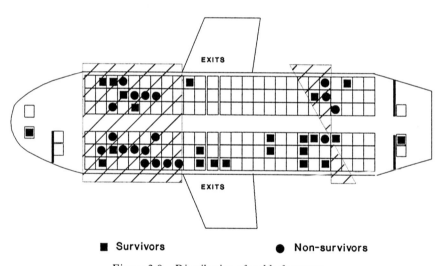

■ Survivors   **● Non-survivors**

Figure 3.9—Distribution of ankle fractures.

dislocations around the shoulder girdle, nine humeral fractures, 21 fractures of the radius and ulna, and 10 fractures or ligamentous injuries affecting the hand. Six of the upper limb fractures were open.

Injuries in non-survivors

Box 3.5 gives the range of injuries found in the 39 passengers who died at

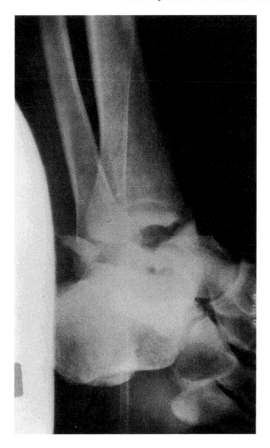

Figure 3.10—Compound talar fracture ("aviator's astragalus").

Box 3.5
Major injuries in the 39 non-survivors
who died at the scene of the accident

Injury	No
Head	39
Thoracic	39
Abdominal	31
Spinal fractures	13
Pelvic/lower limb	95
Upper limb	22

the scene of the accident. It is apparent from the seating plan (figure 3.2) that the majority of the fatalities occurred in those regions of the aircraft that sustained the severest of damage with a loss of the "liveable volume". This is reflected in the severe crushing nature of the injuries seen in the majority of these individuals.

Head injuries

All the 39 passengers who died at the scene of the accident sustained head injuries, ranging from severe bruising and scalp/face lacerations to extensive skull fracture and brain damage.

Chest injuries

Chest injuries were found in *all* non-survivors and represented crush or compression type injuries, with a range of rib fractures, extensive bruising, and/or lacerations to the underlying lungs, heart, and aorta. Younger victims tended to have fewer or no rib fractures, reflecting the flexible nature of their rib cages.

Thus head and chest injury was the leading cause of mortality. This is in keeping with the severe damage sustained by the aircraft in those regions where mortality was high. It is well recognised[1,9–12] that head and chest injuries are the leading causes of mortality in aviation accidents.

Abdominal injuries

Only eight of the on-site fatalities had no evidence of abdominal injury. The abdominal injuries identified were usually fairly extensive and ranged from very severe bruising to lacerated or avulsed organs. This contrasts with the survivors, who sustained few intra-abdominal injuries. This is in keeping with Hill's observation[13] that there is a high incidence of hepato-splenic injuries in fatalities due to aviation accidents and that they are associated with severe multisystem injuries.

Spinal injuries

Spinal injuries in the deceased patients were all of a severe nature. Only one lumbar fracture was found, but there were six thoracic and six cervical spine fractures. All the cervical fractures were combined with dislocations and were of the extension type, resulting either from "whiplash" or from striking the front of the head on the seating or airframe. Thoracic spine fractures were associated with some of the most severe internal injuries, especially aortic transection and sternal fractures.

Pelvic and limb injuries

Upper limb and shoulder injuries occurred in 18 fatalities, with a total of 22 injuries. Fractures of the humerus were the most common, with nine fractures seen. Seven wrist fracture dislocations were also recorded, with the remainder of injuries distributed between the hand, forearm, elbow, and clavicle. One patient sustained a traumatic amputation of an upper limb. Seven of the upper limb injuries were open (compound) fractures.

All but four of the non-survivors sustained lower limb injuries. Nine pelvic injuries were seen, 13 femoral fractures, five knee injuries, 38 lower leg fractures, 24 ankle fractures, and six foot injuries. Forty nine (50%) of these injuries were open (compound) fractures. The distribution of these injuries is demonstrated in figures 3.4 and 3.6–3.9.

Injury scoring in the evaluation of the injuries sustained

With the exception of abdominal injuries, there was little to distinguish the actual types and severity of the injuries sustained by the non-survivors from those sustained by the survivors. Injury scoring techniques as a means of classifying the extent and the severity of trauma has a long history. The abbreviated injury scale (AIS)[14] is a regional threat-to-life scale and has been accepted worldwide as the system of choice for assessing the severity of road related impact trauma; however, the majority of impact injury patients die because of more than one injury. Injuries that in themselves would not be life threatening could have a significant effect on mortality when combined with other injuries. Baker *et al*[15] devised a system, the injury severity score (ISS), as a means of assessing the multiply injured patient.

The ISS has now become an established scoring system for survival prediction and trauma audit. It is an index of anatomical injury but takes no account of the physiological or psychological effects of trauma. The score has been found to be useful as a measure of mortality, survival time, length of hospital stay, and disability.[16] This has now led to a definition of a patient with major trauma as a patient who scores an ISS of 16 or more points. An ISS of 16 is predictive of a 10% mortality.[17]

Abbreviated injury score[14]

Regional AISs were calculated for the occupants on board the aircraft using clinical notes or postmortem findings. In this system, the body is divided into six regions—head and neck, face, chest, abdominal and pelvic contents, extremities and pelvic girdle, and general (external). The injuries are scored in each region with an increasing severity of 1–5. A score of 1 is considered a minor injury, whereas a score of 5 is considered a critical injury—that is, survival uncertain. A score of 6 is possible for any given region but is considered non-survivable.

Scoring injuries in this way demonstrates variations in the severity of

TABLE 3.1 Abbreviated injury scores

Region	Average score		
	Survivors	Non-survivors	p<
Head and neck	1.2	3.7	<0.0005
Face	0.2	1	<0.002
Chest	1.1	4.6	<0·0005
Abdomen and pelvic contents	0.7	2.5	<0.0005
Limbs and pelvic girdle	2.1	2.8	<0.0002
External	1.2	1.7	<0.0002

injuries amongst the survivors and the non-survivors seated in the passenger compartment of the aircraft. From table 3.1 it can be seen that for all anatomical regions scored by AIS, the injuries in the non-survivors were of greater severity, the difference being statistically significant.

Nineteen of the occupants scored the maximum—6—for the AIS for a body region. These included 10 individuals with a maximum score for the head and neck region, and nine for the chest region. Such injuries are not compatible with life, and could be considered immediately fatal.

Injury severity score

The injuries sustained by the occupants can also be assessed using the ISS. This is calculated using the system of Baker *et al.*[15] as the sum of the squares of the three highest AISs. Only the contribution of the most major regional injury is used. The highest ISS attainable is 75 and is scored automatically if any body region scores an AIS of 6. The ISS is a non-linear discontinuous score, with higher values indicating greater severity of injury.

Figure 3.11 demonstrates the ISSs of the passengers and crew. The average ISS of all occupants on the aircraft was 28 (range of 1–75). Survivors of the impact had an average ISS of 16 (range 1–50) and fatalities at the scene an average ISS of 55. Nineteen occupants had a maximum ISS of 75, nine had an ISS ranging between 50 and 74, and 16 between 25 and 49. Furthermore, of the initial 87 survivors, 30 (37%) had an ISS of 16 or greater, and these occupants fulfilled the criteria of a severely traumatised individual according to the definition of Boyd *et al.*[17]

It can be seen from figures 3.2 and 3.11 that the higher mortality values and ISS corresponded to those regions of the aircraft that sustained the most severe structural damage. Survivability and low ISS occurred in those regions that, on the whole, remained structurally intact.

Of the initial 87 survivors to be removed from the wreckage of the aircraft alive, four died within 90 minutes of arrival at hospital. Two died from major head trauma; the other two died of multiple injuries. The ISS

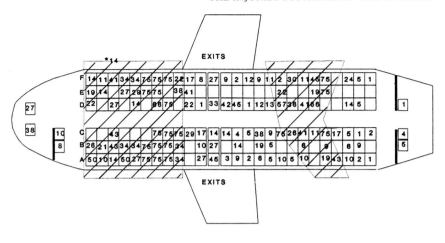

* patient in mother's arms (3F)

Figure 3.11—Injury severity scores of the passengers and crew.

for these early deaths were 26, 36, 45, and 27. A further four patients died during the following weeks, while receiving treatment in hospital. One patient died at 12 hours from head and chest injuries with an ISS of 41. A second died at 11 days after admission with multisystem organ failure with an ISS of 27. The other two patients died from pulmonary embolism at 15 and 22 days with an ISS of 41 and 11.

It is apparent that a number of non-survivors sustained an ISS of a value less than some of the survivors. Severe injuries, however inflicted, will kill one individual but not another, and apparently minor injuries will kill some but not others. The reasons for these variations are unclear in many cases. Factors that contribute to these incongruities include age, sex, physical state, pre-existing disease, drugs, etc. Apart from these individual variations, other external factors may account for these discrepancies, for example entrapment in the wreckage and delay in obtaining medical treatment. It would therefore have been useful to know whether any of those who died at the scene did survive for any length of time after the impact; unfortunately, this information was not directly available.

Fat embolus syndrome

When a bone is fractured the content of the bone, namely marrow and fat, can gain access to the blood stream as microscopic fragments that can be carried to the lungs only if there is an active circulation. These fragments become impacted as fat emboli in the lungs, and the identification of such emboli provides an indication of survival following the infliction of injuries

43

Fat emboli

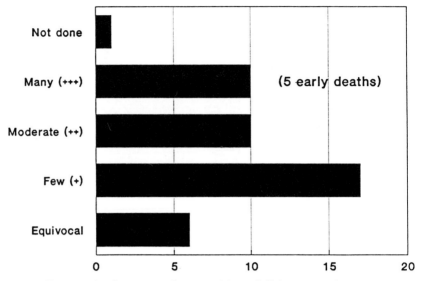

Figure 3.12—Presence and extent of fat emboli in non-survivors.

such as fractures. In can be hypothesised that the greater the length of time an active circulation is present the greater the presence of fat emboli in the lungs.

Histological examination of the lungs in 43 of the 44 early deaths demonstrated the presence of varying amounts of fat emboli in 37 cases and equivocal results in six; the tissues of one passenger were not examined for fat emboli. Thus the majority of those who died at the scene of the accident survived the impact, though the length of survival may have been quite short—indeed, 19 occupants had head and chest injuries that were incompatible with life.

Figure 3.12 illustrates the presence and extent of fat emboli in 44 non-survivors. For those occupants demonstrating greater amounts of fat emboli one can speculate that they survived following the impact for varying amounts of time. Indeed, five of the early deaths away from the scene had many fat emboli in the lungs. For the remaining individuals, the exact length of survival is uncertain but all had a significant head injury that would have rendered them unconscious.

As has been previously stated, entrapment in the wreckage of an aircraft is a cause of mortality in aircraft accidents. Figure 3.13 demonstrates that in some cases occupants were trapped in the wreckage and not transferred to hospital for over 4 hours, with the last occupant to be extracted alive arriving in hospital some 8 hours after the accident. Subsequently he unfortunately died from his injuries, with an ISS of 27.

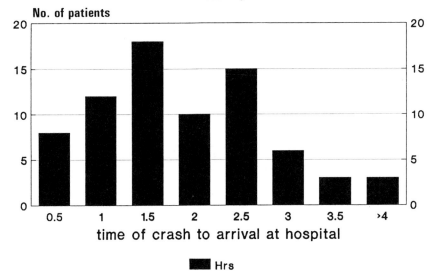

Figure 3.13—Time of arrival at hospital (information was available for only 75 patients).

Summary

The occupants of the M1 aircrash sustained a variety of injuries, from simple bruising to severe crushing injuries. Of those who survived the impact, only 13 patients, as indicated by their low ISS (less than 3), could be considered to be walking wounded and therefore able to help in their rescue. The remaining occupants demonstrated a range of injuries, in particular head and limb injuries, that may have interfered with their ability to escape.

The injuries in those occupants who died at the scene, although in many cases similar to those sustained by the survivors, were of a greater degree of severity. Head and chest injuries accounted for the on-site mortalities, a significant number also demonstrating severe intra-abdominal injuries. Of those passengers who died in the days following the accident, two sustained pulmonary embolism and one died from multisystem organ failure.

The consequences of the injuries to the passengers and crew is immense both in terms of cost of treatment and also human suffering and late disability. The M1 aircrash has demonstrated that, with adequate medical facilities and in the absence of a post-crash fire, survivability is possible in large numbers. The crash also demonstrated that the transmission of forces through the airframe and seats results in serious injuries to the occupants, especially in those regions of the aircraft that sustain catastrophic damage. Even in those areas that remained relatively intact the injuries were significant.

1 Fryer DI. The results of accidents. In: *Gillies textbook of aviation physiology*. Oxford: Pergamon, 1965; 1166–79.
2 White BD, Rowles JM, Mumford CJ, Firth JL. Head Injuries in the M1 Boeing 737 aircrash. *Br J Neurosurg* 1990; **4**: 501–3.
3 Morgon WE, Salama FD, Beggs FD, Firman RK, Rowles JM. Thoracic injuries sustained by the survivors of the M1 (Kegworth) aircraft accident. *Eur J Cardiothoracic Surg* 1990; **4**: 417–20.
4 Rowles JM, Robertson C, Roberts SNJ. General surgical injuries in survivors of the M1 Kegworth aircrash. *Ann R Coll Surg* 1990; **72**: 378–81.
5 Doersch KB, Dozier WE. The seat belt syndrome: the seat belt sign, intestinal and mesenteric injuries. *Am J Surg* 1968; **116**: 831–3.
6 Pedersen S, Jansen U. Intestinal lesions caused by incorrectly placed seat belts. *Acta Chir Scand* 1979; **145**: 15–18.
7 Coltart WD. Aviators' Astragalus. *J Bone Joint Surg* 1952; **34B**: 545–66.
8 Hawkins LG. Fractures of the neck of the talus. *JBJS* 1970; **52A**: 991–1001.
9 Swearingen JJ, Hasbrook AH, Snyder RG, McFadden EB. Kinematic behaviour of the human body during deceleration. *Aerospace Med* 1962; **33**: 188–97.
10 Mason JK. Injuries sustained in fatal aircraft accidents. *Br J Hosp Med* 1973; **May**: 645–54.
11 Mason JK. The mode and cause of death from aviation accidents. In: *Aviation accident pathology*. London: Butterworths, 1962; 106–145.
12 Stephens PH. Reconstruction of events at impact and immediately after an accident. In: *Fatal civil aircraft accidents*. Bristol: John Wright, 1970; 52–60.
13 Hill IR. Hepato-splenic injury in aircraft accidents. *Aviat Space Environ Med* 1982; **53(1)**: 19–23.
14 American Association for Automobile Medicine. *The abbreviated injury severity score.* AAAM, Chicago, Illinois; 1985; revision.
15 Baker SP, O'Neill B, Haddon W, Long WB. The injury severity score: A method for describing patients with multiple injuries and evaluating emergency care. *J Trauma* 1974; **14**: 187–96.
16 Bull JP. The injury severity score of road traffic casualties in relation to mortality, time of death, hospital treatment and disability. *Accid Annal Prev* 1975; **7**: 249–55.
17 Boyd CR, Tolson MA, Copes WS. Evaluating trauma care: the TRISS method. *J Trauma* 1987; **27(4)**: 370–8.

4
On-site management of the victims in the M1 plane crash and the use of triage

MICHAEL J ALLEN

Introduction

Flight BD 92 crashed on the motorway embankment of the M1 on a cold January evening at approximately 2030. The crash site was approximately 10 miles from Queen's Medical Centre, Nottingham, 12 miles from Derby Royal Infirmary and 20 miles from Leicester Royal Infirmary.

As it came to rest on the embankment, the plane split into three sections—the cockpit being some 30 yards from the main fuselage and tail (figure 4.1). By the nature of the impact the tail section had flipped up 90°, to end vertically. Most of the immediate fatalities appeared, at the time of the accident, to have occurred at the junction of the broken rear fuselage and tail, but it later transpired that this was not in fact the case (figure 4.2).

Access to the aircraft was in some ways fortuitous in that it came to rest adjacent to the M1 motorway and the A453 Derby to Ashby road. In other ways, access to the casualties was extremely difficult as the embankment on which the aircraft had come to rest was steeply inclined and wooded. Conditions for the rescuers was worsened by the fact that it was dark and cold, the embankment was slippery, and within 5 minutes of the accident was made worse by foam sprayed over the area to prevent ignition of the 77 000 litres of aviation fuel left in the fuel tanks of the plane. Added to this, many of the casualties were trapped by twisted metal and debris in the cylindrical wreckage, making their extrication extremely difficult.

My abiding memories of the scene were the incredible noise made by the rescue equipment, the 700 helpers, many of whom were nowhere near the wreckage, and the blue sea of flashing ambulance beacons. It would have

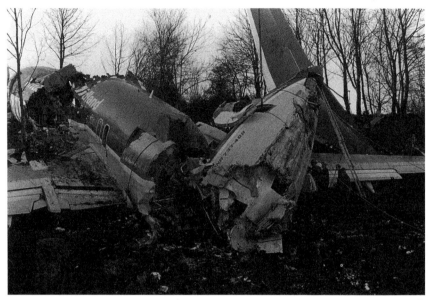

Figure 4.1—The M1 aircrash: it later became apparent that most of the fatalities had not in fact occurred at the junction of the fuselage and tail.

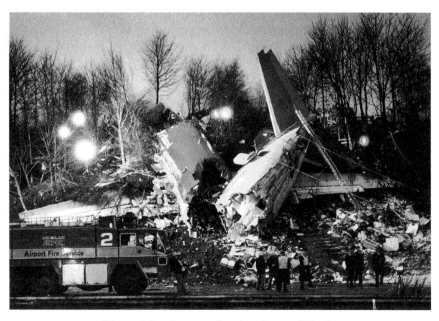

Figure 4.2—Access to the aircraft was difficult.

been better, as in the major accidents protocol, if the ambulance beacons had been extinguished, thus allowing the beacons for the emergency control vehicle to be better visualised. However the most striking feature was the calmness and lack of panic amongst the casualties themselves.

Initial response

At about 2030 the accident and emergency departments of the three main hospitals were alerted to the possibility of an impending incident, and after some initial confusion flying squads from the three main hospitals, and subsequently two back up squads were dispatched to the scene. At no time was official confirmation of the disaster received at any of the three hospitals.

As the crash happened just before peak television viewing time in the winter, the early news flashes prompted the response of most of the staff who came into the departments, thus bypassing the telephone cascade system designed for such events.

Due to the close proximity of, and rapid access to, Queen's Medical Centre in Nottingham and Derbyshire Royal Infirmary, these were declared the designated receiving hospitals (Leicester Royal Infirmary, being some distance away from the scene—20 miles—was designated third on take, in part because access to Leicester appeared to be obstructed by the crashed plane.

The scene

Ambulance and fire crews arrived before medical staff and the first 20 survivors were immediately taken on a "scoop-and-run" basis by ambulance to Queen's Medical Centre. The remaining casualties were trapped by twisted metal in the flipped up tail section and the front and rear sections of the fuselage. Access to the casualties was made even more difficult because the main fuselage floor in the forward section had collapsed into the cargo hold.

Access to the aircraft and thus to the victims was difficult for several reasons. The embankment sloped some 30° to the horizontal and was thickly wooded. The aircraft fire services had sprayed the aircraft with foam, in fear of the remaining 77 000 litres of aviation fuel left in the fuel tanks igniting. This made the embankment extremely slippery, and rescue personnel could only reach the wreckage if helped up the hillside by a human chain of volunteers. As the rescue progressed, steps dug into the hillside by mountain rescue teams helped access, but even these became too slippery after a while. The fact that part of the main fuselage floor had collapsed meant that medical personnel had to be lowered by ropes to the passengers who had been trapped in the cargo hold.

Although the scene was well lit and the aircraft well secured, illumination was extremely poor when working within the wreckage. It would have been extremely useful to have worn miners' type helmets, but these had unfortunately been left behind in the initial haste of departure.

The flying squads from the three hospitals each operated in one section of the aircraft. Derby took one part of the tail section, Nottingham the adjacent tail and rear fuselage section, and Leicester the main fuselage and cockpit. Equipment was limited to what could be carried in the rescuers' pockets and treatment was limited because of the poor access until patients were partially or completely extricated from the wreckage.

Communication between medical teams was extremely difficult, partly due to the incredible noise of the cutting gear and partly due to the nature and location of the wreckage. The only means of obtaining an overall view of the proceedings was to send one of the doctors around the aircraft, a process that took about 20 minutes to complete.

From a medical point of view it was difficult to ascertain the exact number of casualties on board the aircraft, and as the rescue progressed it was even more difficult to tell how many were left. At one stage it was thought there were eight remaining survivors when in fact there were only four. This confusion arose because two separate rescue teams were approaching the same four people from different directions.

It also proved difficult to identify both the profession and rank of personnel working at the scene, which again made communication difficult.

Triage point

This was the base medical station where patients who had been extricated from the wreckage were assessed in order of priority; emergency medical treatment was given, following which they were dispatched to hospital on a priority basis.

Initially the triage point was set up close to the aircraft on the M1 but it was subsequently disbanded and re-established some distance away from the scene. The reasons were firstly that it became overrun by the mêlée of helpers and secondly it was deemed by the fire service to be at risk of being too close to the aircraft were it to explode into flames. Initial medical triage of the victims proved difficult due to the geography of the wreckage. In the early stages of the rescue survivors were simultaneously being extricated from the wreckage at the top and bottom of the embankment. Those taken from the top were transferred by ambulance along the A453 and those from the bottom were transported by the motorway. This made coordinated medical triage nearly impossible. Once the triage point had been re-established and the initial survivors dispatched to hospital the situation became more orderly, with the remaining victims all passing through the triage point. Patients were reassessed at this point prior to hospital transfer, although conditions were less than ideal. The ambulance vehicle that was intended to identify and light the triage point and provide communications unfortunately broke down on its way from Leicester to the site, thus making identification of the medical station to other personnel extremely difficult and making working conditions for those manning the triage point equally difficult.

It proved extremely useful to have one nurse solely in charge of medical equipment at the triage point. As the disaster produced mainly long bone and pelvic injuries, resuscitation was mainly directed at replacing fluid loss, preventing or reversing hypovolaemic shock, and the first aid splintage of broken limbs, along with the administration of analgesia. In fact, 300 litres of plasma expanders were utilised at the scene. By having one person solely in charge made the distribution of equipment orderly in a situation that could otherwise have been chaotic, especially in the poorly lit conditions that prevailed.

Due to the large quantities of fluids, administration sets, etc. required, further supplies were requested from the base hospital, some of which never arrived and have never been accounted for. It is recommended that once the type of disaster is known then the type of equipment most required at the scene is requested from the base hospital and personally brought out by a member of the medical staff and handed over to the triage nurse in charge of equipment.

Transport of the injured

Initially transport was by ambulance to the three designated hospitals, coordinated through their individual control centres. Later, as the rescue became organised, transport was controlled by the chief ambulance officer on site. As information was relayed on the distribution of patients between the three hospitals, further victims were redirected accordingly.

Eventually the roads became congested and Leicester Royal Infirmary, the furthest hospital from the scene, became the designated on take hospital. At this juncture, two Sea King and two Wessex helicopters arrived, which were used to transport the injured to Leicester Royal Infirmary, the flight time being only 9 minutes. This was despite the patients' obvious severe apprehension about further air travel! In all tragedies there are episodes of humour. I will never forget one gentleman who was extricated from the wreckage and then told that he was off to hospital in a helicopter (figure 4.3). His reply was unprintable, but suffice it to say he had a safe and uneventful journey.

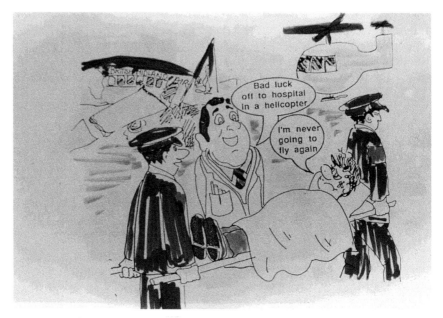

Figure 4.3—Disasters are not without humour.

Documentation

Documentation of casualties proved difficult at the scene. Each hospital used its own system of labelling the casualties in order of priority of treatment. In fact one of the hospitals participating forgot to take their labels and had to use the aircraft luggage labels. The other two hospitals used completely different colour coded labelling systems (figure 4.4) and the labelling is completely opposite; green indicating a dead patient in one system and a walking wounded in another. Despite the difference no catastrophic mistakes were made, but confusion could have arisen. This highlights the need for a nationally agreed labelling system for casualties.

On the night of the disaster it was also found that there was difficulty in completing the labels, due to either lack of writing implements or the fact that the wet muddy conditions meant that the pencils would not write. This implies that the labelling system must be simple, easy to use and water-proof.

Communication

In all previous disasters communication has proved difficult. This disaster proved no exception to the rule. Communication between personnel at the scene of the disaster was difficult due to the very nature of the incident and

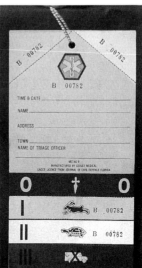
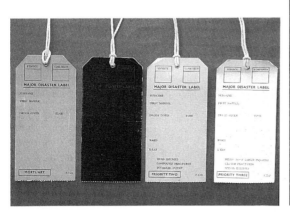

Figure 4.4—Labelling systems for casualties. The system on the left shows green, red, blue, and white labels (from left to right), and that on the right black (0), red (I), yellow (II), and green (III).

also the incredible noise generated by the cutting equipment. As stated previously, communication around the aircraft was also difficult. Communication between the aircraft and the triage point was extremely difficult. Requests for equipment had to be verbally relayed and became distorted.

One of the flying squads had excellent communication between staff at the scene and those at the base hospital because they used cellular telephones. A routine updating call was made every 20 minutes, or sooner if there was important information to relay. However, this did not prevent confusing rumours spreading.

Communication between the site and the other two hosptials was thought to be inadequate, although the cellular telephone was used to ascertain where the injured had been taken and to redirect further casualties accordingly.

Thus, even if communication channels are successfully established, there must be a system by which the information relayed is directed to those people in a position to act upon it.

Conclusion

This particular disaster proved unusual because there were a large number of survivors. Unlike other disasters, medical manpower was not a problem

53

due to the participation of three hospitals. It is doubtful that a single hospital would have been able to cope with a similar situation.

In general, the medical care the patients received at the scene of the disaster was excellent, taking into account the restraints put upon the rescuers by the very nature of the incident. However, lessons can and indeed should be learnt. The most important of these are summarised in the box.

On the night of 8 January 1989 there were many heroes but the greatest credit must go to all the passengers on board flight BD 92, who were all heroes.

On-site management at a disaster site: lessons learned from the M1 aircrash

- Identification of key staff should be improved, making coordination and communication much easier; recommendations arising from the M1 crash have, since the accident, been adopted in major incident plans

- Each rescue service should have its own identification marks on clothing, making recognition and communication easier; this also has recently been adopted in plans

- On arrival of the first flying squad teams, rapid assessment of the pattern and type of injuries requiring treatment should be made and appropriate equipment, accompanied by a nurse, should be requested and transferred to the scene. Specific specialised staff requirements could also be mobilised at this time.

- The triage point, planned after a careful reconnoitre of the site, should be clearly identified and illuminated, with one nurse in sole charge of all equipment

- Provision must be made to allow equipment used in the initial treatment of casualties to be hand carried; this could be facilitated by using rucksacks or belts with pouches

- Climbing (miners' type) helmets should be available, allowing for hand-free illumination when working in dark and confined spaces

- Evacuation by helicopter can be extremely useful; in the M1 accident it allowed in-flight treatment by the accompanying medical staff on the journey to the receiving hospital.

- Use of helicopters can also allow tired medical staff to be replaced by fresh staff and further equipment transferred to the scene

- Provision should be made for the changeover of medical staff if the time required at the scene of the disaster is prolonged (more than 3–4 hours)

- The cellular telephone is invaluable, allowing direct communication between the scene of the disaster and the base hospital; it may be necessary, however, for the police to authorise "access overload control" (giving Home Office registered users priority over other users in the area) to enable cell phone use. When more than one centre is involved, methods should exist for communication between hospitals

- Hand-held radios are possibly beneficial for communication around the aircraft, but personnel must be trained in their use beforehand

- When more than one centre is receiving survivors, patients should be appropriately distributed between centres; this involves regular communication between hospitals as well as between the hospitals and the scene

- Hazardous conditions may exist (in the M1 aircrash, the 77 000 litres of aviation fuel and the slippery terrain): provision should therefore be made for treating injuries to the rescue teams and care should be taken not to close the incident too soon

- A universal patient labelling system for the UK is essential, and steps are being taken to introduce this

5

Dealing with the fatalities of the M1 plane crash

J STEPHEN P JONES

Introduction

When a major disaster occurs the first priority must be to rescue the survivors, to give them immediate supportive treatment, and to despatch them as rapidly as possible to hospital for skilled medical, surgical, and nursing attention. It is worth noting that it is important that non-survivors are labelled as "dead" as soon as this is established by a doctor; otherwise, doctors may be repeatedly called back to the same body. Once survivors have been attended to, it is necessary to focus attention on the care of the dead. This latter consideration is a subject to which relatively little forethought has been given until recent years. Because there is an increasing risk of major catastrophes occurring, and especially those in which there may be multiple fatalities, the time is opportune to study the procedures that should be followed. Many lessons were learnt at the Kegworth aircrash, and it is intended in this chapter to pass on the experience that was gained.

It is a popular misconception that following a major disaster such as an aircrash, once the bodies have been identified, there is no need for any further examination since all can be assumed to have died of "multiple injuries" as a result of the crash. It is worth stating at the outset that there is a great need following such accidents for the most detailed examination on each body (see box).

Practical procedures for the examination of the dead in a major disaster

The legal ownership of the bodies lies with the coroner/procurator fiscal in whose jurisdiction the bodies lie. The responsibility for the care of those bodies, including identification, rests with the relevant county police force.

Objectives of the examination of the dead in a major disaster

- To determine the identity of the body
- To document every injury that has been sustained
- To document any natural disease that may be present
- To establish the cause of death
- To collect such specimens as may be required for further examination (for histology, toxicology, serology, etc.)
- To estimate the time interval between the moment of the crash and death
- To estimate the length of time during which pain and suffering may have been experienced prior to unconsciousness and death supervening
- When two or more members of the same family are travelling together, to ascertain—if possible—the order in which they died
- To obtain forensic, scientific and other evidence in those cases in which criminal involvement is suspected as being a cause of the disaster
- To collect such evidence which may be required for the coroner's inquest, civil or criminal litigation proceedings, national or international inquiry boards

The siting of a major disaster mortuary

In order to carry out an orderly procedure for the identification and examination of the dead it is necessary to designate a site for a major disaster mortuary, usually close to the disaster scene. It is essential that all the bodies are taken to a single mortuary.

Usually, local hospital mortuaries are not used. The reason for this is that if more than one mortuary is used the task of identification and liaison with bereaved relatives is made extremely complex and may be open to error. If there were more than one mortuary, this would necessitate the creation of multiple identification teams and duplication of communications equipment, overburdening a system that would in any case be severely stretched. The reasons for not using local hospital mortuaries can be summarised as follows:

- If the major disaster, as at Kegworth, involves many live casualties as well as dead bodies, it is essential that the approach roads to the local hospitals are kept clear. The traffic routes and reception facilities at the hospitals should not be encumbered by bringing in the dead as well as the live casualties. Additional congestion could be caused by relatives and friends visiting the hospital mortuary, and by potential media involvement

- The arrival of large numbers of bodies at a hospital mortuary would rapidly overwhelm the capacity of that mortuary, thus leading to the use of mortuaries at other sites—a situation already established as being highly undesirable. The influx of a large number of bodies from a disaster would also seriously disrupt the normal routine work of the hospital mortuary for many days and possibly weeks

- Bearing in mind that bodies from a major disaster may be burnt, mutilated, or partly decomposed, it would be undesirable for them to be received and stored in large numbers in a hospital mortuary

- Extensive radiological examinations may need to be carried out and, for the reasons stated in the previous point, use of a hospital radiology department would be quite inappropriate for this purpose.

The requirements for a major disaster mortuary

(1) Ideally the site designated for a major disaster mortuary should have a very large, water-impervious floor space at ground level. It should be large enough to carry out the sequential investigations and procedures of:

  - Identification

  - Pathological and ancillary investigations

  - Embalming

  - Encoffining.

(2) The mortuary should be sited so that there is easy access for the transportation and collection of bodies. The location should be totally secure and it should allow privacy.

(3) There should be adequate lighting, heating, ventilation, water supply, and drainage.

(4) Office facilities, to deal with documentation and communications, must be available. These can be provided by the use of Portakabins and mobile equipment, including telephones, computer link ups, fax machines, etc. Close links with the police casualty bureau, with the coroner/procurator fiscal, and with the criminal investigation department (CID), and other authorities are essential.

(5) Adequate car and lorry parking should be available. It may be necessary to store bodies in refrigerated vans. Space for these and any necessary portable generators needs to be planned.

(6) Storage facilities for the victims' property and clothing will be necessary. Refrigerated space will also be required for the temporary storage of pathological specimens pending further investigations.

(7) Special consideration for the care of the bereaved is of paramount importance. Whereas identification of bodies by visual means is inevitably painful and often unreliable due to their intense distress, there are many relatives and friends who positively wish to view the body. Facilities for the viewing of bodies by the bereaved, with an adjacent quiet waiting area, must therefore be provided. This should, if possible, be physically separated from the mortuary, but easily accessible to it. The area should have a discrete access and it should allow for the viewing of one body at a time. At a later stage, after the examination procedures have been completed and cosmetic restoration has been carried out by the undertakers, more appropriate facilities can be provided to enable the bereaved to spend some time in privacy with the deceased.

The police will set up a relatives or friends reception centre in order to interview the bereaved and to obtain information regarding identification. Ideally, an hotel situated close to the emergency mortuary could be used.

The examination of the dead

If a photographer is available photographs of the dead *in situ* may be taken as long as this does not hamper the rescue procedure. The bodies, having been placed in body bags at the scene and labelled as to the exact site from which they were recovered, are taken to the major disaster mortuary and are placed on the floor in lines at one end of the building. A number is allocated to each body, and this number is used in all subsequent procedures relating to identification and examination. A document file is created for each body.

Identification procedures, such as photography, fingerprinting, description of clothing and jewellery, description of body scars and tattoos, colour of hair, eyes, height, weight, and dental examination are carried out. A checklist is created for each body and each investigator must sign the checklist when each procedure has been completed. The information derived from these identification procedures is fed into the police casualty bureau.

Post mortem examinations: These are carried out by pathology teams (see box on page 60).

An essential and invaluable group—usually consisting of young police officers or cadets—is the bearers, who move the bodies to different parts of the mortuary for the varying procedures to be carried out.

Embalming and encoffining: after the postmortem examinations have been completed each body is passed to the undertakers, who embalm them and prepare them for burial or cremation. If necessary, cosmetic proced-

The pathology team

- A pathologist with forensic experience

- A mortuary technician

- A secretary to whom all information concerning identifying features, details of injuries, and natural disease, and a list of exhibits is dictated contemporaneously

- A photographer from the police scene of crime department, who will photograph all injuries and abnormalities

- A police exhibits officer, who is responsible for labelling and forwarding all the exhibits collected during the investigation; this officer also liaises with the police identification team

- A forensic odontologist, who will chart the dental configuration of the victims, and ultimately will compare the findings with the dental records of the suspected individuals

ures are carried out, as in many cases bereaved relatives and friends wish to see and spend some time with the deceased.

Radiological investigations: a decision will need to be taken at an early stage of the investigation as to whether radiological examination of the bodies is to be carried out. The decision will require joint consultation between the coroner/procurator fiscal, police—especially the CID—and the forensic pathologist.

If the disaster is thought to be due to an explosive device, full radiological examination will have to be carried out on every body. Disintegrated particles from an explosion may have entered the victims. The location and the direction of the traverse of particles through the body may assist in identifying the original site of the explosive device.

Radiological information may also be helpful in identification procedures—for example, by demonstrating old fractures or deformities, or the presence and type of orthopaedic prostheses. This can be especially helpful if disintegration of a body has taken place.

However, radiology is very time consuming and expensive. It requires the transport of mobile *x* ray machinery to the major disaster mortuary; the presence of radiographers, radiologists, and dark-room technicians; and the setting up of protective screening and reporting areas. If it is to be carried out, and in some cases it is essential, the bodies should be *x* rayed as part of the identification process and before the postmortem examination has commenced. Radiological examinations will inevitably increase the time scale of the investigation and will greatly increase the complexity and the cost. However, if they are not instituted, valuable information may be lost. For instance, it is likely the number of spinal injuries in the non-survivors of the Kegworth aircrash has been underestimated because radiological examination were not carried out on non-survivors.

Continuity of evidence: it is of course essential that meticulous attention is paid to the continuity of evidence. The identification number allocated to each body on arrival at the mortuary is the means of coordinating all the information relating to that body. All the property collected from the body, all the identifying features recorded, all the findings at the postmortem examination, which are recorded and charted, and all the fluid and tissue specimens collected bear the designated identification number. A card bearing the number should be included in every photograph taken.

The experience at Kegworth

When the aircraft crashed on the embankment of the M1 motorway in the vicinity of East Midlands Airport it was soon established that there were many survivors and many dead. While the immediate evacuation of the survivors to Nottingham, Leicester, and Derby was taking place a decision was jointly taken by HM Coroner, the Leicestershire police and the Home Office pathologist to establish the major disaster mortuary at the East Midlands Airport. With the full cooperation of the airport authority, the "snowshed" was designated for this purpose. This was a large ground floor shed resembling an aircraft hangar. It normally housed the large snow clearing equipment which was removed from the shed, leaving a completely clear and extensive concrete floor area. The shed was situated in a secure zone of the airport, and it had easy access from the site of the accident. The sides of the shed could be opened by vertical folding doors so that vehicles bringing the bodies from the scene could drive directly into the building. There was ample space within the building for the various stages of the investigation to take place, and ample space in the immediate vicinity of the shed for Portakabins to be placed and for communication equipment to be installed.

The engineering department of the airport authority assembled overhead lighting batons and blow heaters. Temporary mortuary tables were provided by Leicester Royal Infirmary. Forensic pathology teams were assembled from Leicester, Nottingham, and the Royal Air Force Institute, Halton. Forensic odontologists from the Royal Air Force and from Kenyons (undertakers) also attended.

After consultation between the police, pathologists, and the coroner, it was established that this particular disaster was not associated with an explosive device and that from a forensic point of view it was not necessary to embark on a full radiological examination of each victim. While this decision has been criticised by those carrying out research investigations into the details of the injuries sustained by the victims, the justification for considerably prolonging the postmortem investigations and the very high cost of the exercise were not thought to be valid at the time.

One of the features experienced by those who are involved in dealing with the victims of major disasters—a feature not often appreciated by those who have not had this experience—is the enormous pressure by the bereaved and by the media to complete the investigations as rapidly as possible. While it is essential to carry out every examination with meticulous thoroughness, any unnecessary delay has to be avoided, so that the bodies may be released to the relatives promptly.

When the operations at the major disaster mortuary had been completed, the shed was thoroughly cleaned and disinfected. The coordination of documentation regarding identification, cause of death, and details of injuries was carried out within a few days. The coroner was able to issue disposal certificates so that the bodies could be released to the relatives for burial or cremation, as desired.

Number of dead at and after the Kegworth aircrash

Males: 27
Females: 20
Total: 47

39 bodies were recovered from the scene
4 died in accident and emergency departments
4 died in hospital some days later

At the subsequent inquest the pathologists were required to give the cause of death in each case, together with an estimate of the length of time that pain and suffering may have been encountered, from the moment of impact. This information would be required for civil litigation procedures.

Postscript

Many lessons were learned at the Kegworth disaster relating to the organisation for dealing with the dead. Sadly, other major disasters at Hillsborough and Lockerbie occurred within a short space of time. Because no detailed documented guidelines were in existence for the procedures relating to the dead in major disasters, the Royal College of Pathologists commissioned the preparation of a document which was published in July 1990—*Deaths in major disasters—the pathologist's role*. This was written in consultation with the Association of Chief Police Officers who had recently published an emergency procedures manual. The recommendations in

---

Causes of death at the Kegworth aircrash

43 rapid deaths:	Multiple injuries	25
	Severe chest injuries	4
	Severe head injury	3
	Severe head and chest injury	6
	Severe abdominal injury	1
	Severe chest and pelvic injury	1
	Severe chest and abdominal injury	1
	Shock and haemorrhage	1
	Cerebral contusion	1
4 later deaths:	Acute hepatic and renal failure—multiple injuries	1
	Pulmonary thromboembolism	2
	Multiple injuries	1

Main points
- Head injuries, varying from scalp and facial bruising to fractured skull and brain damage, were present in all 43 rapid deaths

- Lower limb injuries were present in all but four of the 43 rapid deaths

- Chest injuries, varying from severe bruising to rib fractures and lacerations of heart and lungs, were present in all of the 43 rapid deaths; the younger victims had fewer or no fractured ribs

- Abdominal injuries: only nine of the 43 rapid deaths were free from abdominal injury; these ranged from severe bruising to lacerated organs

---

these two documents are currently being implemented throughout the United Kingdom.

It is appropriate to place on record the high degree of professional skills and sensitivity that were exhibited in the care of the dead at the Kegworth disaster. Her Majesty's Coroner for North Leicestershire, the Coroner's Officer, the East Midlands Airport Authority, the Leicestershire and Nottinghamshire constabularies, the members of the identification and pathology teams and the staff of Kenyons all worked together in a quiet, efficient, and coordinated way.

I particularly acknowledge the contribution made by Dr Clive Bouch, Home Office Pathologist for Leicestershire, who coordinated the pathology investigations, and who made all the data freely available to me.

I am grateful to Professor Tony Busuttil, joint author of the Royal College of Pathologist's document, *Deaths in Major Disasters—the Pathologist's Role*, and to the College for allowing me to quote freely from the publication.

I wish to thank Mrs Valerie Bolton for preparing the manuscript of this chapter.

Further reading

Association of Chief Police Officers. *Emergency Procedures Manual.*

Busuttil A, Jones JSP. *Deaths in major disasters—the pathologist's role.* London: Royal College of Pathologists, 1990.

Busuttil A, Jones JSP. The certification and disposal of the dead in major disasters. *Med Sci Law* 1992; **32**: 9–13.
Shepherd RT. Planning for disasters [editorial]. *MJL* 1990; **58**: 3–4.
Sivaloganathan S, Green MA. The Bradford Fire Disaster. *Med Sci Law* 1989; **28**: 279–86.
Sturt RMB. The role of the coroner with special reference to major disasters. *Med Sci Law* 1988; **28**: 275–85.

6
Management of the orthopaedic injuries from the M1 plane crash

GAVIN R TAIT

Introduction

The Boeing 737-400 aircraft of flight BD 092 crashed on the embankment of the M1 motorway carrying 126 passengers and crew. The aircraft was attempting an unpowered landing at East Midlands airport but crashed with a velocity of approximately 100 knots, resulting in large vertical and horizontal forces of deceleration and gross disruption of the aircraft. As a consequence, 43 passengers died within the first few hours of the accident, from multiple injuries. The survivors suffered a total of 332 injuries of varying severity. The majority of injuries from this high velocity impact were to the skeleton and locomotor system. This chapter reviews the orthopaedic management of the survivors and their injuries.

After the crash

After the crash, as a consequence of the gross disruption of the aircraft fuselage and cabin, only 13 survivors with minor injuries were able to evacuate themselves from the aircraft. Those remaining were rescued by the emergency services and initially dispatched to hospital on a "scoop and run" basis.[1] Wounds were neither dressed nor fractures splinted. Only later, after a casualty clearing station was established and triage performed, were recognised fractures splinted and open wounds dressed. The supply of available splints and dressings from attending ambulances was limited, however. Only one patient with a compound fracture was given parenteral antibiotics at the site of the crash.[2]

All but two survivors were taken to the three hospitals involved, and at each accident and emergency department triage was performed by the consultant staff. All patients were resuscitated, known fractures splinted, and open wounds dressed with sterile packs.

Operations on survivors of the M1 aircrash (excluding suture of simple lacerations and wound inspections)

Surgical speciality	No of operations	% of total
Orthopaedic	295	85.5
General	13	3.8
ENT	4	1.2
Neurosurgery	4	1.2
Ophthalmology	4	1.2
Thoracic	2	0.6
Faciomaxillary	2	0.6
Plastic	2	0.6
Others†	19	5.5

†Not known.

Each hospital was able to call upon the full consultant complement of their orthopaedic trauma departments, a total of 16 consultants, together with their junior staff. Consequently, all patients had early expert assessment of their orthopaedic injuries and, when possible, surgery without delay. Patients with multiple injuries were admitted initially to the intensive care units to facilitate their resuscitation. Other patients were transferred to theatre reception areas or specially evacuated wards for further assessment and resuscitation.

Within 12 hours of the crash 772 radiological examinations had been performed, including angiograms and CT scans for six patients with head injuries and one patient with a suspected aortic injury.

Eighty per cent of the injuries to the survivors were to the musculoskeletal system, and eventually 85% of the procedures carried out were orthopaedic in nature. On the night of the accident 14 operating theatres in the three hospitals were opened, eight in Nottingham, two in Leicester, and four in Derby. Within 12 hours of the crash 94 operations had been performed; this rose to 136 operations after 36 hours.

The severe and multiple nature of many of the orthopaedic injuries dictated the policy of surgical reduction and stabilisation of many of the fractures. In the first few days 24 external fixators were applied to injured limbs. Such was the demand that fixators had to be borrowed from neighbouring hospitals and dispatched from the suppliers at midnight on the night of the accident. Fifty eight open reduction and internal fixation operations were performed using a variety of techniques, and nine intramedullary nails were inserted. In all, 49 patients (62%) had had some form of orthopaedic implant applied or inserted.

Later orthopaedic procedures were more of the nature of "second look" operations, skin graftings, and refinement of plasters. Fracture stabilisation permitted rapid mobilisation of the injured and early efforts towards rehabilitation.

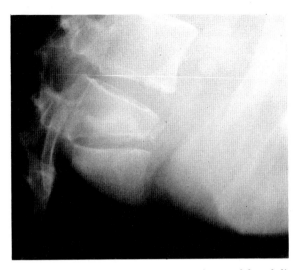

Figure 6.1—Crush fracture of 1st lumbar vertebra; a delayed diagnosis.

The orthopaedic surgery was not without complications.[3] Pulmonary embolus was recognised in four patients and a symptomatic deep venous thrombosis in one other. Two of the emboli were fatal. No doubt many more cases were unrecognised given the severe nature of the injuries present. Only 13 patients received heparin thromboprophylaxis. Two patients required urgent fasciotomies for compartment syndrome. Two patients developed fat embolism syndrome, one requiring ventilatory support. Five cases of septicaemia developed in patients with particularly severe injuries and all five required treatment in the intensive care units.

Thirty per cent of the survivors had significant injuries that were not diagnosed until more than 24 hours after admission to hospital.[4] Overall, in the three hospitals, 9.6% of all the injuries could be classed as delayed diagnosis injuries. Some minor injuries were not diagnosed early while others such as multiple vertebral fractures (figure 6.1) and fracture dislocations of the foot were initially missed. The causes of a delay in diagnosis included failure to complete a comprehensive clinical examination, failure to x ray symptomatic areas, and failure in the interpretation of the x rays. Five patients required surgery following delayed diagnosis of injuries, but in only one case is it likely that the delay influenced outcome.

To avoid medicolegally hazardous and clinically embarrassing delays in diagnosis it is recommended that when a number of patients with multiple injuries are admitted at one time each should be examined thoroughly by two separate clinical teams on two separate occasions. Bone scintigraphy

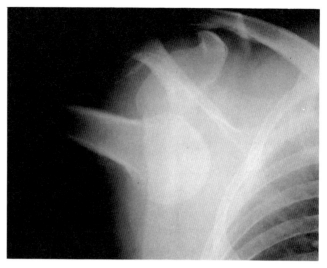

Figure 6.2—"Luxatio Erecta": an inferior dislocation of the shoulder.

(or full radiology of the spine) should be performed on all survivors of serious aircraft accidents. All joints above and below long bone fractures should be *x* rayed and all such investigations should be reported on promptly by a radiologist and communicated to the treating team both verbally and in writing. Finally, all injuries should be accurately documented.

The survivors of the Kegworth aircrash suffered injuries to all regions of the body although the majority were to the pelvis and the lower limbs. A detailed outline of these injuries follows below.

Upper limb injuries

Fifty nine injuries to the shoulder girdle and the upper limb in 36 of the initial survivors represented 28% of all the orthopaedic injuries. Flailing of the arms and impacts with the cabin fittings were thought to account for most of these injuries. However one passenger suffered an irreducible luxatio erecta (dislocated shoulder) when he was released suddenly from his upturned seat in the tail section (figure 6.2). Arm injuries were divided almost equally between the left and right limbs and above and below the elbow. Six (11%) of the injuries were compound. Seven injuries were not diagnosed until after 24 hours.

Shoulder: seven patients suffered eight glenohumeral (shoulder) dislocations, one with an associated fracture of the humeral head. This patient later required open reduction and internal fixation. One other patient required open reduction of a luxatio erecta (dislocated shoulder), which was associated with an axillary nerve palsy. Eight scapular fractures and one acromioclavicular disruption were treated conservatively and did well.

Seven fractures of the humerus were seen. Three minor fractures of the head and neck of the humerus were treated conservatively, as was one four-part humeral neck fracture in a severely ill patient who later died. A three-part fracture was initially treated by manipulation and K-wire fixation, which failed, and the humeral head was later replaced with a cemented Neer II hemiarthroplasty. Two humeral shaft fractures were seen and each was associated with an ipsilateral forearm fracture. One fracture was compound and was treated with wound excision and splintage, while the other was internally fixed and bone grafted with simultaneous fixation and grafting of the forearm fracture.

Elbow: injuries to the elbow were few. Two patients suffered comminuted fractures of the olecranon which were internally fixed with tension band wiring. One undisplaced fracture of a medial humeral condyle was treated conservatively. Three fractured radial heads were seen, one of which was excised.

Forearm: seven patients suffered fractures of the radius and ulna, compound in two cases. One fracture in a 6 month old infant was treated in plaster. The remaining fractures were treated with internal fixation and bone grafting. One compound radius and ulna fracture healed satisfactorily after early debridement and fixation at 7 days. The other compound fracture developed a late infection leading to failure of fixation. Two Galeazzi type fractures and three isolated ulnar fractures were also seen. These were all internally fixed with success.

Wrist and hands: wrist injuries were not common. Six patients suffered seven fractures, two of which were compound. Two undisplaced fractures of the radial styloid and two of the scaphoid waist were treated in a cast. Only one Colles' fracture occurred. This was treated in plaster, requiring remanipulation at 11 days. A Barton's type radial fracture was internally fixed, as was a grade 1 compound Smith's type fracture. One compound comminuted distal radial fracture was treated with wound debridement and external fixation.

There were surprisingly few hand injuries. One fractured fifth metacarpal and two fractured phalanges were treated conservatively. One patient suffered a compound fracture of the fifth metacarpal and several phalangeal fractures with division of tendons. Management was by wound debridement, repair, and external fixation. A further patient suffered a minor sprain of the ulnar collateral ligament of his thumb, treated with splintage only.

Neurological pathology was rare. One patient developed median nerve compression in association with an undisplaced radial styloid fracture and another suffered a reversible C6–7 brachial plexus lesion in association with a fracture of the first rib. One man suffered an axillary nerve palsy as a result of a luxatio erecta (dislocated shoulder). The nerve made an incomplete recovery.

In conclusion, upper limb injuries constituted 28% of all injuries suffered in the aircrash. The diversity and severity of these injuries reflect the high energy of the crash impact. Many required aggressive surgical intervention, but overall the outcome of these injuries was favourable. Early wound debridement, internal fixation, and supplementary bone grafting were the treatments of choice for most fractures. Such principles permitted many survivors with other injuries to be mobilised at an early stage.

The mechanism of the injuries to the upper limb remains unconfirmed. Many of the survivors lost consciousness at the impact and suffered post-traumatic amnesia and could not recall how their injuries occurred. However, it is likely many of the fractures were caused by the impact of flailing limbs on the interior fitments of the aircraft, although some injuries may have been sustained after the crash and during evacuation.

Lower limb injuries

One hundred and forty two major pelvic and lower limb injuries were identified in 57 passengers (average 2.5 injuries per person). Lower limb injuries were by far the commonest injury. There were 23 pelvic fractures or dislocations, 22 femoral fractures, 18 knee injuries, 31 tibial shaft fractures, 26 ankle fractures, and 22 foot fractures. Thirty four of the lower limb fractures were open.

Pelvis: 23 survivors each suffered a pelvic fracture. These included acetabular fractures, some with posterior dislocation of the hip, sacroiliac diastasis, and pubic fractures or diastasis. One patient suffered a fracture of the iliac crest, which required open reduction and internal fixation. The management of the other pelvic injuries involved the application of external fixators and skeletal traction.

Femur: 22 femoral fractures occurred in 19 survivors. Three survivors had bilateral fractures. One diaphyseal fracture was compound grade 2. These injuries were managed with external fixators and interlocking femoral nails as appropriate (figure 6.3).

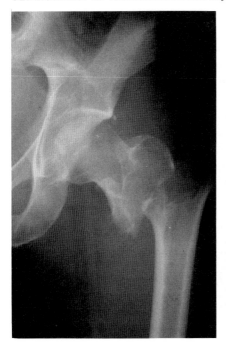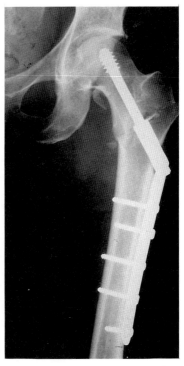

Figure 6.3—Intertrochanteric fracture of the hip (a) treated by internal fixation (b).

Knee: 17 survivors suffered 18 knee injuries, the majority of which were ligamentous in nature.

Tibia: 31 survivors sustained tibial shaft fractures, many of which were segmental or comminuted and compound (figure 6.4). These fractures were managed by wound debridement, reduction, and stabilisation with external fixators.

Ankle and foot: 26 ankle and 22 foot fractures were seen in the survivors. Talar fracture/dislocations, the Aviator's astragalus (figure 6.5), and tarso-metatarsal (Lisfranc's) fracture/dislocations were seen in large numbers. The ankle and foot injuries were managed with debridement of the open fractures, and usually reduction and stabilisation with external fixator frames. Closed fractures and dislocations were immobilised in plaster of paris casts.

71

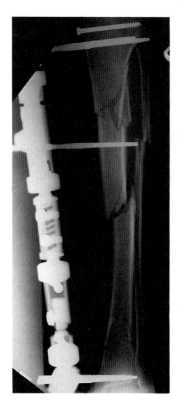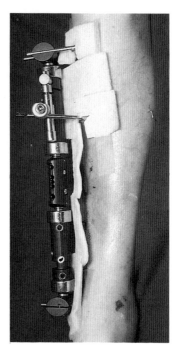

Figure 6.4—Segmental fracture of the tibia (a) treated by external fixation (b).

The lower limb fractures occurred mainly in those parts of the aircraft where there was gross destruction of the floor and displacement of the seats and their supports (see chapter 3).

Open (compound) fractures

Twenty eight of the survivors admitted to hospital sustained a total of 40 open fractures.[2] By the classification of Gustillo and Anderson[5] there were five grade 1, 16 grade 2, and 19 (47%) grade 3 fractures. There were six open fractures of the upper limb and 34 of the lower limb. Half of the most severe grade 3 fractures occurred at or below the ankle.

These compound fractures were initially treated with splintage and sterile dressings, some at the crash site and all on first admission to hospital. All patients received a cephalosporin type antibiotic and tetanus prophylaxis as required. At a mean of 6.25 hours (range 2–14) after the accident all

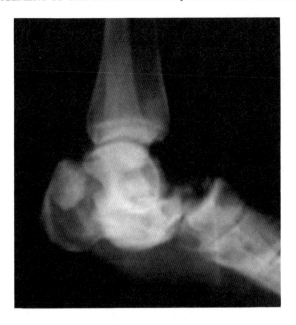

Figure 6.5—"Aviator's Astragalus": fracture dislocation of the talo-naviculor joint.

patients had undergone wound excision, irrigation, and fracture stabilisation.

The five grade 1 wounds were closed primarily, as were 11 of the grade 2 wounds and 10 grade 3 wounds. Five grade 2 and nine of the grade 3 wounds were left open. The grade 3 wounds were mostly large flap lacerations.

All grade 1 fractures were treated with reduction and plaster immobilisation. Seven grade 2 fractures were treated with plaster, three were internally fixed, and five were controlled with external fixators. Five of the grade 3 fractures were treated in plaster, six were internally fixed, and eight were stabilised with external fixators.

There was a 30% incidence of wound problems. There were three (7.5%) cases of delayed wound healing and six (15%) cases of wound infection. Three (7.5%) cases of skin flap necrosis all healed by secondary intention.

Three of the wound infections occurred in one patient who had developed septicaemia and multiple organ failure. His wounds had been left open and both *Enterobacter* and coliform species were isolated from the wounds. A further three cases of *Enterobacter* infection were probably acquired from the hospital environment and occurred in wounds which were closed primarily. The only compound fracture to require eventual amputation occurred after a grade 3 fracture dislocation of the ankle, which was internally fixed and the wound primarily closed. None of the wounds treated by delayed closure became infected.

Of the 40 open fractures identified in the survivors (excluding the one open talar fracture, which required amputation), all but three had united by 9 months after the crash. One of these, an ankle fracture, had undergone surgical fusion. No case of late infection or malunion has been identified in those fractures which have united.

The results of the treatment of the open injuries to the survivors of the aircrash compare favourably with other series. Factors which are important to consider in the management of such injuries include:

- Early resuscitation of patients and administration of broad spectrum antibiotics

- Adequate wound excision

- Early involvement of senior staff

- Delayed closure of contaminated wounds.

Rehabilitation

Despite the number and complexity of the injuries sustained by the survivors of flight BD 092 the early and aggressive stabilisation of their fractures allowed remarkably early mobilisation and rapid rehabilitation.

At 3 weeks after the crash 12 patients had been discharged to their homes and 30 to other hospitals for further care.[3] Fourteen patients had required a further 34 operations for the treatment of their injuries after discharge, and these were carried out in other hospitals. Most of these procedures were orthopaedic treatments for fixation of delayed diagnosis fractures, treatment of delayed or non-union, removal of metal, and reconstructive plastic surgery. One lady required surgical decompression of a missed prolapsed thoracic disc. Ten patients were readmitted to hospital after their initial discharge and required a further 15 operations, including removal of metal, reconstuctive plastic surgery, and treatment of orthopaedic complications. Of the 49 later operations performed on the survivors, 24 (50%) were carried out in only four patients. One patient was readmitted late with a pulmonary embolus and septicaemia.

Long term outcome

The 79 survivors amongst the passengers and crew were reviewed at a minimum of 9 months from the crash to assess (1) their recovery from their injuries, (2) their requirement for continuing hospital care, and (3) their return to work. Such outcomes have been found to be closely related to the severity of the initial injuries suffered in the crash as indicated by the injury severity scores (ISSs) calculated for each patient (page 43).[6]

Nine months from the crash, 49 (62%) of the patients were still attending for outpatient review and 27 (34%) had been discharged. Three patients remained in hospital, two with paralysis as a result of a spinal injury and one patient in a persistent vegetative state following a traumatic craniotomy.

Forty six (58%) of the survivors were judged to have made a good recovery from the injuries, having only minor discomfort and being able to function at a similar level to that present before the crash. Twenty five people were found to be moderately disabled with pain, limp, or joint dysfunction. These survivors were, however, functionally independent in their activities of daily living. The remaining eight (10%) survivors were severely disabled and dependent, six as a result of neurological injuries and two as a result of severe fractures to the pelvis and limbs. As previously mentioned, one young man remained in a persistent vegetative state.

Sixty per cent of the survivors who had been in work prior to the accident had returned to work at 9 months. These survivors had had an average ISS of 11. Their recovery seemed to have been augmented by their age, low ISS, and the optimal primary treatment of their injuries as well as their rehabilitation programme. Those patients who had not returned to work by 9 months had an average ISS of 22. Data on the return to work are given in figure 6.6.

In conclusion, it can be seen that from the Kegworth aircrash 58% of survivors made a satisfactory recovery from their injuries and returned to work by 9 months. However, 62% of the survivors still required hospital supervision and 10% of survivors were severely disabled and dependent.

The orthopaedic lessons from the Kegworth air crash

The NLDB study (the Nottingham, Leicester, Derby, Belfast crash study group) has been the first in-depth contemporary investigation of the management of a major aircraft accident. Lessons learnt can be applied to any future transportation disaster. Such accidents will invariably result in many survivors with multiple injuries as a result of a high velocity impact. The majority of injuries will be orthopaedic in nature and will include many contaminated fractures. The immediate involvement of senior staff and the management of fractures by surgical stabilisation should provide

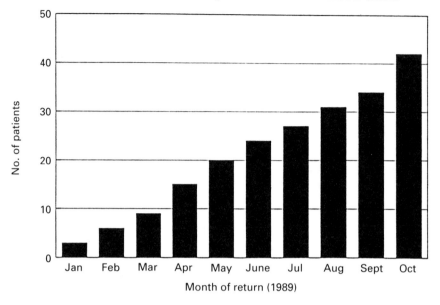

Figure 6.6—Cumulative data for the 42 survivors who returned to work within 9 months of the crash.

for optimum fracture treatment and early recovery.[3] Later procedures and the requirements of rehabilitation will require further orthopaedic resources. There will be an initial great demand for external fixators and implants, and pooling of National Health Service and commercial resources may be required rapidly. The army medical services should be able to provide large numbers of devices at short notice, but their administrative machinery makes it unlikely that their help could be prompt.

The demands on an orthopaedic service of a major disaster are such that the normal routine workload will be disrupted for some time, maybe weeks, and allowances must be made for this ongoing problem. Appropriate pacing of the nursing and senior medical staff will be needed to accommodate the workload over such a period. Repeated accurate reassessment of the patients and their injuries will be necessary to avoid potentially damaging delay in diagnosis.

Further major transportation disasters are inevitable. However, the outcomes of the physical injuries for the majority of the survivors of the Kegworth aircraft accident have been favourable. This can only reflect well on the immediate and later care and attention from the emergency staff involved, particularly the orthopaedic staff of Queen's Medical Centre Nottingham, Leicester Royal Infirmary, and Derbyshire Royal Infirmary. The ongoing care from the Belfast team ensured good continuity of care, and the collaboration of members from each of the centres in the NLDB group has ensured that the lessons learned from this accident may be used for others in the future.

1 Kirsh G, Learmonth DJA, Martindale JP. The Nottingham, Leicester, Derby aircraft accident study: preliminary report three weeks after the accident. *BMJ* 1989; **295**: 503–5.
2 Learmonth DJA, Martindale JP, Rowles JM, Tait GR, Kirsh G, Sheppard I. Initial management of open fractures sustained in the M1 aircraft disaster. *Injury* 1991; **22**: 207–11.
3 Rowles JM, Learmonth DJA,Tait GR, Macey AC. Survivors of the M1 air crash; outcome of injuries after one year. *Injury* 1991; **22**: 362–4.
4 Tait GR, Rowles JM, Kirsh G, Martindale JP, Learmonth DJA. Delayed diagnosis of injuries from the M1 aircraft accident. *Injury* 1991; **22**: 475–8.
5 Gustillo RB, Anderson TJ. Prevention of infection in the treatment of one thousand and twenty five open fractures of the long bones. *J Bone Joint Surg* 1976; **58A**: 453–8.
6 Rowles JM, Kirsh G, Macey AC, and the NLDB Study Group. The use of injury severity scoring in the evaluation of the Kegworth M1 aircrash. *J Trauma* 1992; **32**: 441–7.

7
Management of spinal injuries from the M1 plane crash

RAYMOND MORAN, WILLIAM CURTIN

Introduction

Most experimental information on spinal injuries that result from air disasters has been obtained from anatomical studies on cadavers subjected to controlled impacts and from sensor data retrieved from crash simulations. Research at the National Aeronautical Space Agency (NASA) base at Edwards Airforce Base had demonstrated that the negative G forces acting on the cockpit floor during experimental crashes at fixed impact speed depended upon the angle subtended by the aircraft at impact as well as on the terrain over which the aircraft had decelerated.[1] As the angle of impact increased from 18° to 27°, peak G forces increased fivefold. Similarly, very high peak decelerations were encountered when an aircraft hit a solid stationary object, and less abrupt decelerations were noted when the aircraft slowly decelerated over a long distance on soft ground.

Fortunately, not all the kinetic energy of a crashing aircraft is transmitted to its occupants, because much is absorbed by serial crushing and collapse of parts of the fuselage. Even so, the spinal column as the principal loadbearing structure of the torso is frequently injured during such sudden violent decelerations. It has been estimated that in the sitting position the spinal column of the average person can withstand a 20 G force for a fraction of a second before vertebral fracture will occur.

In order to appreciate the pattern of spinal injuries noted in the M1 aircrash it is first necessary to review some aspects of spinal anatomy and the classification of spinal trauma.

Functional anatomy of the spine

The vertebrae that form the spinal column, while generally similar, display specific adaptive features that characterise the cervical, thoracic, and lumbar segments. Anteriorly, each vertebra possesses a cylindrical body composed of a thin rim of cortical bone enclosing an inner core of cancellous bone. Cartilaginous end plates cap the body on its superior and inferior surfaces at the boundaries of the intervertebral disc spaces. On each side of the superolateral aspects of the vertebral body, pedicles project dorsally and together these form the lateral walls of the spinal canal. The posterior wall of the spinal canal is formed by the spinal laminae, which are continuous across the base of the spinous process. At the junction of the laminae and pedicles, superior and inferior articular facets articulate with the respective inferior and superior facets of adjacent vertebrae.

The cervical spine consists of seven vertebrae. The articulations between the occiput, C1, and C2 principally allow for flexion, extension, and rotation. Between the third and seventh cervical vertebrae the facet joints lie in a coronal plane and subtend an angle of 45° to the horizontal, allowing lateral flexion and rotation between adjacent vertebrae but less antero-posterior motion.

In the thoracic spine, paired ribs articulate with demifacets on contiguous vertebrae at the level of the intervertebral disc. Although the articular facets allow free motion in all planes, the rib cage limits lateral flexion, flexion, and extension. Rotation is therefore the least constrained motion in this segment of the spinal column. Several anatomical features, including thickness of the intervertebral discs, horizontal alignment of the splinous processes, and non-overlapping laminae, facilitate free motion in the lumbar spinal segments. The orientation of the facets within the lumbar spine restricts lateral flexion and rotation but allows a relatively wide arc of flexion and extension.

Injury to the spinal cord arises most commonly when displacement of part or all of a vertebra compromises the dimensions of the spinal canal. The spinal cord in the midthoracic spine is most at risk in this regard, as at this level it occupies most of the spinal canal. By contrast, fractures that encroach on the spinal canal below the level of the conus medullaris frequently escape neurological sequelae. These anatomical factors help explain fracture patterns and neurological loss in patients with spinal trauma.

Classification of spinal injuries

Nicoll[2] is credited with one of the earliest and most enduring classifications of spinal fractures. He classified fractures into stable and unstable types. Stable fractures included anterior and lateral wedge compression fractures and all laminar fractures. Unstable fractures included fracture dislocations and subluxations associated with ligamentous disruption. Holdsworth, who pioneered the management of spinal injuries in the United Kingdom this century, noted that five mechanisms gave rise to the majority of spinal fractures—that is, flexion, flexion/rotation, extension, axial compression, and shear.[3]

While the classification of spinal injury through the description of the deforming force is desirable, it is often not practical to apply this type of classification in situations in which high velocity trauma may produce extremely complex fracture patterns. Denis evolved a three column concept of the spine.[4] The anterior column comprised the greater portion of the vertebral body, the anterior longitudinal ligament, and the anterior annulus. The middle column included the posterior wall of the vertebral body, the posterior longitudinal ligament, and the posterior annulus. The posterior column contained the facet joints, posterior vertebral arch and associated ligaments. Instability in the context of spinal injury correlated with trauma to more than one column. The compression fracture was viewed essentially as a stress fracture of the anterior column. The burst fracture implied failure of the anterior and middle column, while fracture dislocations suggested failure of all three columns. Although this classification was developed for thoracolumbar fractures it may nevertheless be applied to the cervical spine for the formulation of treatment strategies.

Treatment of spinal injuries

The most appropriate treatment for unstable spinal injuries remains contentious. Guttmann[5] proposed non-surgical treatment for such injuries, using postural reduction and prolonged recumbency. The premise that optimal conditions for neurological recovery will be facilitated by adequate reduction of displaced spinal fractures and dislocations is generally accepted by proponents of both methods of treatment. Many of the arguments in favour of non-surgical treatment have been based on the poor results obtained by early methods of surgical stabilisation and are not directly applicable to the rigid fixation offered by the more modern implants.

Holdsworth advocated the use of spinous process plates such as the Meurig-Williams system but noted that a potential to develop late spinal deformity still existed.

The Harrington system of distraction rods was first applied to thoracolumbar fractures in 1958. This technique proved easy to apply and gave satisfactory results in many studies.[6] Recurrence of deformity, however, has been reported with this system,[7] and the necessity to immobilise at least two segments above and two segments below the fracture level means that a minimum of five and often seven segments require fusion over the instrumented area. The risks of displacing sublaminar hooks with this technique have been decreased by applying adjacent sublaminar wires as described by Luque for the treatment of scoliosis.[8]

Magerl[9] developed a technique of external spinal fixation using percutaneous transpedicular Schanz screws in the vertebrae immediately above and below the injured segment or segments. Displaced fractures could be manipulated into position and immobilised by connecting the Schanz screws to an external frame. This system was modified by Dick who inserted open Schanz screws and applied an internal fixation system.[10] This mode of treatment was particularly effective in treating unstable thoracolumbar fractures and allowed early patient mobilisation. Roy-Camille used pedicle screw plates for unstable thoracic and thoracolumbar fractures with similar favourable results.[11]

Anterior cervical instability, particularly associated with multiple level spine defects may be treated by anteriorly placed plates, which do not require screw purchase in the posterior vertebral cortex. Spinal stabilisation in the presence of posterior instability may be achieved with posterior plates, or sublaminar or trans-spinous wiring. Recently the AO (Arbeitsgemeinschaft für Osteosynthesefragen) group have introduced plates that incorporate a hook that is placed beneath the lamina of the vertebra immediately below the injured segment and screws that obtain purchase in the lateral masses of the unstable vertebra.[12]

The management of all significant spinal injuries that resulted from the M1 aircrash of 1989 depended to a large extent upon the philosophy of the institution in which the patient was treated. We did not attempt to compare the results of the surgical and conservative methods applied to these patients, as the numbers in each category were too small to make statistically valid comparisons.

The M1 aircrash

Of the survivors of the M1 aircrash, 24 significant spinal fractures (excluding minor avulsion fractures) in 21 patients were documented. Six patients (28%) sustained major neurological loss and three patients sustained spinal injuries at more than one level. There were two late fatalities in those who had spinal injuries.

Patients with unstable spinal injuries were among the most severely injured patients who survived the crash. The mean injury severity score (ISS) for all patients surviving the disaster was 15, while the mean score for patients with spinal injury was 25. There were six cervical spine injuries, six thoracic spine injuries, and 12 lumbar spine injuries.

TABLE 7.1 Cervical spine injuries

Number of injuries	Type	Presentation	Treatment	Outcome
6	C7 Compression	Acute	Conservative	Satisfactory
	C7 Compression	Acute	Conservative	Satisfactory
	C5 Compression	Acute	Conservative	Satisfactory
	Atlanto-axial subluxation	Acute tetraparesis	C1–C2 Fusion	Partial recovery
	Fracture-dislocation C5/C6●	Acute paraplegia	C5–C6 Fusion	Subtotal recovery
	Dislocation C6–C7	Acute tetraplegia	Conservative	No recovery

● Injuries pertain to same patient as table 7.3

Cervical spine injuries

Of the six cervical spine injuries (table 7.1) there was one anterior atlantoaxial dislocation with disruption of the transverse ligament, thought most likely to be produced by an acute flexion of the head. Two compression injuries of the body of C7 were noted, one identified from standard radiography and one from isotope scanning. These injuries were consistent with a flexion deformity of the cervical spine without rotation or axial compression.

One patient demonstrated a comminuted fracture of C7. Computed tomography (CT) of this particular fracture did not demonstrate any encroachment of bone fragments on the spinal canal. The force most likely to produce this fracture was an axial loading of the cervical spine in the neutral position. An extension distraction force in another patient caused a fracture of the pedicle of C5 and an associated fracture of the C6 lamina best demonstrated on CT. Flexion associated with axial loading of the cervical spine was the presumed cause for a vertebral body fracture of C5, with a teardrop fracture and minimal retrolisthesis.

The incidence of appendicular injuries amongst patients with cervical spine trauma was high. Although one patient with a C5 fracture did not have any other injuries the remaining patients all had severe peripheral injuries, which included fractures of the femoral shaft (two patients), compound fractures of the tibia (two) and forearm fractures (two). In addition, two patients had severe head injuries and two had sustained blunt chest trauma. Not surprisingly therefore, the ISSs for this group of patients ranged from 8 to 50.

Four patients were managed conservatively. The patient with atlanto-axial subluxation presented with tetraparesis. This association is common, as the intact odontoid is likely to abut directly on the spinal cord in the subluxed position. This patient underwent a C1/2 Gallie type fusion (see

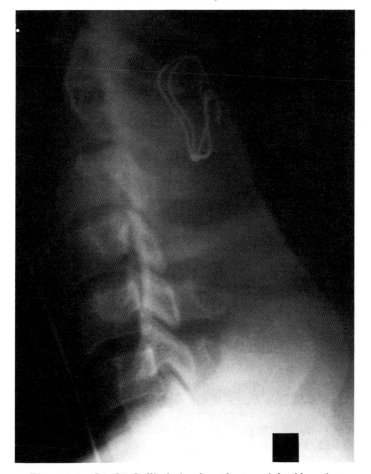

Figure 7.1—C1–C2 Gallie fusion for atlanto-axial subluxation.

figure 7.1), because ligamentous healing at this level cannot be relied upon to provide sufficient stability to the upper cervical spine. Fortunately, this patient made a significant neurological recovery, although he did require an amputation of the left leg because of an open comminuted tibial fracture. It was decided that the extension fracture of C5 spanned all three columns of the spine, the patient therefore underwent anterior fusion of C5 to C6 with an anterior H plate and posterior hook plate stabilisation and bone graft fusion over the same segments (see figure 7.2).

Thoracic spine injuries

All the fractures of the thoracic spine (table 7.2) occurred as a consequence of indirect trauma. There were three hyperflexion injuries that produced

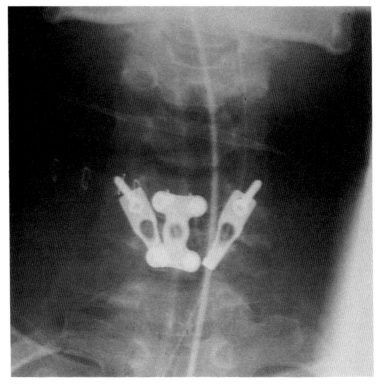

Figure 7.2—Anterior and posterior stabilisation of three column fracture C5.

wedging of the affected vertebral segments (see figure 7.3). In addition there was one extension injury at the level of T4. Although there was no evidence of vertebral fracture on standard radiographs a magnetic resonance imaging (MRI) scan demonstrated a recent extradural haemorrhage at the level of T4 and T5 in this patient. One patient died shortly after admission to hospital because of multiple severe injuries. His radiographs demonstrated a fracture/dislocation of T4 on T5 due to a rotational stress at this level. One traumatic disc rupture was diagnosed late, at a follow up examination for persistent low back pain with a mild paraparesis. Curiously this patient was the only one of the group of thoracic spine injuries who required surgery, and was treated by delayed transthoracic discectomy but regrettably is left with a significant paraparesis.

The ISSs of patients with thoracic spinal trauma ranged from 19 to 41. Curiously, injuries to the feet were common in this subgroup. Lisfranc fracture dislocations were noted in two patients and a fracture of the os calcis was identified in another. One patient sustained bilateral tibial fractures and there was one instance of blunt chest trauma associated with a myocardial contusion.

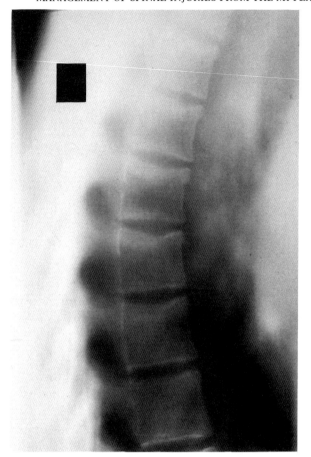

Figure 7.3—Minor compression fractures of T5–T9.

Lumbar spine injuries

Of the 12 documented lumbar spine fractures (table 7.3) seven were of the wedge compression variety (see figure 7.4) and five were burst fractures.

Two of the patients with burst fractures presented with major neurological loss. One patient who presented with a burst fracture of L1 was managed conservatively and has shown no signs of neurological recovery, the other patient who had a burst fracture of L5 was treated operatively with an Olerud fixator and secondary anterior vertebrectomy with tricortical strut grafting (see figure 7.5). This patient made a partial neurological recovery to the point where she is now independently mobile with a frame but still requires intermittent self catheterisation. The patient with the extension fracture of C5 also had a three column axial loading type fracture

TABLE 7.2   Thoracic spine injuries

Number of injuries	Type	Presentation	Treatment	Outcome
6	T7 Compression	Acute	Conservative	Satisfactory
	T12 Compression	Delayed	Conservative	Satisfactory
	T5 Compression	Acute	Conservative	Satisfactory
	T4–T5 Fracture/ dislocation		Died from associated severe injuries	
	T4–T5▲ Extensions/ Distraction	Acute paraplegia	Died 2 weeks post injury	
	T4 Herniated disc	Delayed	Trans thoracic discectomy	Poor

▲ Injuries pertain to same patient as table 7.3

of L1 which was treated surgically using the Olerud fixator. Similarly, the patient with the extension injury to the thoracic spine at T4 had a coexistent three column fracture at L4. This fracture was treated operatively, again using the Olerud fixator, but unfortunately there was no early neurological recovery and tragically the patient died from a massive pulmonary embolism 2 weeks after surgery.

TABLE 7.3   Lumbar spine injuries

Number of injuries		Type	Presentation	Treatment	Outcome
12	1 Burst fracture 5	L1●	Acute paraplegia	Olerud fixator	Subtotal recovery
		L1	No neurology	Conservative	Satisfactory
		L1	Acute paraplegia	Conservative	No recovery
		L4▲	Acute paraplegia	Olerud fixator	Died 2 weeks post injury
		L5■	Delayed	Conservative	Satisfactory
		L1■	Delayed	Conservative	Satisfactory
		L4	Delayed	Conservative	Satisfactory
		L1	Delayed	Conservative	Satisfactory
		L5	Delayed	Conservative	Satisfactory

■ Injuries pertain to same patient
▲ Injuries pertain to same patient as table 7.2
● Injuries pertain to same patient as table 7.1

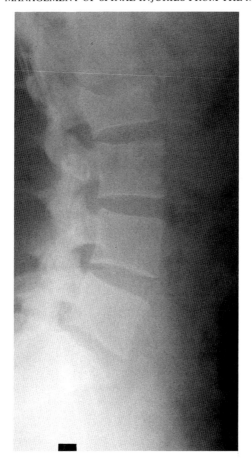

Figure 7.4—Wedge compression fracture of L2 involving anterior and middle columns.

Discussion

Among the initial survivors of the M1 aircrash there were three patients who sustained separate (non-contiguous) spinal fractures. As these patients also had severe peripheral injuries, it is important to emphasise that a thorough examination of the entire spine is mandatory even when one fracture has been identified.

Nine patients who had spinal fractures were not diagnosed on initial presentation. All of these injuries were minor axial compression or flexion fractures. These fractures might have been diagnosed earlier had routine radiography of the whole spine been applied to all victims. Alternatively, isotope bone scanning can be employed to detect areas of increased osteoblastic activity within the spine, which may then be further assessed by localised radiographs. In this small series of spinal injuries MRI

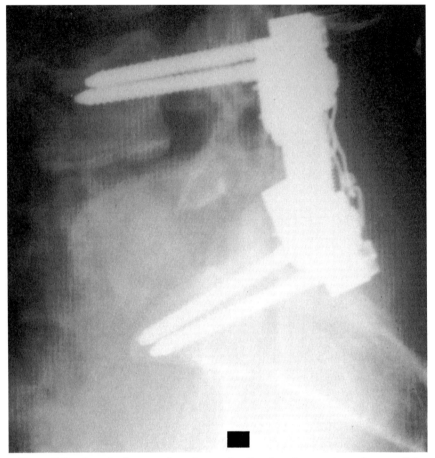

Figure 7.5—Anterior bone graft and posterior fixation of severe burst fracture L5.

identified one extradural spinal haematoma. While MRI is unnecessary in the routine assessment of spinal trauma, it is particularly useful in cases of spinal cord injury without obvious vertebral fracture and in the diagnosis of disc prolapse.

Six patients presented with major neurological deficits. Of these, three survivors were treated surgically and have made satisfactory neurological recoveries, while two patients who were treated conservatively were left with major residual neurological deficits. As the types of injury were so variable, however, no conclusion as to the relative efficacy of surgical and non-surgical treatment can be drawn from the results of this study.

Conventional aircraft design employs forward facing seating. The spine of a passenger in this position will experience a flexion moment during sudden deceleration. This is especially true if a simple two-point restraining belt is used as it potentiates the natural tendency of the upper torso to jackknife unless the braced position is adopted. The high numbers of flexion and flexion/compression fractures in the M1 aircrash are explained in this manner. Improved passenger restraint could be achieved with the routine use of five-point harnesses. These provide far greater stabilisation of the torso and have been used extensively in aerobatic aircraft. The airbag is another method of protecting passengers from sudden impact against the bulkhead. It is constructed from woven nylon and is fed compressed air through a deceleration sensitive valve mechanism. Inflation occurs rapidly, and simultaneous leaking of air through a porous zone prevents entrapment of the passenger after landing.

Rear facing seating may have a theoretical advantage in frontal impact situations, as the relatively weak cancellous bone of the anterior column is unloaded in favour of a stronger pathway through the articular facets and posterior column. While this form of seating has been made standard on many forms of military aircraft, its adoption by commercial aircraft has been slow because of cost and most particularly an apparent lack of acceptance by passengers.

Summary

- Study of spinal injuries in the M1 aircrash emphasises the vulnerability of the spinal column to serious injury in high speed impact trauma

- Most fractures were defined by x ray; CT was useful for coronal reconstruction of complex fracture patterns

- Certain vertebral fractures were detected at a late stage; earlier diagnosis might be faciliatated by bone scintigraphy (isotope scanning)

- Magnetic resonance imaging was helpful in assessing spinal injury associated with disc injury

- Factors that lead to aircrashes are unlikely to be completely eliminated, thus research must continue into prevention of deceleration trauma

- Safer restraint systems in commercial aircraft, such as the five-point harness, and rear facing seates would be of significant benefit

1 Hayduk J. *Full scale transport controlled impact demonstration.* National Aeronautics and Space Administration; Washington, DC, 1986. (National Aeronautics and Space Administration Publication 2395.)
2 Nicoll EA. Fractures of the dorso-lumbar spine. *J Bone Joint Surg* 1949; **31B**: 376–394.
3 Holdsworth F, Hardy A. Early treatment of paraplegia from fractures of the thoracolumbar spine. *J Bone Joint Surg* 1953; **35B**: 540–394.
4 Denis F. Spinal instability as defined by the three column concept in acute spinal trauma. *Clin Orthop* 1984; **189**: 65–76.
5 Guttmann L. Surgical aspects of the treatment of traumatic paraplegia. *J Bone Joint Surg* 1949; **31B**: 399–403.
6 Yosipovitch Z, Robin G, Makin M. Open reduction of unstable thoracolumbar spine injuries and fixation with Harrington rods. *J Bone Joint Surg* 1977; **59A**: 1003–1014.

7 Myllynen P, Bostman O, Riska E. Recurrence of spinal deformity after removal of Harrington fixation of spinal fractures. *Acta Orthop Scand* 1988; **59**: 497–502.
8 Luque ER, Cassis N. Segmental spinal instrumentation in the treatment of fractures of the thoraco-lumbar spine. *Spine* 1982; **7**: 312–320.
9 Magerl FP. Stabilization of the lower thoracic and lumbar spine with external skeletal fixation. *Clin Orthop* 1984; **189**: 125–141.
10 Dick W. The "Fixateur Interne" as a versatile implant for spine injury. *Spine* 1987; **12**: 882–900.
11 Roy-Camille R, Saillant G, Mazel C. Internal fixation of the lumbar spine pedicle screw plating. *Clin Orthop* 1986; **203**: 7–17.
12 Jeanneret B, Magerl F, Ward EH *et al*. Posterior stabilization of the cervical spine with hook plates. *Spine* 1991; **16**: 556–563.

8

Management of the head injuries and investigation of the causes of head injury from the M1 plane crash

BARRIE D WHITE, JOHN L FIRTH

Introduction

Major disasters characteristically overwhelm the normally available resources of hospitals serving the area involved. Major disaster plans often include recommendations for the dispersal of casualties to a number of units and the provision of back up equipment and manpower from outside the area. The problems facing regional services, such as neurosurgery, differ from those posed to other specialties in a number of respects.

Outside London, neurosurgical centres are widely separated in order to serve geographically distinct catchment areas. Only one, or at most two, could be expected to provide convenient cover for any single major incident. The average British neurosurgical unit comprises four consultants with supporting staff and facilities, which include two dedicated operating theatres and shared intensive care space. The provisions to care for a sudden large influx of patients with severe head injuries are clearly limited and easily exceeded. Additional non-dedicated operating theatres with extra staff to man them may be required.

Provided that good resuscitation facilities including intubation, ventilation, and blood pressure support are available at the scene of the disaster, those patients thought likely on initial triage to require neurosurgical care should be transferred to the regional centre rather than to a primary hospital, which will have less than ideal facilities. It is wasteful of resources and dangerous to the patient to have to undergo a secondary transfer.

The best compromise under these circumstances is likely to be between the concentration of all available neurosurgical manpower in a regional centre where the best facilities are readily available, and the need to provide neurosurgical care to some patients who have been initially transferred to outlying hospitals. Additional problems are faced by those neurosurgical units which are physically separate from the general theatre suite or hospital site, and which may have to import surgeons from other specialties to allow synchronous surgery on those survivors with severe multiple injuries.

Although surgery for cranial trauma is possible in most district general hospitals, many of which now have CT scanners, it is increasingly rare for neurosurgical procedures to be performed away from specialist centres. This lack of exposure and practice reduces the efficiency with which severe head injuries can be managed. The problem is exacerbated during a disaster, when these same general staff may already be overstretched by injuries more relevant to their specialty. The alternative—sending trained neurosurgeon to an outlying hospital to perform emergency surgery—is possible but requires him to operate with an unfamiliar team and will dilute the effort in the regional centre, which may be left dangerously under-manned.

In practice, what is possible or actually achieved depends to a degree upon prior planning of the response options to a number of potential disasters, efficient communications with all those concerned during the crisis, the flexibility to deal with unexpected events as they occur and, as always in these circumstances, an element of good luck.

Neurosurgical management of the M1 aircrash survivors

Preparations

In the initial response to the M1 aircraft accident, the neurosurgical unit in Nottingham prepared itself to receive directly all those survivors with neurological injuries. Wards were emptied, intensive treatment unit beds were prepared, theatres were opened, and off duty staff were alerted.

Problems were immediately encountered when the hospital switchboard became jammed with calls. The request that all identified head, spinal, and paediatric injuries be brought directly to Nottingham was only made possible by the duty neurosurgical consultant using his car phone from outside the casualty department. Only later were formal neurosurgical communications established via the ambulance network.

On impact the aircraft fuselage broke into three sections, with areas of major structural failure on either side of the wing box. The forewarned emergency services were on the scene almost immediately, preventing the left engine fire from spreading and ensuring rapid high quality medical care for the many severely injured survivors.

Management

Ambulances began arriving at University Hospital, Nottingham, within 35 minutes of the accident. Later congestion on the M1 and roads south and east was overcome by helicopter evacuation from the site to Leicester Royal Infirmary. The first wave of survivors comprised the most readily accessible seriously injured passengers, taken largely from the intact central section of the aircraft. Among this initial group were four of the six most severely head-injured adults admitted to hospital. All were unconscious with Glasgow coma scores (GCSs) between 4 and 7. Each, quite unexpectedly, had injuries to the back of the head and none had any serious extracranial injuries.

On their arrival, they were intubated, hyperventilated, given an intravenous mannitol infusion, and CT scanned. All displayed marked brain swelling and were transferred to the intensive treatment unit for further general resuscitation and cerebral stabilisation prior to intracranial pressure monitoring or wound debridement. By delaying surgery temporarily it was possible to leave the neurosurgical theatres empty, ready for the possible arrival of an acute extradural or other intracranial haematoma that would require immediate surgical evacuation.

Two of these initial survivors died of uncontrollable cerebral swelling shortly after admission and a third died in a similar fashion the following morning. The fourth had sustained a traumatic posterior parietal craniectomy with a major dural tear and brain herniation. Early death due to uncontrollable cerebral swelling was probably prevented by this traumatic "decompression".

By this time, the plan to centralise the treatment of neurological injuries in Nottingham seemed to be working so the off duty members of staff were called into the regional unit rather than dispersed to other hospitals in the area. This provided a complement of three consultants, one senior registrar, two registrars, and two senior house officers to care for the neurological injuries. The duty consultant and senior registrar remained in the accident and emergency department to assess and prioritise all new arrivals and to coordinate their management with other surgical teams. A second consultant was based in the CT scanner suite to reassess those patients sent for scanning and arrange their transfer to wards, the intensive treatment unit, or theatre, as appropriate. The third consultant was ready in the intensive treatment unit to ensure optimal treatment of those head-injured patients with cerebral swelling but without an intracranial haematoma. The registrars covered the routine neurosurgical inpatients while reassessing those aircrash victims who had been sent from the accident and emergency department to a separate ward designated for their care and those taken directly to theatre under the primary care of orthopaedic and general surgeons.

Two further patients with severe head injuries were admitted to Nottingham within the first hour. Both were extricated from the forward section of the fuselage. One had a major basal skull fracture with temporal lobe contusions, a Le Fort III facial injury, atlantoaxial subluxation, a C6 cord contusion, and limb injuries. The other was the only infant passenger on the flight. His injuries included a closed head injury with bicoronal skull fractures, cerebral swelling and fits, bilateral femoral and lower leg fractures, and a right ulnar fracture.

At one stage, when University Hospital, Nottingham, believed they had admitted around 40 casualties and were becoming overwhelmed, incoming ambulances were diverted to another district hospital as laid down in the major incident plan. This was detected and the diversion of neurological injuries countermanded by the duty neurosurgeon, thus enabling their continued evacuation to Nottingham, where the capacity of the regional neurosurgical unit was not exhausted.

As the influx of casualties slowed and no further severely head-injured survivors were identified either at the site of the crash or in the other hospitals, it was judged safe to commence neurological surgery on those patients already admitted.

The patient with a parietal craniectomy and dural tear was taken to theatre for wound toilet and pressure monitoring. The man with Le Fort III fractures and temporal contusions underwent pressure monitoring during the course of his other procedures. The infant received volume replacement and limb splintage, his epilepsy was controlled, and an intracranial pressure monitor inserted. All three patients underwent intensive intracranial pressure control with deep sedation, circulatory support, hyperventilation, and cooling.

As the duty neurosurgical team began operating, the two off duty consultants made contact with Derbyshire and Leicester Royal Infirmaries to ensure that no previously undetected neurosurgical problems were developing elsewhere.

In Derby, a consultant neurologist had taken on the task of neurological surveillance, and though no head injuries required neurosurgical attention, two otherwise unsuspected spinal cord injuries were detected and treated appropriately. In Leicester, a young woman who had been fully conscious on release from the wreckage deteriorated to a coma score of 10 and was found on CT scanning to have an extradural haematoma. One of the off duty neurosurgical consultants travelled to Leicester (a distance of 30 miles), where the female patient was successfully treated surgically without further transfer.

Helicopter transfer: The evacuation of the aircraft site was performed under almost ideal circumstances with easy access to both the site and three major local hospitals with all the necessary facilities. Manpower, equipment, and transport were never limiting factors but, despite this, many hours were necessary before the wreckage was fully cleared of casualties, many of whom were seriously injured as well as trapped.

The use of helicopters in such a situation should be considered.

Where the site is inaccessible to road vehicles, airlift of personnel, rescue and resuscitation equipment is clearly mandatory, with evacuation of casualties by the same route. Where there is road access, the benefits of air transport are less clear but in the abscence of good roads the ability of helicopters to reach otherwise inaccessible sites can potentially shorten transfer times significantly.

In this crash, helicopters were used to transfer a few seriously injured casualties rescued late in the evening, by which time the serving roads were congested. One of these patients was the young lady with an expanding extradural haematoma, which was expeditiously removed on her arrival in Leicester.

Helicopter transfer clearly has a role but there are drawbacks which must be weighed against the benefits. Our previous experience with helicopter transfer has shown that urban transport is not necessarily quicker because, unless the helicopter is readily available and properly medically equipped, its departure time is often delayed. In addition, transfer to and from the helicopter often requires short ambulance journeys at either end, adding to the overall transfer time.

As with ambulances, resuscitation must be established prior to transfer because of the difficulties of clinical intervention in flight. For practical purposes, with evolving head injuries this may well mean intubation and anaesthetic support.

In summary, helicopter transfer is neither panacea nor short cut to good care, which must commence prior to transfer. It is purely an alternative form of transport which may be a useful adjunct to conventional means when, because of accessibility or physical distance to necessary facilities, road transfer time is likely to exceed 1 hour. Low altitude unpressurised flight is not contraindicated and does not need to be avoided for head injuries when effective rapid transport is the only consideration.

Overview

Most passengers had some degree of head and facial trauma. More than half the survivors were rendered unconscious by the impact. Despite head injury being a major cause of death, there were fewer survivors with moderate or severe head injuries than expected. Only seven occupants with severe head injuries survived long enough to reach hospital. Six of these arrived in the neurosurgical unit within the first hour of the crash. None of them required immediate surgery, which meant that the anticipated deluge of head injury surgical workload did not occur.

Follow up of the survivors

Routine review of all the surviving patients during the succeeding days identified four with mild persistent headaches or suspicious clinical signs, but CT scans were either negative or showed only minor subcortical contusions. No further surgical intervention was necessary and no later scans were performed. All of the initial survivors who later died, at up to 3 weeks after the crash, had macroscopic brain injuries ranging from mild cerebral swelling and contusions to a clinically "silent" subdural haematoma. It is likely that many other survivors suffered subclinical cerebral damage without obvious consequence.

Of the six adult initial survivors with severe head injuries, five had injuries to the back of the head and four had no significant extracranial trauma. Three of these patients died of their head injuries. A fourth patient survives with permanent severe neurological disability. One remains disabled by spinal cord and limb injuries. The sixth patient has made a good recovery.

Organisational constraints

At an early stage in the neurosurgical management of this disaster, several features of the medical response to the disaster became apparent which were related to dispersing the patients to a number of hospitals.

The need and ability of the generalists to limit the overall number of admissions and spread the patient load to other hospitals contrasted with the regional neurosurgical unit's need to centralise its admissions in order to provide optimal care. The administration of this dual policy was difficult, but these conflicting requirements must be recognised. Operating in this fashion required the regional specialty to remain in direct contact with the disaster site and all serving hospitals and to tailor its responses and advice appropriately. Efficient communications are vital to success in these situations and the initial absence of communication between the hospital and the accident site could have been embarassing had it not been for the availability of a portable phone. Direct access to the hospital bleep system and national telephone networks without going through a switchboard is necessary. Provision of shortwave radio communications within the hospital and an open frequency to the disaster site greatly facilitate such openings.

Until the success or otherwise of the attempt to centralise neurological care remained uncertain, it seemed better for the off duty staff to remain at home so that they could make use of uncongested roads clear of accident traffic should they need to travel to outlying hospitals. Once centralisation had been achieved, they were able to quickly join the unit and provide maximal specialist staffing with the full support of the regional facilities.

The key to providing the best cover on the night was the ability to remain flexible in the face of uncertain and changing circumstances.

Clinical reviews of the survivors

During the first hours of the crisis the most striking clinical observations were the quite unexpected incidence of severe posterior head wounds sustained during a deceleration accident, and the remarkable similarity of injuries sustained by all the occupants but an apparent random pattern of fatality with uninjured and dead sitting in adjacent seats. In an effort to understand the mechanism of these posterior injuries and also to explain the wide range in the severity of head injury, it seemed appropriate to undertake a detailed clinical review of the survivors. This clinical study[1] has subsequently been enhanced by postmortem reports made available by the coroner and detailed structural analysis of the wreckage provided by the Air Accident Investigation Branch. Using a seating plan compiled from boarding passes, together with passengers' and rescuers' recollection, it proved possible to relate each individual's injuries to a particular seat and damage environment within the aircraft.[1a]

Comparison of each individual's injury severity score with the aircraft's structural damage demonstrated a positive relationship between local damage and degree of trauma sustained. The worst injured victims were recovered from rows 6–9 and 22–24, which corresponded with the two major fuselage fracture sites. Here the main cause of death was overwhelming crushing trauma affecting all parts of the body.

Away from the fracture sites in the aircraft, the injury pattern among the fatalities was different. Although aircraft structural damage was significantly less and extracranial injuries were less severe, head injuries were almost as bad as at the fracture site. Of the 14 fatalities away from the aircraft sites, only three had systemic injuries that might have been the prime cause of death. Ten died with brain swelling and four had acute subdural haematomas. Nine of these victims had injuries to the back of their head. It is possible that some of these passengers with isolated head injuries survived the initial impact and might have benefited from neurosurgical attention but died whilst trapped and inaccessible in the wreckage.

Victims with pulmonary oedema and brain swelling were said to have died of asphyxia. Without detailed neuropathological examination it is not safe to assume that the pulmonary oedema was not neurogenic in origin and thus secondary to a cerebral injury. The importance of obtaining specialist neuropathological opinion on those who had died on site cannot be overstressed and it is a matter of great regret that it was not allowed in this incident.

Even without detailed neuropathology, away from the areas of major airframe structural damage the most potent cause of death or disability

97

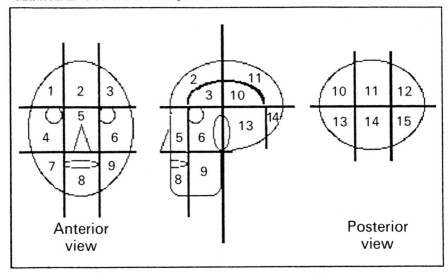

Figure 8.1—The grid used for recording the superficial head and facial injuries.

appears to have been posterior head injury. In their turn, these injuries appear to have been caused by cabin furniture becoming detached on impact and raining forward as a hail of debris as the aircraft decelerated. The evidence for this is that 42 of the 118 passengers had posterior injuries and some of the recovered seats had indentations in the headrests suggestive of impact from above and behind. Several areas were identified where passengers or seats arranged sequentially one behind another suffered similar damage of this type.

All but one of the overhead bins were torn from their mountings by the crash. Each had a load limit of 80 kg, although it is estimated that the average loading for such a bin during a commercial flight is closer to 25 kg.[2] This flying debris was considered by us to be the cause of death for nine of the fatalities at the scene and three of the initial survivors, all of whom had injuries that otherwise were compatible with survival. The most severely injured survivor remains permanently disabled, mute, and tetraparetic as the result of such an isolated posterior head injury.

In order to explore the possible causes of the wide range of severity of individual head and facial trauma among adjacent survivors, each was interviewed at length during the first 3 days following the accident and all their injuries recorded and photographed. Head and facial injuries were plotted on an empirical grid dividing the head into 15 sectors (figure 8.1). Injuries to the back of the head were noted and a superficial injury score (SIS) was calculated by scoring one point for each area containing a cut or contusion.

The recollections of each individual of events leading up to and through the crash and rescue were recorded. In particular, they were asked whether and how they had braced themselves for landing. Any gaps in memory were noted and an estimate of duration made. Where recall was complete, the patient was asked for an account of the actions of other passengers during the crash.

During these early interviews it was noted that those passengers who had no recollection of the crash suffered little psychological disturbance as a result of the event and their injuries, whilst those who had remained conscious throughout were greatly disturbed by nightmares, intrusive thoughts, and heightened anxiety. These observations were subsequently incorporated into a separate longitudinal psychological study of the post-traumatic stress suffered by the survivors (W. Gregg *et al.*, personal communication).

Of the 77 initial survivors included in the study (those in *passenger* seating, wearing lap belts), 73 (95%) had evidence of head and facial trauma ranging from minor bruising to traumatic craniectomy. Forty two passengers (55%) had no recollection of the crash and this was closely related to the degree of head and facial trauma as assessed by the SIS. None of the 11 survivors with minor facial bruising (SIS $\leq$ 1) lost consciousness. Above SIS = 1, there was a direct linear relationship between the extent of superficial trauma and the likelihood of unconsciousness. No passenger with SIS $\geq$ 6 recovered with their memory for the incident intact. There was a similar significant trend towards prolonged amnesia and more severe head injury with increasing SIS.

The importance of brace position

Ten seconds before impact, a cabin announcement ". . . prepare for crash landing! . . ." was made and repeated by the aircraft's captain.

Of the 77 surviving passengers, sitting in forward facing passenger seats, analysed in detail, 26 gave a clear history of being tightly braced for landing (head right down with hands clasped behind the head and elbows outside knees). Their mean SIS derived from the anatomical grid was 2.1. Only one of the group (3.8%) was amnesic for the event (retrograde amnesia of seconds; post-traumatic amnesia of minutes). Two (7.7%) had posterior injuries but neither of these lost consciousness.

Ten passengers were part braced (leaning forward over lap luggage or semiflexed holding the back of the seat in front). Their mean SIS was 3.0 and their mean abbreviated injury score (AIS) 1.6. Five (50%) had no recollection of the crash, whilst three (30%) had posterior head injuries.

The "unbraced" population included those too frightened to move on the pilot's crash warning, those confused or unaware of the proper position and those who were attending to companions at impact. These 23 unbraced passengers had a mean SIS of 3. Eighteen (78%) lost consciousness on impact and six (26%) received posterior injuries.

The remaining 18 passengers were classified as of unknown brace position because no reliable account of their position at landing could be established. The mean SIS in this group was 5.0, suggesting head and facial trauma at least equivalent to the unbraced population. All of these passengers lost consciousness during impact and 10 (56%) had posterior injuries.

Statistical analysis of the data confirmed significant trends towards reduced superficial head trauma (SIS), unconsciousness, duration of amnesia, and severity of head injury (AIS) with increasingly braced posture at landing. Full bracing also conferred significant protection against posterior injuries.

No statistical difference in aircraft structural or seat damage was seen between each of the brace groups. A fully braced position for crash landing provided real protection against head injury, unconsciousness, and injuries from behind irrespective of the degree of local damage.

Bracing (with legs forward) gave some protection against chest injury but less against abdominal injury and none against limb injury, which was more closely related to the degree of local floor disruption than brace position.

Using the crash pulse for the accident (derived by Cranfield Institute of Technology under contract to the Air Accident Investigation Branch) a computer model of the sequence of events at crash landing was developed by a commercial firm of engineering analysis consultants (HW Structures Ltd).[3] The results were presented as freeze frame graphics and in terms of absolute loads and acceleration. In addition a head injury criterion[4] (HIC) score was calculated for each brace position and with possible alternative harness and seat configurations.

The HIC score is a single figure derived from an integrated head-acceleration/time history used in the automotive industry when designing for occupant safety. American Federal Regulations for car design require this figure to be below 1000. Although injury and concussion might be expected to occur at lower levels, this value is felt appropriate as fire is relatively rare in automobile accidents, and so the preservation of consciousness is not essential to survival. Similar criteria may not be applicable to aircraft accidents, in which fire is more common, water landing is possible, and preservation of consciousness is vital for rapid evacuation.

The unbraced HIC score of 974 (table 8.1) is compatible with significant head injury and unconsciousness, and is close to the Federal Regulations' limit of acceptability for automobile design.

The HIC score for a braced occupant in this simulation was 278, affording almost as much protection against head injury as a lap and diagonal seat belt (HIC = 266). At this score, minor abrasions might be expected but consciousness would be preserved, and death should not

TABLE 8.1 Predicted head injury criterion (HIC) score, loads, and acceleration for each brace position (from occupant modelling in aircraft crash conditions, CAA paper 90012[3])

		Acceleration			
	HIC score (at 36 ms)	Head (m/s² max)	Chest (m/s² max)	Pelvic load (N)	Tibial load (N)
Unbraced	974	798	586	8024	1152
Braced	278	534	332	5394	0
Three-part belt	266	462	321	6005	1560
Rear facing	152	369	448	5597	1807

occur. The lowest recorded score was with a rear facing seat, but at these levels it is unlikely that any real survival advantage would be gained when compared with a braced posture for crash landing.

Comment

Despite the reducing incidence of aircraft crashes during the last 30 years,[5,6] the risk of death or serious injury in any individual crash has not altered.[7] This is partly because improvements in aircraft cabin safety design have lagged behind increasing aircraft reliability. This contrasts with the situation in the automobile industry, which accepts that car crashes are commonplace and therefore designs for occupant safety with accidents very much in mind.

Most aircraft accidents occur during take off or landing, so that help is often at hand and the relatively low impact velocities favour survival.[8] Ninety per cent of all accidents are survivable by at least some of the occupants,[7] but on average in fatal accidents 35% of passengers and 40% of crew die.[9] The major causes of death in aircraft accidents have remained the same for many years. They include being crushed within the collapsing airframe, failure of passenger restraint, being struck by unrestrained cabin contents, and being trapped or otherwise unable to escape (as by unconsciousness) from the wreckage.[10,11]

It is clear that in this crash overall injury was proportional to aircraft damage and death was most likely where fuselage fracture occurred.

A fundamental goal for engineers and materials scientists is to devise economical ways of improving floor, fuselage, and seat design so that aircraft strength exceeds human tolerance levels and cannot therefore contribute to the excess mortality known to be caused by structural failure in relatively low G force fields.

101

Restraints and harnesses

The head is more often seriously injured than any other part of the body in aircrashes.[12–15]

Lap belt restraint has limited efficacy in preventing head injury in deceleration accidents.[10,12,16] The upright passenger flails forward in an arc of more than 1 m radius,[14] subjecting the brain to high radial acceleration, then striking the seat in front, frequently to sustain a fatal head injury.[12,17,18] Pleas to make the area traversed by the flailing head safer have been made since 1956.[13,17]

A clear advantage is afforded by shoulder harness in pure deceleration accidents,[16,19] but vertical forces may be high in aircrashes.[10,13,14] Forces in this direction are poorly tolerated[12] and if the occupant remains sitting upright, thoracolumbar fractures may result.[10,13] In this crash, neither pilot nor co-pilot, who would have been exposed to the highest impact forces at the front of the plane, escaped head injury or concussion despite full harnesses, whilst both sustained lumbar spinal compression fractures, one with permanent neurological disability.

Rear facing seats

Rear facing seating with adequate head support offers considerably increased protection in test crashes[16,18,19] and has been fitted to Royal Air Force and US Air Force transport fleets since 1947.[12] It is undoubtedly safer in pure deceleration accidents on the test track, but its application to the real situation in commercial aircraft has been hotly debated for 40 years.[12,13,17,18,20] In this crash it would not have saved lives at the major structural fracture sites and, in areas of structural integrity, rear facing seats would have exposed many more passengers to the hail of overload bins, with a consequent increased risk of death by decapitation or severe head, neck, and upper trunk injury.

Flying debris

Flying debris is recognised as a potent cause of injury in aircrash[10,11,17,18] and elimination of this hazard has to be a priority. Ideally, the overhead bins should be removed or replaced by low level storage. It is estimated that passengers take an average of 6 kg hand baggage on to flights.[3] This could be accommodated in underseat storage space.

Bracing

In this crash, even with the current forward facing seats and lap belts, the incidence and severity of head injury, concussion, and injuries from behind were all reduced in those survivors who adopted a tightly flexed brace position for crash landing.

Bracing, by limiting head flailing, decreases brain acceleration and minimises impact with the seat in front. Reduction of sitting height reduces exposure to the hail of flying debris and maximises the cover provided by the passenger's own seat back.

Escaping from fire

Once having survived a crash landing, the main subsequent factor affecting occupant mortality is fire.[11,12,16,18] Attempts have been made to improve this aspect of survival by the introduction of fire blocking materials, floor proximity lighting, smoke detectors, and additional access to overwing exits,[9] whilst provision of smoke hoods has been suggested, but ignore the importance of preserved consciousness.

Consciousness

All of the methods described depend for their success upon calm, conscious, cooperative survivors making an orderly escape from the wreckage.

Alteration of consciousness following actual crash landings and in simulated accidents has been documented, but its contribution to the loss of life of potential survivors has been underemphasised.[12,18] Up to 60% of survivors lose consciousness on impact.[19] "Inability to escape" is a potent cause of mortality.[11,14,21] Among the survivors of this crash, 45 (52%) were unconscious for variable times following the crash. All of these survivors had moderate to severe facial bruising and the seat backs in front of them bore witness marks of head and facial impact. An overlapping group of 50 survivors (57%) had lower limb injuries that prevented unassisted escape. Had the left engine fire spread, only 13 of the initial 87 survivors could have escaped, leaving the remaining 74 (85%) unconscious and unaware of the danger or, worse, conscious but unable to escape due to lower limb injuries. This must, in accidents complicated by fire, flood, or toxic fumes, call into question the efficacy of smoke hoods or other safety devices dependent on passenger effort. Passive extinguisher systems could be safer and more effective in this situation, although their design may be difficult and they still depend on individuals' ability to extricate themselves.

Bracing has been shown in our studies to preserve consciousness, thereby allowing escape, whilst in addition the computer simulation suggests that limb injuries could be minimised, providing floor damage does not occur,[3] by positioning the feet on the floor slightly behind the knees.

Recommendations of the crash report

Many of the 31 recommendations of the official crash report are technical and intended to prevent a similar aircraft failure in future.[2] The final six recommendations call for research into cabin safety design, including improved seat back padding, evaluation of upper torso restraint and rear facing seats, re-evaluation of floor strength and overhead bins, and the provision of purpose designed child seats rather than supplementary lap belts.

Summary

- A good braced position during crash landing provides the best opportunity to remain conscious, limit head injury, and stay below the hail of flying debris

- Loose or unstable cabin furniture, which is the source of this debris and a potential cause of unnecessary injury, should be removed or upgraded

- Removal of overhead bins and other potential sources of flying debris could markedly improve the survivability and reduce the mortality of aircrash, even with present seat and harness arrangements

- Passive fire/flood safety systems should be investigated

- Redesign of aircraft should have regard to the strengthening of cabin floors so that floors are more likely to remain structurally intact with good seat fixation points

- Alteration of seat design, orientation, and harnessing may be of value but is still unproven and they must be considered in conjunction with the other associated factors

- Potential effects of any design alteration should be fully evaluated prior to its introduction; hasty change may not produce the hoped for improvements in survival

- Computer-generated design will allow more accurate prediction of structural and occupant behaviour in real crash situations, and will allow exploration of infinite theoretical design changes, with respect to the many interrelated factors, to limit passenger injury

- The inadequacy of passenger protection during crash landing has been recognised for many years, but change has been slow (standards are lower than those of the automobile industry); standards could be greatly raised by simple and economical precautions

- Many passengers, when warned of imminent crash landing, were unsure of the correct position to adopt. This should be clearly demonstrated as part of pre-flight instructions and all passengers should practise bracing if a precautionary landing is proposed, thus maximising the number of conscious survivors in good condition and improving evacuation of the wreckage

- Public, market, media, and government pressure will have to be maintained to ensure the application of even more radical re-evaluation required to apply present knowledge to future aircraft design and operation

I would like to acknowledge the Nottingham, Leicester, Derby, Belfast study group, The Air Accident Investigation Branch, HM Coroner, and HW Structures Ltd.

1 White BD, Rowles JM, Mumford CJ, Firth JL. Head injuries in the Boeing 737 aircrash. *Br J Neurosurg* 1990; **4**: 503–10.

1a White BD, Firth JL, Rowles JM. The effects of structure failure on injuries sustained in the M1 Boeing 737 Disaster, January 1989. *Aviat Space Environ Med* 1993; **64(2)**: 95–102.

2 Air Accident Investigations Branch, DTp. *Aircraft accident report 4/90—report on the accident to Boeing 737-400-G-OBME near Kegworth, Leicestershire on 8 January 1989.* HMSO, London; 1990.

3 Civil Aviation Authority. *Occupant modelling in aircraft crash conditions.* Gatwick: Civil Aviation Authority; Oct 1990. (CAA Paper 90012.)

4 US Department of Transport. Federal Motor Vehicle Safety Standard 208. Occupant Crash Protection. The head injury criteria score. *Federal Register* 1989; **54**: 211 (s6.2.2).

5 Veale JB. Foreword. In: Stephens PJ, ed. *Fatal civil aircraft accidents.* Bristol: John Wright; 1970.

6 Safety: nowhere [comment]. *Flight Int* 17–23 Jan 1990: 3.

7 Muir HC, Marrison C. Human factors in cabin safety. *Aerospace* 1989; **April**: 18–21.

8 Rutherford WH. An analysis of civil aircrash statistics 1977–1986 for the purposes of planning disaster exercises. *Injury* 1988; **19**: 384–8.

9 Learmount D. The arrogant decade. *Flight Int.* 17–23 Jan 1990: 48–50.

10 Moseley HG, Zeller AF. Relation of inquiry to forces and direction of deceleration in aircraft accidents. *Aviat Med* 1958; **Oct**: 739–49.

11 Fryer DI. The results of accidents. In: Gilles JA, ed. *Textbook of aviation physiology.* Oxford: Pergamon Press; 1965: 1166–79.

12 Stapp JP. Crash protection in air transports. *Aeronaut Eng Rev* 1953; **12**: 71–8.

13 Hasbrook AH. Crash injury research: a means of greater safety in aircraft accidents. *J Aviat Med* 1957; **28**: 541–52.

14 Swearingen RR, Hasbrook AH, Snyder RG, McFadden EB. Kinematic behavior of the human body during deceleration. *Aerospace Med* 1962; **33**: 188–97.

15 Mason JK. The mode and cause of death from aviation accidents. In: *Aviation accident pathology.* London: Butterworths; 1962: 106–45.

16 Mason JK. Other relevant safety equipment. In: *Aviation accident pathology.* London: Butterworths; 1962: 45–57.

17 Hawkes R. Aircrash death or injury may be prevented by sound detail design. *Aviat Week* 1956; **65**: 61–79.

18 Stephens PJ. Reconstruction of events at impact and immediately after an accident. In: *Fatal civil aircraft accidents.* Bristol: John Wright; 1970: 52–60.

19 Fryer DI. The preventive medicine of accidents. In: Gillies JA, ed. Textbook of aviation physiology. Oxford: Pergamon Press; 1965: 1202–12.

20 Mason JK. Injuries sustained in fatal aircraft accidents. *Br J Hosp Med* 1973; **May**: 645–54.

21 Mason JK. Reconstruction of a fatal aircraft accident from the medical findings. *Proc R Soc Med* 1968; **61**: 1079–84.

9

The M1 plane crash—managing the hospital response

NIGEL J CLIFTON

Introduction

Preparing for and rehearsing the response to an accident involving numer-ous live casualties is a fundamental aspect of emergency planning and training in the United Kingdom. The emergency services—police, fire, and ambulance—hospital trusts and health and local authorities, along with a range of voluntary organisations, are required to have coordinated plans that can be implemented quickly and effectively.

National Health Service (NHS) emergency planning aims to ensure that health care services are prepared to make an effective response to any major incident. Current guidance from the Department of Health states:

There is no standard definition of a "major incident" which would satisfy the health service and other agencies likely to be involved, as each tends to determine such incidents in the light of its own responsibilities. For the purpose of this guidance, however, a major incident arises when any occurrence presents a serious threat to the health of the community, disruption to the service, or causes or is likely to cause such numbers of casualties as to require arrangements by the health service.

The M1 aircrash at Kegworth in January 1989 demonstrated the value of careful planning and preparation by many organisations, which had taken account of the special risk of an aircraft accident at or on approach to East Midlands Airport. Demands placed on services emphasised the need for exceptionally thorough coordination, intelligent management, and flexible responses.

The effect of mass casualties on health care services may be substantial and prolonged. Following the Kegworth aircrash, the four East Midlands hospitals involved received a total of 87 survivors, and 36 were still in hospital 3 weeks after the accident. The emergency plans for these hospitals focused on the immediate response, but Kegworth produced serious long term effects on the working of at least one hospital. These included disruption of clinical activity, with scheduled work postponed; coping with the demands of an unusually large number of highly dependent patients, and providing support to their relatives. Special arrangements were made to provide counselling for patients, their families, and staff.

This chapter describes the key elements for planning and managing the whole hospital response to a major accident, and draws on the lessons learnt from the Kegworth aircrash and its effects on University Hospital, Queen's Medical Centre (QMC), Nottingham.

Disaster planning

The general principles of National Health Service disaster planning are well documented, and in the United Kingdom are set out in circulars issued by the Department of Health to health authorities and trusts.[1] Essentially, hospital major accident plans are concerned with the arrangements for mobilising staff and running the hospitals so that patients can be assessed and treated as they arrive, and how, once admitted, those patients will be cared for. These plans describe the arrangements for command, control, and communication, and for coping with the needs of relatives. At QMC our plans also covered support for staff and volunteers, dealing with the media, and for managing the aftermath.

In the United Kingdom, Regional Health Authorities (RHAs) are required to assess the capacity of different hospitals to deal with various types and severity of casualties, and their ability to supply medical and nursing teams if required. At the scene of the incident, the local ambulance service is responsible for managing the distribution of casualties, taking into account local circumstances and conditions such as traffic routes and the location of clinical specialties, (for example, burns units). Suitable hospitals are termed "receiving hospitals" during an incident.[1]

Following Kegworth, two hospitals, QMC and Derbyshire Royal Infirmary (DRI), were immediately identified as receiving hospitals, because of easy road access to the crash site, with a clear motorway return, and both a distance of around 11 miles from the crash site. Leicester Royal Infirmary (LRI) 20 miles from the crash site was also designated to receive casualties; two patients were taken to Mansfield General Hospital (north of Nottingham), immediately after the QMC made a decision to admit no more emergencies.

The essential elements of a major accident plan are designed to concentrate resources on the response to the incident, releasing staff, facilities, and equipment to cope with the sudden influx of casualties, while maintaining emergency services for the local resident population. The four hospitals involved in the Kegworth incident together provide services for just over 2 million people. Just because there had been an aircrash on the M1 didn't stop people fighting in pubs, crashing their cars on the A46, or having a coronary, and an essential feature of the major accident plans in use at the time was the ability to channel all accident and emergency cases, from whatever source, through a single triage point, where patients could be assessed and resuscitated.

Coordination, control, and communication

Department of Health instructions to listed receiving hospitals emphasise the importance of coordination, control, and communication. Hospitals alerted by the ambulance service may be asked to supply mobile medical and nursing teams, although the decision about which hospital should send a team does depend on the initial assessment of the situation and the resources available at the receiving hospital.

Once casualties arrive at the hospital, priorities are rescusitation and identification. An enormous range of skills and facilities is needed, and it is essential that these are managed effectively—the organisation of resources depends on clearly defined coordination, control, and communication arrangements.

At QMC, the hospital control team is responsible for managing the whole hospital response to an incident and is based in a central control room for the duration of the incident. Following the aircrash at Kegworth, the QMC control team was led by the general manager, supported by the professor of medicine, designated as medical director because his medical skills were not required immediately, and the director of nursing. Essentially, the job of the control team was to ensure the effective management of the whole hospital response, using information from the emergency services at the scene, and staff within the hospital, to make decisions about the deployment of staff and resources, and anticipating likely needs.

The plan used was based on the assumption that specific activities would cease immediately. Scheduled operating, fracture, and orthopaedic clinics planned for the following day were cancelled immediately, and the hospital control team had to decide whether activities in other outpatient and diagnostic departments would have to be suspended. Early on, the team concluded that the hospital would remain under pressure for the next 24 hours and decided to cancel many routine activities.

Notification

Normally, warning of an accident will come through the emergency services, and the ambulance control has NHS responsibility for selecting and alerting the most appropriate receiving hospitals. However, it is not uncommon for patients to arrive at hospital before the major incident plan is implemented, one example being the arrival of walking wounded at St. Bartholomew's Hospital Accident and Emergency Department in London within minutes of the April 1993 Bishopsgate bombing.

A fundamental feature of the QMC plan is the delegation of authority and responsibility to accident and emergency staff on duty to decide whether to implement the whole hospital plan. The decision doesn't have to wait until a manager is contacted.

Uniquely, an aircraft in difficulty may be able to give advance warning to emergency services. At Kegworth, ambulance and other emergency services were notified more than 10 minutes before the British Midland Airways Boeing 737 crashed, although local hospitals were not told until after the incident occurred. The NHS Management Executive recommends that hospital major incident plans (HMIP) should clearly state the action to be taken when an alert call is received or cancelled, and includes provision for hospitals and emergency services being placed on standby without being fully mobilised. Airborne emergencies are not uncommon, and by going to standby as soon as an aircraft is known to be in difficulties, hospitals could be ready to activate the full plan in the event of a major incident, or alternatively to stand down when further instructions are received from the ambulance service.

Enormous disruption occurred immediately after the accident, and continued for several hours, as casualties began arriving at the same time as staff were being mobilised. In the first 15 minutes after ambulances arrived on the scene, 20 casualties were dispatched to the accident and emergency departments at QMC and DRI and within the first 2 hours, these two hospitals alone received a total of 76 survivors, of whom 70 were seriously injured. The first journalists arrived at the hospitals within 30 minutes of the accident being announced, almost simultaneous with the first admissions, and telephone enquiries from relatives started soon after. At QMC, seven operating theatres were opened up within an hour and remained in use throughout the night.

Leicester Royal Infirmary was the last to receive patients, and the control team there had more time to consult and initiate patient transfers from the intensive therapy unit (ITU). Because more was known about the incident by this time, it was possible to make a reasonable estimate of the likely number of patients and range of injuries the LRI would be receiving. With this information the LRI was able to adjust its major incident plan appropriately.[2]

Cascade call out and communications facilities

One of the objectives of the QMC major incident plan is to limit the load on the hospital telephone switchboard, and to keep communications open and flowing, and largely this was achieved during that night. The switchboard team contacted key personnel in each department, who in turn began the internal call out procedure using a cascade system. The first person contacted at home was responsible for telephoning others, who in turn then called in their colleagues. Even though it was a Sunday evening, the high proportion of successful contacts made through the cascade reinforced the importance of requiring each department to keep an up to date call out list, available for key personnel to use from home. Departments that have a member of staff on duty or on call in the hospital should not expect that person to work through a lengthy call out list, because they may be too busy with patients.

At QMC, the staff use various commercial paging systems to keep in touch with the hospital, which works well in normal circumstances. However, because there was no standard system that could be used to broadcast a general message, there were delays communicating with some staff. The QMC hospital switchboard has a facility to block out incoming calls during the call out sequence, which meant that staff who relied on long distance tone pagers which required them to call back to base were unable to get through to the hospital to respond. This experience underlined the need for standardisation, and the disadvantages of using tone pagers in an emergency. The news was carried very quickly on local radio and TV stations, and in one case, an on-duty orthopaedic registrar was telephoned at home by a relative living in Australia, who saw the news on TV and informed him of the accident before the cascade call out reached him.

The rapid availability of staff, free from other commitments that they might have had on a busy weekday, undoubtedly contributed to the success and speed of the overall response, but also demonstrated the importance of being able to identify staff and the need to keep the control team informed of any changes in staff deployment.

At QMC each department works with detailed internal plans and with action cards for individuals, describing specific responsibilities and the sequence of actions in priority order. Medical and other volunteers who do not have specific duties as part of the plan are sent to the volunteer base. Such offers of help require tactful and sensitive management. The under-standable wish of skilled people to help, and for some, the need to be involved, has to be balanced against the need to cover services possibly for several days afterwards, while tired staff recuperate.

The Kegworth accident occurred just before 2030 on a Sunday evening. QMC was notified of the incident as shifts were changing, with both day and night staff present in the hospital. The operating theatres were unusually quiet, and it was possible to contact staff on call at home. Staff responded rapidly and effectively—many who were off duty came in and worked throughout the night and then completed their rostered shifts the following day. The speed and volume of the response produced some operational difficulties. Instead of reporting to the volunteer centre, many staff went straight to the accident and emergency department, which became extremely crowded.

While this was a natural reaction by staff who wanted to use their skills, it could have produced an imbalance in the allocation of staff at a critical stage during the implementation of the plan, and it created practical problems because of the difficulty of identifying eveyone working in the area.

This experience emphasised the importance of ensuring that all staff are given training in the basic principles of the major incident plan as part of their introduction and induction to the hospital.

Clinical workload in the first 12 hours

During the first 12 hours, 33 out of the total of 83 survivors actually admitted to East Midlands hospitals underwent immediate or urgent surgery, involving a total of 92 procedures. At QMC, which received 39 patients, 11 patients were operated on during the night with 38 procedures being performed. Several other patients with multiple injuries were taken to the Intensive Therapy Unit for resuscitation and monitoring and, in all, 12 patients were accepted by the ITU. In all, 409 radiological examinations were performed during that night, including CT and angiograms; and in the first 12 hours, 248 units of blood had been used—209 were cross-matched within 150 minutes of the crash.

Demand on facilities and staff in Leicester and Derby was on a similar scale. At LRI, on the first night, two operating theatres in the main theatre block and the operating theatre in the fracture clinic were opened. Ten patients required 23 surgical procedures, including the evacuation of an extradural haematoma and the repair of a ruptured bladder, from 2245 hours on Sunday through to 1100 hours on the following Monday morning. A further six patients were stabilised in splints and plaster and their surgery planned for later that week. Only four patients had minor injuries—metatarsal fractures, cuts, and bruises—and did not require surgery. The 21st patient arrived at 0500 but died in casualty.[3]

The DRI received 25 patients from the crash site over a 90 minute period. In the first 12 hours, 11 patients underwent surgery, with 31 procedures being performed.

Demand for specialised equipment and supplies

The QMC plan calls in supplies staff from the outset. Like most hospitals, QMC maintains stocks of items such as plasma volume expanders, dressings, and instrumentation likely to be required in quantity immediately. However, the type of injuries caused at Kegworth produced exceptional demand for highly specialised external fixation equipment. The value of having supplies specialists on site immediately was confirmed; and, by extraordinary coincidence, the local representative of a company that manufactures external fixation equipment happened to be on the M1 at the time of the accident and made immediate arrangements to supply additional equipment to the hospital.

The clinical aftermath

The accident at Kegworth had immediate effects on scheduled services, effects that continued for several weeks afterwards. Surgeons at the three main hospitals involved worked throughout the night, and the following morning. The increased level of theatre activity at QMC was sustained throughout the next 2 days. In the first 36 hours, 64 operative procedures were performed and two operating theatres remained in use from 0900 until late evening for the remainder of the week in order to treat those needing surgery. The position at LRI and DRI was similar—at DRI, over the first 48 hours, a total of 49 procedures were completed on 21 patients, and elective orthopaedic admissions planned for the following week were cancelled, largely because of the high bed occupancy. However, DRI was able to continue routine orthopaedic emergency treatment on the day following the accident.

Even though QMC had more than 1200 usable beds, the impact on the inpatient services were so severe that much of the non-urgent trauma related surgery arranged for the next 3 weeks had to be postponed. The number of beds taken up by highly dependent patients was exceptional and the ITU could only accept selected elective surgical patients such as neurosurgical and life threatening vascular cases.

The consequences of the length of time patients needed to recover or become fit enough for transfer had not been anticipated and had a knock-on effect on services. After 21 days, only 12 of the 35 patients who survived at QMC had been discharged or transferred. At LRI, 13 out of 21 had been discharged home or transferred to hospitals nearer their homes for rehabilitation. During the week after the accident, LRI theatre lists had to be arranged so that closed injuries could be treated, soft tissue wounds inspected, and fracture treatment reassessed, involving a total of 25 procedures on 15 patients. In particular, surgeons at LRI reported that soft tissue problems, such as devitalised skin areas requiring skin grafting, continued to occupy surgical time. At DRI, four of the 25 patients admitted remained in the hospital's care after 21 days.

As a proportion of the total acute beds available in the three hospitals, the number of patients remaining at the end of 3 weeks (34) may seem small, but within the specialties primarily affected—trauma and orthopaedics, and neurosurgery—their presence in the receiving hospitals meant a series of lost opportunities to treat local people already waiting for admission to hospital.

The importance of negotiating repatriation arrangements, and the willingness of medical teams and hospitals in the districts of residence of survivors to accept transferred patients cannot be overstated. Without these offers of help, and speedy and efficient transfer, the hospitals that responded to the M1 accident would have remained under even greater pressure and services for local people would have been significantly reduced.

Availability of specialist staff

Vital lessons about the mobilisation and deployment of key staff were learned. Although the development of specialised centres of excellence in the United Kingdom concentrates expertise and scarce resources, an event such as a survivable air accident is likely to require the resources of several hospitals. Decisions had to be made about the best way of deploying specialist teams, with patients needing their skills in hospital up to 30 miles away from base. Kegworth demonstrated the effectiveness of triage and assessment at the scene, with patients being directed to the centre with the most appropriate facilities. The neurosurgical team at QMC was able to advise colleagues at the crash site, and at hospitals in Leicester and Derby, with the result that nearly all the patients with severe head injuries were brought direct to QMC—the only hospital with an on-site neurosurgery unit. The subsequent review of the management of the incident reinforced the view that when assigning medical resources, specialist teams should remain at their base hospitals. While moving patients to the specialist hospital may place the individual at increased risk, dividing clinical activity between sites may adversely deplete these highly specialist teams.

The number and severity of the head injuries that occurred at Kegworth meant that all three consultant neurosurgeons based in Nottingham were required at QMC. One LRI patient underwent evacuation of extradural haematoma in Leicester during the first night, resulting in the diversion of one of the QMC neurosurgeons, who was much needed, to another hospital (LRI).

Identification of casualties

Booking and loading procedures for air transport, unlike bus or rail travel should mean that a manifest or passenger list is available from the operator almost immediately. This aids identification and reconciliation of lists of survivors, deceased, and missing with the information held by hospitals.

Easy access to comfortable mass travel may mean that passengers travel lightly dressed and are easily separated from their identification. In June 1975 a coach carrying elderly people crashed on the A74 at Johnstone Bridge, Dumfries and Galloway. Travelling on a warm day, passengers had already discarded their coats, and became separated from their handbags, with the result that the shocked and very ill survivors could not be identified immediately by the team at the the receiving hospital. In some cases, positive identification depended on the police using casualty bureaux techniques normally used to identify the dead.

International air travel, with overflying passengers, also poses the additional problem of casualties being unable to speak the language of the host nation where they are being treated.

The importance of following agreed procedures for the identification of patients was very clearly demonstrated when wards began to substitute major incident record numbers with patients' names, without checking back to hospital control or to medical records. This increased the risk of misidentification of patients, particularly those with similar sounding names or members of the same family.

After the M1 accident, proposals were put forward to standardise identification systems used by each agency in order to ease reconciliation of hospital documentation to information received from relatives enquiries, police casualty bureaux and other sources.[3] Even so, can the travel industry be persuaded to standardise listings and ensure that manifests are listed alphabetically as well as by seat order? Our problems in identifying and crosschecking patients would have been much reduced if such listings had been available.

Continuity and coordination

Coordinated emergency planning, and multiple agency involvement in a major incident means it is essential to rehearse and review systems for coordinating numerous organisations, and communicating between them. Even though we had had an exercise 3 months beforehand, the M1 accident highlighted a lack of familiarity with certain procedures and, in some crucial aspects, departures from the plan. The QMC control team, which was established and working within 20 minutes of notification, had difficulty keeping up with and recording information as required by the plan, and some early decisions were not logged. This made handover and briefing arrangements unnecessarily complex as new members joined the team, and demonstrated the importance of recording actions and decisions both for the sake of continuity and to support the "post mortem" to review the way in which the plan was implemented.

Following Kegworth, QMC plans have been extended to designate a clinical controller—a consultant orthopaedic surgeon—based on the receiving ward, to take over the care of patients as they are admitted, working in conjunction with the medical controller and the theatre manager.

The original QMC plan did not include a "post mortem" to assess whether the objectives of the plan were achieved. Information and experiences gained were applied to improve the plan for the future. The QMC plan now includes provision for comprehensive debriefing as soon as possible after the event, requiring everyone involved to take part, serving the dual purpose of checking whether procedures worked as planned and giving staff the opportunity to share their feelings with one another. We also found it was important to include those staff who felt left out because they were out of town or not contactable at the time.

Managing staff resources to cope with the prolonged aftermath is a major task, with the need to match staff and skills to particular types of patients, as staff became more and more tired. At QMC, following the crash, a significant number of the day staff, who were about to go off duty when the hospital was notified of the crash, stayed on to work through the night and reported for duty the next day. A review of reports published following major accidents in other parts of the United Kingdom during the last 5 years confirms that the number of staff who volunteer for extra duties at the outset frequently exceeds the numbers required. Considerable management time, tact, and skill may be needed to reallocate and assign these staff to make a contribution in the days that follow.

Following Kegworth, demands on staff created short and medium term effects across the hospital, with the cancellation of routine elective surgery and orthopaedic clinics on the first full working day after the accident. A backlog of routine surgery built up because of the priority that had to be given to those injured in the accident. While managers anticipated the effects of the sudden influx of highly dependent patients, and their requirements for postoperative and intensive care, there were some unexpected consequences such as staff in other areas of the hospital having to cope with patients who were waiting for major elective surgery whose operations had to be cancelled because there were no beds available in the ITU.

Handling the media

An aircraft accident is undoubtedly national news, but it usually attracts international interest as well. Following Kegworth, the response by the media was immediate and sustained, and demanded enormous managerial resources. The first journalists arrived at QMC within half an hour of the incident, by which time the hospital control room was in operation and a senior member of the management team had been assigned to act as press officer. Escorting and controlling journalists within the hospital tied up senior staff for several days, and one of the major lessons we learnt included the need to site the press room well away from both the hospital control room and the areas where relatives were being received, but to keep up the flow of detailed and accurate information. From the outset, we decided to hold regular scheduled press conferences, and the media were told that there would be no statements by any members of hospital staff except the duty press officer. Other agencies and visitors to the hospital made their own arrangements to speak to the press, and some well intentioned volunteers caught up in the emotion and intensity of the event spoke to the media:[4]

> There is always a risk that spontaneous remarks could cause distress to patients and their relatives, as well as creating organisational difficulties for the hospital.

On the whole, the story was not sensationalised—the journalists were largely preoccupied for the first couple of days trying to work out which of the engines had failed, and what the passengers had seen. Even so, there were some difficult experiences. In one case, two survivors did not wish to comment to the media but a relative at home made a series of statements without reference to the patients. Several others sought help from the hospital press office to deal with press enquiries and pressure on relatives. In another case, a local radio station carried a story without first checking with the hospital press office that blood donors were required, with the consequence that both the hospital and the Blood Transfusion Service telephone switchboards received dozens of enquiries from potential blood donors. This well intentioned response to an unverified story could have jeopardised communications, as well as taking up the time needed to sort out and correct the story. On the other hand, the local media responded very quickly to a request to broadcast and repeat announcements that outpatient clinics on the following working day had been cancelled.

Each of the hospitals involved in the response to Kegworth reported some local difficulties with controlling and coordinating the response to the media. Journalists at one hospital, "attempted to film through a window, and eventually, police assistance had to be obtained to control some of the nuisance press."[2]

Initially, journalists concentrated on basic information such as the number, ages, and sex of the survivors. Enquiries were received from all over the world—the QMC press office received more than 200 calls during the first night. The following morning, breakfast TV and national radio and TV news requested facilities to speak to medical staff and those patients who were fit enough to be interviewed. One of our jobs was to ensure that patients' privacy and dignity were protected and that public relations specialists were on hand to provide advice and guidance to interviewees. Press interest only declined gradually and it was not practical to close the press office until 6 days after the event.

VIP visitors

One aspect of the aftermath of the incident which was not anticipated was the series of visits by politicians and religious leaders. Patients at QMC received 12 VIP visitors within 6 working days. Some VIPs arrived unannounced; a request from the Prime Minister was declined, and the arrangements for the visit by HRH The Prince of Wales were discussed and agreed 48 hours in advance. Inevitably, VIP visits require a great deal of organisation and are particularly demanding if they take place during the first 24 hours after the incident, when services may be only just beginning to settle down and staff are very tired or still fully occupied by clinical work. It is difficult and probably inappropriate to turn down requests from community leaders to visit seriously injured patients and talk to hospital staff, but the internal organisation involved, the need for media briefing, and in some cases the security are considerable. Emergency planners may need to consider assigning extra staff to the press and public relations team to handle the organisation of VIP visits.

Military security requirements following Kegworth placed additional pressures on the local hospitals. Several of the injured patients were service personnel based in Northern Ireland, for whom special security arrangements were made, and this added to the clinical and organisational complexity of the response to the incident.

Psychological effects

The Trent report[2] on the Kegworth accident concluded that:

> The experience of people faced with terrible events is always personal and deeply disturbing but those involved as casualties, relatives, witnesses or other local people may need to be helped to overcome the enormous shock, numbness and extreme distress, which can also apply to the rescuers.

The social and psychological effects of a major disaster on survivors, relatives, and those involved in their rescue and care are widely recognised. After Kegworth, professional confidential counselling as an aid to recovery was offered. There is still vigorous debate about the need for counselling, and who should receive it, but it is increasingly accepted that counselling to cope with the psychological effects, and the disruption to normal life is beneficial for some individuals. The Trent report[2] commented:

Social work counselling is becoming increasingly regarded as a valuable part of the process of helping people to come to terms with a major crisis. However, while counselling is the most important skill required on these occasions, it is not the only form of support provided by social workers. They offer assistance in practical ways by maintaining links with friends and relatives, by arranging transport, by liaising with other services and by organising volunteers and other forms of support. People also need help in confronting the terrible reality of their experience and social workers can assist in this process by arranging for attendance at funerals, accompanying people who wish to visit the scene, helping to gather together belongings and preparing people who may have to identify severely injured or dead relatives and friends.

This type of support was offered by social services departments in all three counties where patients, relatives, rescuers and carers all had access, and most importantly was continued by social services departments in those areas to which the survivors returned after discharge from hospital.

One particular feature of an aircrash is that survivors are likely to be some distance from home, adding to the practical difficulties that distressed relatives have to face. Major incident plans should assume that relatives will arrive at the receiving hospitals very soon after the incident, although in the case of Nottingham the first relatives did not arrive at QMC until midnight—$3\frac{1}{2}$ hours after the aircrash. They were received in the relatives' waiting area, which had been set up close to the hospital control room and was staffed by outpatient nursing staff and the hospital chaplain.

With the large number of patients being cared for in the ITU, many relatives preferred to stay close to the hospital, using overnight accommodation, and taking over an empty ward. The initial contact with many of the relatives was when they telephoned for information and provided descriptions to help identify passengers. At QMC, a small team of social workers began the detailed and meticulous process of locating and identifying passengers, sharing information with the other two major receiving hospitals and the police and returning calls to relatives and friends who had been enquiring about passengers. The team coped with an enormous volume of calls for the next 48 hours, only closing down the relatives' information service at 0900 on Wednesday 11 January.[2]

The assistance offered to relatives and friends included counselling, emotional support and practical assistance, such as arranging accommodation and organising financial support. The role of British Midland Airways in supporting the hospitals and in helping with the care and comfort of relatives and friends was exemplary. Mr Michael Bishop (now Sir Michael), Managing Director of British Midland, instructed his ground staff to help all the hospitals with caring for the relatives and they set up centres in each of the hospitals, which then became contact points for the relatives. They also provided transport for relatives between Belfast and all the hospitals looking after the injured. Mr Bishop had previously been involved in the management of another aircraft accident, and from his experience then he was aware of the tremendous contribution that his company could make in easing the distress of all those affected by the accident.

Effective response to an emergency depends on teamwork—but allowance should also be made for the effects on individual members of staff who are away or not called in for an incident and subsequently express feelings of having been excluded from the teams that coped so well.

> The professional and personal impact of Kegworth on staff must not be underestimated. It had a psychological and emotional effect on hospital staff who were involved in the rescue, and those providing care and support for patients and their relatives. At all three hospitals Social Services staff and psychologists were involved in counselling and support for many of the staff involved with the incident and its aftermath.[2]

The report[2] of the Trent Regional Health Authority into the Kegworth disaster concluded that:

> . . . account should be taken of the need for an independent counselling service to be made available to support staff who have been involved professionally in a major disaster. Staff are not necessarily the best judge of their own counselling needs, given the pressures that such situations inevitably create.

The revised major incident procedure for QMC, produced after Kegworth, includes a commitment to provide formal counselling for any staff who require it and also advises departmental managers to be sensitive to the needs of those not involved, because indirect "complex emotions are generated in all those who work in a hospital which has been involved in a major accident and if these are not recognised, destructive divisions may appear."[4]

Conclusions

The immediate task after the Boeing 737 crash landed on the M1 at Kegworth was to rescue survivors and to ensure that they were transferred as quickly as possible to hospital, where their injuries could be assessed and treated.

The QMC major accident plan worked as intended, but vital lessons were learned about the effects of mass casualties on a local hospital from a survivable aircraft accident.

Managing the hospital response to a disaster: lessons learned from the M1 aircrash

- The demand for resources, staff, materials, and facilities was immediate and intense, and was underestimated in the plans

- Trauma and orthopaedic services for the local population were disrupted for several weeks

- Triage and assessment at the scene ensured that casualties were directed to the most appropriate hospital

- Specialist teams should stay at their base hospital

- Coordinated planning, review, and rehearsal are all-important; training and familiarisation with the principles of the major incident plan should be an essential aspect of induction of all hospital staff

- Command and control arrangements must be clear and simple, and the people in that role must have the authority and experience to respond flexibly and pragmatically

- Cascade call out systems are effective, provided that managers ensure that information is kept up to date and available to those who need it

- Spiritual, emotional and practical support for patients, their families, and staff should be built into the plan, and the resources assigned to make sure that that support is available for as long as it is needed after the incident

- Plans must ensure that sufficient experienced staff are assigned to dealing with the media, and VIPs, leaving the control team free to get on with the business of running the hospital

- If the people involved come from outside the immediate area, it is important to make early contact with their local hospitals, medical teams, and social services to negotiate repatriation and continuing medical care

---

References

1 NHS Management Executive. *Emergency planning in the NHS: health service arrangements for dealing with major incidents*. London: HMSO; November, 1990.
2 Trent Regional Health Authority. *Report—Aircraft Accident BD092—M1 Motorway*. Sheffield: Trent Regional Health Authority.
3 *Civil Protection*, issue 18. London: The Home Office; Spring 1991.
4 Queen's Medical Centre. *Major accident procedure*. Nottingham: Queen's Medical Centre; 1990.

General reference

Clifton NJ, Bradford A. *Aircraft accident at Kegworth—University Hospital response: internal management report*. Nottingham: Queen's Medical Centre; 1989.
Trent Regional Health Authority. *Guidance on major accident procedures*. Sheffield: Trent Regional Health Authority; 1985.

10

The Nottingham, Leicester, Derby, Belfast (NLDB) studies

W ANGUS WALLACE, JOHN M ROWLES, PETER
BROWNSON, CHRISTOPHER L COLTON

8/9 January 1989

During the night of 8 January most of the consultant orthopaedic surgeons in Nottingham were working in the operating theatres treating the survivors. By the early hours of the morning of 9 January most of the emergency operations had been completed and the surgeons were "relaxing" in the coffee room. Discussions turned to the accident and why so many of the occupants of the plane had been so severely injured.

We had been horrified at the severity of the lower limb injuries, particularly those injuries occurring below the knee. In addition the number of head injuries that the passengers had sustained, coupled with their severity, gave grave cause for concern.

During our discussions the topic of rear facing seats was raised by two of our anaesthetic colleagues who had travelled in rear facing aircraft seats while in the Royal Air Force. It was postulated that rear facing seats might have reduced the number and severity of the injuries.

This being the only recent passenger aircraft accident in which a large number of passengers had survived but with severe injuries, two of us (WAW and CLC) relalised the unprecedented nature of this crash. Over the subsequent 24 hours it became even clearer that this accident was indeed unique. The impact forces were high but because there was no post-crash fire many of the severely injured had survived. How had these severe injuries been sustained?

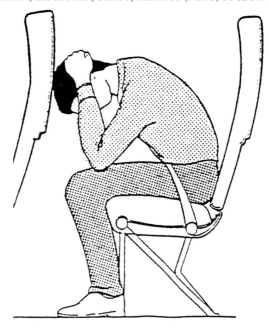

Figure 10.1—The NLDB "brace for impact" position for forward facing passengers. The accompanying instructions are: adopt a crouched position like a ball. Apply both hands to the top of the head without interlocking the fingers. Pull head down and bring elbows down towards the knees. Head can rest on the seat in front which may move forward (break over). Legs should be positioned firmly on the floor with feet together slightly behind the knees.

We were to learn later that survivability in aircraft accidents had increased over the previous 10 years due to improvements in aeroplane crashworthiness. For example, aircraft fuel had been modified to make it less flammable in the event of an aircraft accident. We learned subsequently from the Air Accident Investigation Branch (AAIB) that it was now possible to throw a lighted match into a pool of aviation fuel without it igniting. Neither we, nor apparently the fire service, were aware of this at the time of the accident. It did become clear, however, that although in the past an accident of this type would commonly be followed by an engulfing fire, this was no longer the case and therefore the pattern of survival following future aircraft accidents might well be changed.

We soon realised that this aircraft accident presented a unique opportunity to study the injuries sustained and to identify areas where occupant protection could be improved in the future. At that stage we had no idea that later research would lead to a standard "brace for impact position" (figure 10.1) which would be used by *all airlines flying into and out of the UK and illustrated on safety cards for aircraft passengers.*

9 January

During Monday 9 January we continued to contemplate a research project on the survivors of the aircraft accident but were unsure as to how this might be carried out.

The media had descended on the hospitals in Nottingham, Leicester, and Derby, and great demands were made on the hospital administration to provide facilities for the families of the injured and to provide information for the press, radio, and television. We became increasingly aware of the tremendous support that was being offered to the relatives by British Midland and in particular by Mr (now Sir) Michael Bishop, Chairman of British Midland. He demonstrated by his presence and accessibility to the media, and by his honest responses, that he was an extremely able and compassionate businessman. British Midland were exceptional in the speed of their response to this aircraft accident and in the organisation of their ground staff, who were directed to the three hospitals to help the hospital administration.

The 39 injured patients in Nottingham had been distributed between the 10 consultant orthopaedic surgeons, each surgeon taking responsibility for a number of cases. The heaviest load had fallen on Mr John Webb, who has a special interest in spinal injuries, and he was summoned from the operating theatre on the night of 9 January for a brief television interview, when he publicly raised the question of the causation of the injuries and whether rear facing seats would have resulted in a reduction in the severity of the injuries. Some of the surgical teams retired to bed late that night knowing that tomorrow would be another full day of operating.

10 January

On the morning of Tuesday 10 January each consultant orthopaedic surgeon reviewed his own group of injured patients. The soft tissue injuries (represented by cuts, bruising, and skin damage) were becoming very apparent. Mr Brian Holdsworth, the consultant orthopaedic surgeon on call on the night of the air crash, suggested that the soft tissue injuries be documented and so arrangements were made to photograph all of the soft tissue injuries over the next few days. Also it was announced that His Royal Highness the Prince of Wales would be visiting the next day to see the injured and assess for himself the work that was being carried out in looking after them.

His visit took place on the morning of 11 January and was a great morale booster not only for the patients but also for all of the members of the hospital team—doctors, nurses, management staff, blood transfusion staff, porters and cleaners. We were impressed by the dramatic effect that the royal visit had on all of us in such a difficult situation and we discovered the tremendous value of such impromptu visits.

Inevitably, however, the visit of Prince Charles was associated with much standing around and waiting, and it was during one of these lulls on one of the trauma wards at Queen's Medical Centre that the feasability of proceeding with the research project emerged. We knew that we needed a doctor with a background training in orthopaedic surgery (a research fellow) and sufficient funds to allow the extensive investigation that would be needed—photography, full x ray investigation, identification of injuries, and the collation of all the information and its interpretation. This would be a vast undertaking.

While waiting, we met our district general manager, Dr David Banks. We explained to him the unique nature of this accident and our plans for the vital research to identify the cause of the injuries involved. Spontaneously, he responded by agreeing to underwrite the salary of a research fellow to be appointed immediately. This turned out to be the springboard from which the Nottingham, Leicester, Derby, Belfast study group was launched.

Within 72 hours we had appointed one of our previous orthopaedic junior surgeons—Mr John Rowles—who at that time was working in Bristol. He started officially on 1 February 1989.

11 January

During the next 24 hours a document was prepared outlining the investigations planned to be carried out by the collaborative study group. The centres involved were those treating the injured patients—Nottingham, Leicester, and Derby—and the centre to which most of the injured would be returning—Belfast.

The aims of the NLDB study group as identified on 11 January 1989 were:

(1) To identify and document all soft tissue and bony injuries to crash victims.
(2) To analyse the mechanical forces generated by the crash at each seat position.
(3) To investigate the likely cause of the injuries sustained.
(4) To document the immediate and definitive management of all injuries sustained.
(5) To follow up all injured patients for at least 6 months and establish the outcome.
(6) To carry out an internal audit of our own performance in looking after the crash survivors.

A few days later we added a seventh aim because we had noted delays in the diagnosis of some of the injuries:

(7) To identify the nature and number of "missed" injuries.

Because of the difficulties involved in documenting all the soft tissue and bony injuries, the next 48 hours involved frenetic activity by the members of the university department of orthopaedic and accident surgery. Two research assistants—Vicki Price and Cathy Elliott—who had been working on another project, were seconded to the plane crash study and were asked to visit and document the injuries of every survivor in all four hospitals—Nottingham, Leicester, Derby, and Mansfield. Orthopaedic registrars were identified in the three main receiving hospitals to act as the local coordinating doctors and were asked to arrange for photography of all the injured in order to document the soft tissue injuries (This was a matter of urgency as the evidence, provided by cuts and bruises, would last for only a few days). Photography started on 11 January, 60 hours after the accident had occurred, and continued until the fifth post-accident day.

We were very grateful at this point to Wing Commander David Anton, who had been appointed by the AAIB at RAF Farnborough as the accident inspector to investigate the survivability aspects of the accident. Wing Commander Anton discussed with Professor Wallace the proposed research project, and it became clear that he strongly supported the concept of collaboration. However, he had reservations about the feasibility of our research plans, as outside parties are not normally allowed access to accident investigation information until the final accident report is produced. Never before had a research group worked closely in this way with the AAIB, and it was feared that there would probably be obstructions to our establishing any cooperation between the research group and the AAIB investigators.

12–16 January

Within the next week a research grant application had been submitted to the Medical Research Council and other charitable sources of research funding. On Saturday 14 January we had the first meeting of what was initially called the NLD study group. This brought together the coordinating orthopaedic registrars from the three hospitals, the research assistants from the Department of Orthopaedic and Accident Surgery, and other specialists, particularly the neurologists and neurosurgeons. The plans for the next 2 weeks were laid down and the need for approval from the AAIB became clear. On Monday 16 January we learned that the AAIB had agreed to recognise our research group but they could not yet agree full collaboration.

8 February

On 8 February, Professor Wallace, Mr John Rowles (research fellow), and Mr George Kirsh (Nottingham coordinating registrar) were summoned to the AAIB headquarters in Farnborough for a discussion of the proposed research project. The interrogation was intense. For about 20 minutes the AAIB members fired questions at us, clearly trying to identify whether the research work proposed was the result of a genuine interest in improving safety in aircraft or whether we were a lightweight organisation likely to cause trouble and interfere with the AAIB investigation. We heard later that the interview went well, and it was interesting that after 20 minutes the confrontation became more friendly: by the end of the meeting we appeared to have won the seal of approval from the AAIB. The emphasis throughout the interview had been on the necessary confidentiality surrounding AAIB investigations and the need for absolute secrecy during the period of the investigation until the publication of the final report. WAW assured the AAIB that the whole research group would be bound by a confidentiality agreement and that we would not publish or divulge any information without prior permission from the AAIB or until after the final report was in the public domain.

We were able to fulfil our promise throughout the period of our studies but in the late summer of 1990 there were repeated leaks of parts of the AAIB reports by other parties to the press.

A number of people were responsible for helping the research to get off the ground—particularly Mr Eddie Trimble, inspector of accidents at the AAIB, who gave unreserved support to the NLDB research group. In addition to John Rowles, who was the first NLDB research fellow, Peter Brownson was appointed the second NLDB fellow in 1992, and he has compiled additional studies on the "brace for impact" crash position.

Progress of the research programme

The collaborative research programme continued for a period of $4\frac{1}{2}$ years. Mr Peter Brownson succeeded Mr John Rowles as research fellow. In January 1992 the research entered a second phase and concentrated upon identifying a crash brace position that would minimise head and lower limb injuries. This research culminated in a report submitted to the Civil Aviation Authority (CAA) in May 1993 which recommended a modified passenger crash brace position. This is the crash brace position now described in airline passenger safety cards.

Charitable donations for the research were provided by a number of organisations (listed in Appendix 1), in addition to two grants from the Medical Research Council and a number of contracts between the CAA, the RAF Institute of Aviation Medicine, and the engineering firm Hawtal Whiting (previously HW Structures).

Appendix 2 lists the timetable of the activities surrounding the NLDB group and Appendix 3 is a bibliography of those publications produced by members of the NLDB study group or in association with the study group. We remain indebted to all those who helped us complete the research programme.

Appendix 1—Donations to the NLDB study group

Donations were received from:

AO Foundation, Switzerland
Barclays Bank PLC
Bonfab, Nottingham
British Airways
British Midlands Airways Ltd
CSM Systems, Nottingham
Howmedica (UK)
Leicester Area Health Authority
M1 Kegworth Air Disaster Appeal
Northern Ireland Office
Nottingham District Health Authority
Nottingham University Trust Fund

Private Patients Plan
Rainbow Ball
Special Trustees for Nottingham University Hospital
St John Ambulance Association, Derby
Straumann (GB), Welwyn Garden City
Tandon (UK)
Thackray Orthopaedic, Leeds
The Medical Research Council, UK
The Civil Aviation Authority

We sincerely thank all those who contributed and made the research work possible.

Appendix 2—Timetable of the NLDB study group

8.1.89	2025 Kegworth aircraft accident
9.1.89	0300 Research project conceived
10.1.89	Mr Brian Holdsworth suggested photography of soft tissue injuries
11.1.89	Royal visit by Prince Charles Photographs of soft tissue injuries
14.1.89	First meeting of the Nottingham, Leicester, Derby (NLD) study group
25.1.89	Second meeting of the NLD study group
28.1.89	Third meeting of the NLD study group
8.2.89	Professor Wallace, John Rowles and George Kirsh visit the Air Accident Investigation Branch (AAIB) Headquarters at Farnborough

22.4.89	NLD becomes NLDB study group (to include Belfast) Fourth meeting of the NLDB study group
17.6.89	Fifth meeting of the NLDB study group
4.7.89	Professor Wallace meets the Civil Aviation Authority (CAA) at Gatwick CAA funding supported for the NLDB group to commission computer simulation research
17–19.7.89	NLDB group members visited Farnborough and analysed structural damage to the plane
19.8.89	Sixth meeting of the NLDB study group
14.10.89	Seventh meeting of the NLDB study group
25.11.89	Eighth meeting of the NLDB study group held at HW Structures Ltd, Leamington Spa, to view computer simulation
3.2.90	Ninth meeting of the NLDB study group
6.6.90	Tenth meeting of the NLDB study group
19.9.90	Presentation of some of the NLDB findings to a European Cabin Safety Conference run by the CAA at Gatwick
15.10.90	Release of the NLDB report Release of the AAIB report
15.11.90	BBC documentary *Midlands Report*
8.1.91	Second anniversary of the M1 Kegworth aircraft accident, and "The M1 Kegworth air accident" meeting on "Engineering and medical aspects of survibability" at the Institution of Mechanical Engineers, London
Feb 1992	Appointment of Clinical Research Fellow Mr Peter Brownson to the NLDB study group for phase 2 of the studies—further biomechanical evaluation of the crash brace position used on passenger aircraft
May to Sept 1992	Impact testing at RAF Institution for Aviation Medicine, Farnborough. This work done in conjunction with Hawtal Whiting, Leamington Spa, who used computer simulation techniques to further investigate the crash brace position
13.10.92	Air operators committee, Gatwick, meeting Results of impact testing and computer simulation discussed. Decision made to proceed to further investigation of the crash brace position
Apr 92	Presentation to NATO Advisory Group for Aerospace Research and Development in Turkey (AGARD)
Apr 92	First repot on "Brace position study—impact testing" (Mr JM Rowles) submitted to the CAA
May 92	Second report on "Brace position study—correlation study between impact testing and computer simulation" (Hawtal Whiting) submitted to the CAA

May 93	Third report on "Brace position study No 2—impact testing" (Mr P Brownson) submitted to the CAA
Jul 93	Professor Wallace, Dr Anton, Mr Brownson, Mr Haidar, and Mr Rock meet with the CAA to discuss the findings from phase 2 of the studies
Aug 93	Draft notice to air operators prepared to advise of new standardised brace position
Oct 93	Notice to air operators circulated advising that all safety cards should have the new "brace for impact" position illustrated by April 1994
Nov 93	Fourth report on "Brace position study Phase 2—correlation between impact testing and computer simulation" (Hawtal Whiting) submitted to CAA
Dec 93	"Advances in Passenger Safety" Meeting, Holme Pierrepont, Nottingham
Jan 94	Fifth report on "Brace position—spine model development and analysis" (Hawtal Whiting and P Brownson) sumbitted to CAA
Feb 94	Research on the brace position presented to the US Federal Aviation Authority (FAA)
Apr 94	All UK air operators have brace position on Safety Cards

Appendix 3—Publications produced by members of the NLDB study group or in association with the study group

Wallace WA. Personal view—the M1 plane crash: the first twenty-four hours. *BMJ* 1989; **298**: 330–1.

Kirsh G, Learmonth DJA, Martindale JP and the NLDB study group. The Nottingham, Leicester, Derby Aircraft Accident Study: a preliminary report three weeks after the accident. *BMJ* 1989; **298**: 503–5.

Staff of the Accident and Emergency Departments of Derbyshire Royal Infirmary, Leicester Royal Infirmary and Queen's Medical Centre, Nottingham. Coping with the early stages of the M1 disaster: at the scene and on arrival at hospital. *BMJ* 1989; **298**: 651–4.

Costley JA. *Aircraft accident BD092—M1 motorway/East Midlands Airport—Sunday 8th January 1989*. Sheffield: Trent Regional Health Authority; 1989. (The Report of the Trent Regional Health Authority: Emergency Planning JAC/C17/24.)

Colton CL. The night of miracles. *Fragments* 1989; **8**: 1–5.

Martindale JP. Response to the M1 aircrash. *BMA Newsletter* Mar 1989: 20.

Rowles JM. Three cities combine to analyse M1 crash injuries. *Univ Nottingham Newsletter* Mar 1989: 1.

Harris T. Kegworth: an ICU experience. *Intens Care Nursing* 1989; **5**: 129–33.

Rowles JM and NLDB study group. The injury severity score as a predictor of hospital stay. *Health Service J* 7 June 1990: 848–9.

Busuttil A, Jones JSP. *Deaths in major disasters—the pathologist's role*. London: Royal College of Pathologists; July 1990.

Morgan WE, Salama FD, Beggs FD, Firmin RK, Rowles JM and the NLDB Study Group. Thoracic injuries sustained by the survivors of the M1 (Kegworth) aircraft accident. *Eur Cardiothorac Surg* 1990; **4**: 417–20.

Rowles JM, Robertson CS, Roberts SNJ and the NLDB study group. General surgical injuries in the survivors of the M1 Kegworth air crash. *Ann R Coll Surg* 1990; **72**: 378–81.

The NLDB study group. *NLDB report on the M1 aircraft accident.* Nottingham: University of Nottingham; 1990.

HW Structures and the NLDB study group. *Occupant modelling in aircraft crash conditions.* Gatwick: Civil Aviation Authority, 1990. (CAA Paper 90012.)

McConachie NS, Wilson FMA, Preston BJ, *et al.* The impact of the M1 aircrash on the radiological services at Queen's Medical Centre, Nottingham. *Clin Radiol* 1990; **42**: 317–20.

White BD, Rowles JM, Mumford C, Firth JL and the NLDB study group. A clinical survey of head injuries sustained in the M1 Boeing 737 disaster: recommendations to improve air crash survival. *Br J Neurosurg* 1990; **4**: 503–10.

Wallace WA. The conception of the Nottingham, Leicester, Derby, Belfast (NLDB) study group. In: *The M1 Kegworth air accident—engineering and medical aspects of survivability.* London: Institution of Mechanical Engineers; 1991: 1–5.

Allen MJ. A description of the accident scene. In: *The M1 Kegworth air accident—engineering and medical aspects of survibability:* London: Institution of Mechanical Engineers; 1991: 31–3.

Rowles JM, Learmonth DJA, Martindale JP. The injuries sustained by the survivors. In: *The M1 Kegworth air accident—engineering and medical aspects of survivability.* London: Institution of Mechanical Engineers; 1991: 35–46.

Bouch C. Injuries sustained by the non-survivors. In: *The M1 Kegworth air accident—engineering and medical aspects of survivability.* London: Institution of Mechanical Engineers; 1991: 49.

Kalyan HK, Colton CL, Webb JK. Biomechanics of external fixation. In: *The M1 Kegworth air accident—engineering and medical aspects of survivability.* London: Institution of Mechanical Engineers; 1991: 51–61.

Kalyan HK, Webb JK, Colton CL. Biomechanics of spinal fixation. In: *The M1 Kegworth air accident—engineering and medical aspects of survivability.* London: Institution of Mechanical Engineers; 1991: 63–73.

Haidar R. The use of computer simulation to determine the injury mechanisms of the Kegworth air crash. In: *The M1 Kegworth air accident—engineering and medical aspects of survivability.* London: Institution of Mechanical Engineers; 1991: 75–82.

Anton DJ. The role of crash simulation impact testing. In: *The M1 Kegworth air accident—engineering and medical aspects of survivability.* London: Institution of Mechanical Engineers; 1991: 85–7.

White BD, Rowles JM, Mumford CJ, Firth JL. Head injuries in the M1 Boeing 737 disaster—suggestions to improve crash survival. In: *The M1 Kegworth air accident—engineering and medical aspects of survivability.* London: Institution of Mechanical Engineers; 1991: 89–94.

Hall DJ, Rowles JM, Webb JK. Spinal injuries from the M1 air crash. In: *The M1 Kegworth air accident—engineering and medical aspects of survivability.* London: Institution of Mechanical Engineers; 1991: 97–102.

Rock NIC. Injury prevention through occupant analysis of the Kegworth air crash. In: *The M1 Kegworth air accident—engineering and medical aspects of survivability.* London: Institution of Mechanical Engineers; 1991: 105–15.

NLDB study group. The findings and recommendations of the NLDB Study Group. In: *The M1 Kegworth air accident—engineering and medical aspects of survivability.* London: Institution of Mechanical Engineers; 1991: 117–33.

Kalyan HK. The M1 Kegworth air accident: engineering and medical aspects of survivability. *Biomed Eng News* April 1991: 1–2.

Wallace WA, Rowles JM, Haidar R and the NLDB study group. Computer simulation of impact and correlation with bodily injuries. *Proceedings of the European Cabin Safety Conference 1990.* London: Civil Aviation Authority; 1991: 211–24.

Learmonth DJA, Martindale JP, Rowles JM, Tait GR, Kirsh G and the NLDB study group. Initial management of open fractures sustained in the M1 aircraft disaster. *Injury* 1991; **22**: 207–11.

Fulford P. Meeting report—an aircraft accident: how to survive. Symposium at the Institution of Mechanical Engineers, London, 8 January 1991. *J Bone Joint Surg* 1991; **73B**: 694–5.

Rowles JM, Learmonth DJA, Tait GR, Macey AC and the NLDB study group. Survivors of the M1 air crash: outcome of injuries after one year. *Injury* 1991; **22**: 362–4.

HW Structures. *Report No 5422A.) Aircraft crash victim simulation.* Submitted to the Civil Aviation Authority, Gatwick; Dec 1991.

Tait GR, Rowles JM, Kirsh G, Martindale JP, Learmonth DJA and the NLDB study group. Delayed diagnosis of injuries from the M1 aircraft accident. *Injury* 1991; **22**: 475–8.

Rowles JM, Kirsh G. The management of major disasters. *Recent Adv Orthopaed* 1992; **6**: 133–43.

Rowles JM, Wallace WA, Anton DJ. Can injury scoring techniques provide additional information for crash investigators? *Agard Conference Proceedings 532—Aircraft Accidents: Trends in Aerospace Medical Investigation Techniques.* 12.1–12.0.

Rowles JM, Brownson P, Wallace WA, Anton DJ. Is axial loading a primary mechanism of injury to the lower limb in an impact aircraft accident? *Agard Conference Proceedings 532— Aircraft Accidents: Trends in Aerospace Medical Investigation Techniques.* 1992; 13.1–13.8.

Rowles JM, Kirsh G, Macey AC and the NLDB study group. The use of injury severity scoring in the evaluation of the Kegworth M1 aircrash. *J Trauma* 1992; **32**: 441–7.

Rowles JM. Impact biomechanics of the pelvis and lower limbs in occupants involved in an impact air crash. Doctor of Medicine Thesis, University of Nottingham.

White BD, Firth JL, Rowles JM. The effects of structural failure on injuries sustained in the M1 Boeing 737 disaster—January 1989. *Aviat Space Environ Med* 1993; **64**: 95–102.

White BD, Firth JL, Rowles JM and the NLDB study group. The effect of brace position on injuries sustained in the M1 Boeing 737/400 disaster, January 1989. *Aviat Space Environ Med* 1993; **64**: 103–9.

Brownson P. *Report No 1: brace position study—impact testing.* Civil Aviation Authority, Gatwick; May 1993.

HW Structures. *Report 5483. Report No 2: brace position study—correlation study between impact testing and computer simulation.* Civil Aviation Authority, Gatwick; May 1993.

Brownson P, HW Structures. *Report No 3: brace position study—spine model development and analysis.* Civil Aviation Authority, Gatwick; Aug 1993.

Brownson P. The brace position for passenger aircraft—a biomechanical evaluation. Doctor of Medicine thesis, submitted to University of Nottingham.

Brownson P. A modified crash brace position for aircraft passengers. In: *Proceedings of the International Aircraft and Cabin Safety Symposium,* Long Beach, California, February 1994.

11

Managing people's social and psychological needs after a disaster—experiences from Belfast and the M1 plane crash

MARION GIBSON

The acute disastrous circumstances of major catastrophes represent much of our struggle to deal with the stresses of existence. As such, they symbolize and condense many factors important to understanding human behaviour and alleviating human suffering. The death and devastation of disaster represents the worst of human fears.

Beverley Raphael[1]

Introduction

This chapter deals with the social and psychological needs of people following a disaster. These needs must be recognised by all personnel involved, and provision of support for all people involved in a disaster should be included in disaster plans. Experience from disasters over the last decade has led to a growing body of knowledge on this subject. Post-traumatic stress reactions, which were first identified in the victims of the holocaust, the survivors of concentration camps, and war veterans, can be used to understand the reactions of those affected by other types of disaster. A greater awareness and understanding of such needs has not always been matched by an enthusiasm to plan for an appropriate network of "helpers" trained to respond in the event of a disaster. "Helpers" can include friends, family members, professional groups, or members of voluntary organisations. Different stages in the reaction of those involved will require the support of different helpers. The generic term "Helper", used in this chapter, does not diminish the role of the professional in the tasks outlined but is used to promote a greater understanding of the psychological and social needs of people who have sustained a trauma in their lives.

This chapter draws on relevant theory and my professional experience as a social worker involved with the victims of trauma and as the manager of a crisis counselling team established within a community unit in Belfast. Following the M1 disaster in 1989 I was one of the two social workers sent from Northern Ireland to East Midlands to work with social work colleagues in Derby, Nottingham, and Leicester to help with the support given to the bereaved, the injured, and their relatives, 70% of whom originated from Northern Ireland. I believe that we must learn from the experiences we have had to enhance any future response we will make. Experiences that may appear devastating and overwhelming at the time can provide opportunities in the planning and organisation for future disasters. I pay tribute to the many victims who have allowed me to share in their struggle to become survivors.

Organisations that have plans for their response to a disaster or a traumatic incident usually include in these plans arrangement for the evacuation of staff and mechanisms for contacting the emergency services. In addition, it is important for commercial companies to include plans for limitation of damage to their business and arrangements for continuing with their normal work as soon as possible. These factors are actually some of the most important aspects required for an organisation or community to achieve speedy recovery following such an event. Emergency planning may be required for legal reasons, as with airports, or it may be seen as a desirable precaution to take, "just in case". Plans are made with varying levels of commitment, as they plan for incidents which it is hoped will never happen.

In many such plans, provision for the psychological care of those who may be involved with the disaster may be absent or, more often, is given a low priority. Crashed aircraft are disposable, bombed buildings can be rebuilt, and burned out football stadia can be reconstructed. These results of disaster are visible, but the psychological trauma and effect on peoples' lives is less visible and may impede their normal functioning for a long period of time.

Loss is an inescapable result of disaster. There may be loss of life or there may be injuries that result in the loss of personal life plans. The loss of buildings may mean the loss of jobs, and this can disrupt a sense of community. Loss of homes can lead to a crisis of identity, as cherished photographs and irreplaceable memorabilia are destroyed. When older people have to move from their homes, they can lose their links with places where family history was made. They may experience grave difficulties in establishing attachments in a new area. Disasters can cause people to lose a sense of security in normal things. A city shopping area in Warrington, a place for a pleasant Saturday outing, was turned in to a place of terror when a bomb exploded in March 1993, claiming the lives of two young boys and injury to 55 passers-by. People can lose hope for the future and become depressed. Some question their religious faith, while for others such faith can provide the way of making some sense out of the pain caused by such senseless happenings.

Factors that determine social and psychological outcome

The people affected by a disaster or other traumatic event may be divided in to three categories:

- The bereaved

- The injured and their families

- Others traumatised by the event. These may include members of the emergency services, bystanders, those who could have been involved if circumstances had been different, those who have experienced a similar trauma in the past. Also, helpers themselves may be affected by their involvement.

To consider how the psychological needs of these different groups may be met it is necessary to consider what are the elements in any incident which will affect the outcome. All incidents are unique, and experience has shown that there are patterns in the psychological reactions of those affected. These reactions may vary in relation to the type of incident and in relation to the period of time that has elapsed since the incident.

Type of disaster

The grid shown in figure 11.1 can be used by those who have to plan provision for the psychological needs of those affected. The grid identifies some of the main variables that are common to all incidents, and yet consideration of these variables can determine elements that contribute to the uniqueness of a single event.

Why did it happen?

The perceived cause of an incident can have a significant effect on how the categories of people listed above will react. The classical division of man-made or natural disasters can provide a valuable starting point for causal analysis. If the perceived cause of the disaster is the weather, a failure of a harvest, or an earthquake, then God or the elements themselves can be

	Natural			Man-made		
Personal						
Local	Small	Medium	Large	Small	Medium	Large
National						
International						

Figure 11.1—Elements of disasters. From Gibson[6] with permission.

blamed. Early civilisations would have sought protection against such happenings through rituals which appeased the "mighty forces".

Following natural disasters the loss experienced can result in great feelings of helplessness. Television coverage of a major earthquake, such as that in Armenia in 1988, shows many people standing around shocked and apparently frozen into a state of inactivity in the face of such overwhelming devastation. Psychological support to such victims must recognise this aspect of their reaction. Anger against the cause of a natural disaster is more generalised than the anger generated by a man-made disaster, in which a person or an organisational system can be blamed.

Following a disaster, people look for who is to blame in their search for an answer to the question "Why?". The media can quickly influence such perception by speculation even before the full impact of the disaster has been assessed. Such debate, often with diagrams and photographs, can have a powerful influence on the reactions of those affected. Following the M1 aircrash, pilot error, engine failure, and aircraft design were widely debated as possible causes. While such debates are necessary for future air safety and are vital issues with respect to compensation, they can cause additional stress for those who are trying to make sense of and come to terms with the loss of a loved one. Following an act of terrorism the organisation that carried out the act may publicly claim its responsibility as a method of advancing its cause—hollow words to those whose homes or businesses have been devastated or who have had to identify mutilated bodies. Anger in these cases has a focus that is accessible, punishable, and available for retaliation. After such events, however, many immediate

135

family members call for no retaliation. Their pain is so great that they do not want any other family to have to undergo a similar experience. In many cases, the shared pain of loss transcends divisions in community or ideologies.

Those providing psychological support to people affected by man-made disasters must be sensitive to possible reactions to the causal agents. If an organisation is perceived to have been negligent it may affect the way in which practical help from them is received. Some may view it as an admission of guilt, demand more help as a right, or refuse such help as totally inadequate "blood money" in relation to the loss being experienced. These reactions occurred to a minor extent after the M1 plane crash, when British Midland ground staff did so much to help the hospitals and relatives of those injured.

Natural and man-made factors can both be present in some disasters. The collapse of buildings following an earthquake can be viewed as the result of natural forces, but illegal cost cutting building practices can also be a significant cause in the total loss incurred.

Where did it happen?

Aspects of the geographical location of an incident also need to be considered. Transport disasters may happen in a location far removed from the homes of those most affected. Help will be needed at the location of the accident but longer term help may be needed in the home towns of those affected. This can have major implications in terms of resource allocation in areas not seen to be the site of the incident. Those who were the recipients of help at the site may have difficulty in accepting help from those who were not involved at the time of crisis. These features were experienced by the helping agencies in Northern Ireland following the M1 aircrash. Thus the local, national, or international nature of the disaster is a significant determinant in the type of response that will be required. Personal disaster is added to this grid as a reminder to those who are involved in the provision of psychological support that the needs of these victims are equally important: family members bereaved through a road traffic accident, a single murder, or an industrial accident will have similar reactions to those affected by a larger incident but may receive less attention from helping agencies or society.

In 1987, the Hungerford shootings and the bomb explosion at the Remembrance Day service in Enniskillen were local incidents. These local communities were deeply affected. Local people were involved in the rescue and had to deal with victims they had known as neighbours and friends. Community anger had to be coped with, as the communities themselves have had to recover on many levels while still finding that the very names of their towns remain associated with these tragic events.

Local disasters, such as that at the Hillsborough football stadium, can be considered as a national disaster, when a wider community is affected and the circumstances could be replicated nationwide. The cause of such incidents and the rescue and support services available may receive nationwide media attention and those affected may receive practical support in the form of a disaster fund. Media coverage may result in positive help in terms of financial support but it can also bring the negative effects of national voyeurism through media attention on the injured or the bereaved, not only at the time of the incident but at the inquest, anniversary, or subsequent court proceedings.

When Pan-Am flight 109 exploded over Lockerbie on 21 December 1988, killing all 270 on board and 11 local residents, the implications of such an international disaster became apparent. Thirty three different nationalities were involved and the multiplicity of cultural aspects of grieving, as well as different legal systems, had to be sensitively accommodated.

How many people were involved?

The size of an incident is also an important aspect in the planning of any response. The number of those directly involved must be seen as a starting point only. The number of people affected by any disaster can be compared to the effect of dropping a pebble into a still pond of water. The ripples created in the water spread out in rings from the centre. The effect of a disaster on people can also spread far beyond its epicentre.

Stages of recovery

The needs of those affected also vary in terms of time from incident. Any consideration of such needs must be based on the up to date information available from research and experience. The identification of the possible stages in human reactions for so many different groups of people can only be carried out in general terms. Just as each disaster has elements that make it unique, people are also unique and their reactions are affected by past experiences, the support they receive, and how they view their own world in the light of the trauma to which they have been subjected. Figure 11.2 shows a time continuum as a guide for those who have to manage any response. The stages are suggested as a general guide to some of the reactions which may be observed. These stages are not exclusive and they may not be experienced in a sequential way. A late crisis time, such as giving evidence at an inquiry, can make the person feel that any progress they have made has been destroyed and that they are forced back to a more painful and earlier reaction.

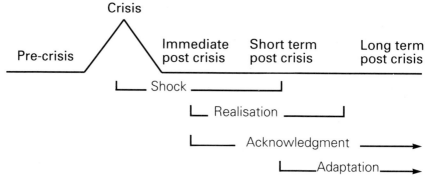

Figure 11.2—The time continuum of psychological rehabilitation. From Gibson[6] with permission.

It should be noted that the pre-impact stage is significant when providing support to any of the categories of those affected. Pre-crisis circumstances may shape an individual's reactions in the post-crisis period. The diagrammatic representation in figure 11.2 can be used in relation to the bereaved, the injured, and their relatives or others traumatised by the event.

Pre-crisis stage

Warnings may have been given of impending disaster. How people react at this stage may have a significant bearing on how they react later. Lack of such warnings or failure to take action that might have avoided the disaster can provide a focus for subsequent anger and recrimination. Following the M1 disaster, work with one bereaved family included help to come to terms with the fact that, due to their late arrival at the departure gate, their relatives missed the flight on which they were booked and were given seats on the flight that crashed. Relationships before the disaster can also have an influence on later reactions. Much distress can be caused by an unsaid farewell or unresolved family friction. A mother can feel guilty that her action in sending her children to the shops contributed to the fact that they were involved in a major road traffic accident. Pre-crisis events can form the basis for the "if only . . ." syndrome that occurs after the event. Others traumatised by the event may be those who are regular users of an ill-fated ferry or train but were not travelling when the disaster happened.

Crisis stage

The physical need for rescue and damage limitation are paramount at this stage. It is important to remember that all emergency services personnel are involved in the psychological management of an individual at the very beginning of the recovery process. The way that they talk to victims or organise the rescue procedures can influence the way in which a victim will react to future offers of help. Methods of rescue that preserve the dignity of those being rescued or the handling of bodies can have a significant influence on the psychological recovery process for all involved.

Immediate post-crisis stage

Chaos may exist at this stage. There may be lack of information on how many people have been injured or killed. Shock dominates the reactions of those directly affected and of their relatives. Shock can mean that there is a psychological numbness, an inability to concentrate or to comprehend information. To provide support to relatives at this stage will require a team who can be proactive in their approach but do not overwhelm highly vulnerable people. At this stage those involved with the victims may lack information on whether their relative is alive or dead. Support at this stage has been described as psychological first aid, with a need to address practical issues. Their needs can be remembered under the eight "T's": tears, tissues, talk, tea, time, telephones, toilets, transport. The provision of a helpline, with trained personnel to deal with the calls, can be of vital importance at this stage. The use made of this helpline will subsequently change over time. Initially it will be used to gain information and to receive offers of help. Later it will be used to access counselling support.

People need to have confidence that those who are available to help them are organised. Whitham[2] details how a collaborative and structured approach by the social workers, chaplains, nurses, and British Midland Airlines staff, in the Queen's Medical Centre, Nottingham, was appreciated by the relatives of those injured in the M1 crash. Relatives recall how they felt reassured as each family group was allocated a helper to accompany them to the first, emotional meeting with their family member in the wards. This helper had been briefed on the current medical condition and was able to prepare the relatives as to what to expect of the visual condition of the patient. After a brief meeting the relatives were escorted to a ward that had been cleared for their use as a "safe space", where they could deal with their emotional reactions.

When planning to respond at this stage it is necessary to have devised, with all agencies, a protocol that provides adequate and personalised help to each family group. It is necessary, in the pre-crisis stage, to plan for a method of call out. Pre-planning can enable possible organisational resources, both statutory and voluntary, to be assessed in terms of volume and specialism. The aim should be to provide a response that is coordinated and avoids duplication. Initial help should be proactive but people must still have the opportunity to reject help at any stage. There should be a preplanned method of recording those with whom contact has been made. The confidentiality of such information should be protected and shared with other agencies only on a pre-agreed basis.

Short term post-crisis stage

Information should be more available at this stage. Feelings of shock can give way to the pain of harsh reality. The identification of bodies may have to be undertaken. Support to the bereaved at this stage has been found to be particularly helpful. In contrast, bodies may not be recoverable, as was the case following the Piper Alpha oil rig disaster in 1988. This can be extremely distressing for relatives and can have a major effect on their grieving process.

The use of information leaflets that identify where help is available and the range of possible feelings that may be experienced can be appropriate at this stage. Following the M1 aircrash visits to the site of the disaster were organised for those bereaved or injured who wanted to make such a pilgrimage. Such visits have been found to help both relatives and survivors in many recent disasters. The bereaved may use the visit to aid their process of understanding as they struggle to face the reality of their loss. The use of floral tributes can help people to express emotions and begin the grieving process. Such visits must be efficiently and sensitively organised, with a due sense of reverence and with privacy from the media. Differing cultural needs must be respected in the funeral rituals that have to be arranged.

Those who have been injured may experience an initial feeling of euphoria at their survival. These feelings can give way to feelings of guilt that they survived when others perished. The numbness of initial shock gives way to the reality of their own injuries and how their future lives may be affected. The initial interest by the media may lessen and the support of friends and relatives may diminish quite quickly after the event. Those affected may experience sleep problems, intrusive dreams about the incident, feelings of anger at their inability to change the situation, and the "if only . . ." syndrome. Much has been written on the effects of post-traumatic stress disorder (PTSD). For some people it is a reality and requires skilled psychiatric help. For the vast majority of people, however, their reaction is one classed as post-traumatic stress reaction (PSTR). Symptoms may be similar those experienced in PTSD but are less intense and of shorter duration. Leaflets or helpers, advising people that their feelings are within the "normal" range of reaction to an "abnormal" situation, are beneficial at this stage. Many suffer great fear that they are losing their sanity and fail to share their feelings in case others will confirm their worst fears. In addition to the natural network of family, friends, doctors, and clergy, access to support from voluntary or statutory agencies may be especially helpful at this stage. This is important because the person most directly affected can still feel alone and overwhelmed by his or her emotions, when friends or relatives may be ready to get back to normal activity.

Long term post-crisis stage

Realisation is replaced by an acknowledgment of the change that the crisis has brought to a person, a family, or a community. Family anniversaries have to be lived through without the loved one. Future life plans may have had to be altered because of injuries. Legal proceedings associated with the disaster will have to be coped with.

Adaptation can be described as the end of the recovery process and the beginning of living life in a way that acknowledges the past and integrates the changes in a way that causes less pain. Coping with the loss of a person is recognised as a grieving process, but there can also be loss through injury: before being able to adapt to the person he or she has become, the injured person may have to grieve for the person he or she once was. Recovery from loss is like the healing of a scar. The scar remains but as it heals it opens less easily and causes less pain.

To manage a longer term response, to the needs of those affected, it is necessary to ensure that they are advised where they can get access to help when they feel it is necessary. Helping agencies should be able to relate to the incident, and continuity of helper is most desirable.

Helpers' needs

The most important resource of any organisation is its staff, yet few plans deal adequately with this aspect of a disaster.

Support to staff should be included as a significant part of all plans if total recovery is to be achieved. No organisation can recover unless its "people" are supported in such a way that they too can achieve damage limitation in their personal lives. Helpers will cope if they feel that the organisation cares for them as people who may experience feelings that mirror those of the bereaved or injured. All involved have to live the rest of their lives with the psychological experience of the incident integrated in to their personality in such a way that it does not make them emotionally disabled in their personal or professional life.

Helpers can also experience the cumulative effect of trauma work even when such work is part of their normal role. This phenomenon is often found when working with nursing staff in areas such as accident and emergency departments. Traumatic events are coped with, but there can be a build up of stress which manifests itself only after many incidents. The incident that triggers the reaction may in itself be relatively minor but some element of the incident may have particular personal meaning for the staff member involved.

Training for helpers in the pre-crisis stage can minimise the initial feelings of being de-skilled and inadequate when confronted with a disaster. This training needs to be skill based to ensure that helpers can fulfil their role, but it should also include awareness training on the management of the stress they may experience. Helpers can experience abnormal levels of energy, which enables them to work extra hours at an intense level. They can experience feelings of attachment to the people affected and this can lead to overinvolvement with "their" victims in "their" disaster. These feelings can create problems that lead to physical and emotional exhaustion. The helpers can, in these circumstances, become dysfunctional in their response and in dealing with the very people they are trying to help. The effects of such stress can cause friction in the workplace or in personal relationships. Helpers may have sleep problems and experience an inability to distance themselves from the event when they return to normal working practices. Return to work may bring changes in their motivation as a result of their ability to value less intense work patterns. Some find that they increase their alcohol or nicotine intake, experience changes in their eating patterns, and increasingly rely on drug therapy. Unresolved emotional reactions can cause physical or mental ill health, which results in absenteeism.

If an organisation invests resources in the training of helpers, it makes good commercial sense to minimise the effects of the stress they may experience. Critical incident stress debriefing should be carried out as soon as possible after the experience. It is most beneficial when a period of work has ended and helpers are leaving the scene of the disaster. This enables the helpers to share experiences and to discuss their feelings with those who have fulfilled a common task. Further group or individual sessions may be necessary. Access to a confidential counselling service, beyond the organisational structure, should also be considered as an option.

A study by Alexander and Wells,[3] with the Grampian police involved in the handling of bodies after the Piper Alpha oil rig disaster, produced a number of important findings that confirmed the value of good organisational and managerial practices in combating the potentially adverse reactions to harrowing and distressing duties. Such findings suggest that support to staff should not be something designed for disaster situations only but should be an integral part of good everyday management practice.

Not all the effects on helpers, or indeed organisations, are negative. Helpers may develop new skills that can enrich their future practice. As a result of the expertise gained at the time of a major incident, organisations may establish counselling services to help people who have had to cope with personal disasters. On a personal level, helpers may re-evaluate their life goals and consider their own mortality, having glimpsed death and destruction.

Children's needs

Following disasters the needs of children are often underestimated or neglected. Adults, struggling to come to terms with effects of trauma, may be unable to give their usual attention to children. Children can only comprehend the long term effects of the disaster at their own level of experience and understanding. Care must be taken to explain bereavement or the implications of injury in terms that they understand. Truthful explanations are necessary, even if they are painful to the care giver. Questions from the child will seem searching and difficult to answer. Children who have to make sense of their changed world will need the reassurance that there will be someone who will continue to love them and who will try to minimize the effects of the changes. Schools have a very significant role to play in these circumstances. Teachers should be trained in responding to the needs of the traumatised child in the classroom environment.

Planning

> A major disaster is the classical "ambush" situation; we plan, prepare, and exercise with great care and attention to detail and "out of the blue" the situation that presents itself is almost always a total surprise which does not quite "fit" the exercise pattern . . .
>
> JA Costley[4]

The dynamics of providing a response to the psychological needs of those people affected by a disaster are multiple and complex. The needs, as detailed earlier, are also variable. Planning must therefore be flexible, adhere closely to normal practice, and use established communication networks. Plans need to be "owned" by those who will have to enact them. This can be achieved by enlisting their help at the design stage and in the updating process. Good practice is the best insurance that any disaster response will be adequate.

The Disasters Working Party report *Disaster—planning for a caring response*[5] highlights the need for a forum at which all agencies and voluntary organisations can meet on a regular basis to share plans and agree procedures that avoid duplication. The report suggests that the director of social services should have this coordinating responsibility. Duplication causes added distress to the people affected, is wasteful in terms of human resources, and can cause destructive competition between helping agencies. Joint training, which raises the awareness of the psychological needs of those people affected, should be encouraged. Lessons learned from one response should be recorded and shared to allow future plans to be refined.

Conclusion

Provision of support for all people involved in a disaster must be integrated into all levels of planning for the response to the aftermath of any disaster. It must be remembered that disasters can affect people of all ages, all ethnic backgrounds, and all social classes. Some people may never have experienced an episode of trauma in their lives before. Some will have past experiences that may reawaken painful memories. Others will have had experiences that have enabled them to develop coping skills that they can utilise in a new situation. Just as disasters are unique, so are the reactions of the people affected by them.

Helpers can become "experts" in responding to perceived needs as defined by theory, but they need to become expert in listening and responding to the needs as defined by those they seek to help. It is a humbling and enriching experience to share the pain and recovery process of another human being. Helpers cannot make the recovery happen, they can only support a person to achieve his or her own recovery.

An elderly survivor of the M1 aircrash, in which his wife died, was present at the unveiling of the memorial stone in the graveyard at Kegworth many months after the crash. He commented to a helper, "Even the weather was right. At the start of the service the black clouds were thick overhead but at the end the sun began to break through." In providing a response to the social and psychological needs of people affected by disasters we cannot take away the black clouds, but we can aim to help make the sun break through more quickly.

Summary

- The psychological needs of people affected by disasters are variable and are influenced by the type of incident, its causes and its location

- The psychological impacts of disaster can be divided into a number of stages before and after the incident: different types of help will be needed in the different stages

- Children have special needs, which should not be overlooked

- Helpers—from professional or voluntary organisations—will benefit from critical incident stress debriefing following an incident. They may also need access to counselling services. Better provision should be made for training them to cope with their own reactions to the psychological impact of their task

- Planning for management of disasters does not always pay sufficient attention to psychological aspects and should be improved

1 Raphael B. *When disaster strikes*. Hutchinson; 1986: 4.
2 Whitham D, Newburn T. *Coping with tragedy*. Nottingham: Nottingham County Council, National Institute for Social Work; 1992.
3 Alexander DA, Wells A. Reactions of police officers to body-handling after a major disaster; before and after comparison. *Br J Psychiatry* 1991; **159**: 547–55.
4 Trent Regional Health Authority. *Report on the M1 Aircraft Disaster*. Sheffield: Trent Regional Health Authority; 1989.
5 Disasters Working Party. *Disaster—planning for a caring response*. London: HMSO; 1991.
6 Gibson M. *Order from chaos—responding to traumatic events*. Birmingham: Venture Press; 1991.

12

Planning medical services for air disasters

TERENCE E MARTIN

Introduction

In the past decade, emergency services in the United Kingdom have dealt with over 20 major disasters. These include the Bradford and King's Cross fires, gas explosions in Putney and Edinburgh, the Clapham, Cannon Street, and Purley rail crashes, the Manchester, Lockerbie, and Kegworth aircraft incidents, the Piper Alpha and Ocean Odyssey oil rig fires, the sinkings of the *Herald of Free Enterprise* and the *Marchioness*, the Hillsborough stadium tragedy, and the Hungerford shooting incident. Over and above these large scale tragedies, there have been civil riots, terrorist bomb explosions, hurricane force gales, and a number of major accidents on the motorways and in the waters surrounding the UK.

Overseas, major disasters have included the earthquakes in Turkey, Iraq, Japan, Mexico, Armenia, China, San Francisco, and Australia; hurricanes in the Caribbean (Gilbert), Nicaragua (Miriam), and Florida (Andrew); floods in the American mid-west, Bangladesh, the Sudan, and Rio de Janeiro; the Heysel stadium disaster; toxic gas clouds in Cameroon; the sinking of cruise ships in the Aegean and in the Baltic; and the explosions at Chernobyl, in the Siberian Tundra, and in Addis Ababa. Aircrashes have occurred in western Germany (the Ramstein airshow), the USA (Fokker F28 in New York, Tristar and Boeing 727 in Dallas, DC-9 in Denver, MD-80 in Detroit and DC-10 in Sioux City), Hawaii (Aloha Boeing 737), France (Airbus A320s at Habsheim and Strasbourg), the Netherlands (El Al Boeing 747 near Amsterdam), Nepal (Pakistan International Airlines Airbus A300 at Kathmandu), Portugal (Martinair DC-10 at Faro), South Korea (Asiana Airlines Boeing 737), Russia (Korean Air Lines Boeing 747), Thailand (Lauda Air Boeing 767), the mid-Atlantic (Air India Boeing 747), and the Persian Gulf (Iranian Airbus A300). Civil unrest, revolt, and war have also caused enormous strain on the world's medical and emergency resources (Yugoslavia, the Middle East, Somalia, Ethiopia, Afghanistan, Tiananmen Square, Beirut, Panama, Albania, and Romania, to name but a few).

By definition, a disaster exists, at least in the medical sense, when the number of casualties exceeds the capability of the emergency services to manage them. Perhaps, more properly, this mass casualty situation should be called an *uncompensated disaster* when the responding services are overwhelmed. The response of these services and their ability to cope is a function of the size and quality of the resources available. A small number of seriously injured patients might significantly overload a small district general hospital, but will have little consequence in a city with several large facilities. Many authors have attempted to classify disasters according to a number of criteria, such as by the number of casualties, by the cause (that is, natural or artificial), by location (urban or rural), and by the integrity of resources (roads, telephones, hospitals, etc.), which may be intact or disrupted.

A major incident that results in large numbers of casualties and stretches the emergency services to their absolute limit but is within their capabilities to manage is, by convention, called a multicasualty situation. It is, in effect, a compensated disaster. Regardless of these semantics, the same essential planning is needed for any major incident, since ability to cope with the number of casualties will be unknown in the early stages.

The facility to plan for and manage a major incident will depend on many factors, and it should be remembered that the resources and infrastructure possessed by many Third World nations will differ significantly from those of the so-called developed countries. Nevertheless, many of the problems that will be encountered will be much the same, despite the fact that those countries with adequate resources will best be able to compensate.

A significant number of all disasters involve aircraft and, although planning for all incidents must adhere to basic principles, those which involve aircraft have certain specific peculiarities and problems. Areas to be considered include the following.

The falling aircraft, which may land in urban areas (for example, the A10 Thunderbolt in Remscheid), in mountains (for example, the Airbus A320 near Strasbourg and the DC-10 on Mount Erebus), in wooded rural areas (for example, the Airbus A320 at Habsheim), in thick jungle (for example, the Lauda Air Boeing 767 in Thailand), in the sea (for example, the Air India Boeing 747 in mid-Atlantic), and occasionally into dense crowds (for example, the Italian national aerobatic team at Ramstein) (figure 12.1).

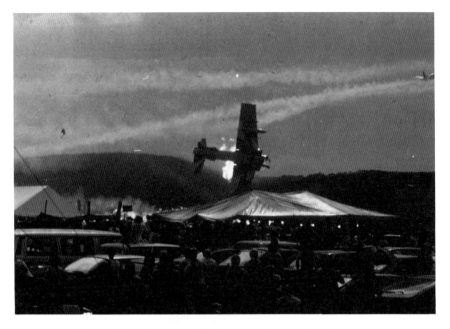

Figure 12.1—Jet aircraft falling into the crowd at Ramstein.

Wreckage may spread over a vast area (as was the case for the Pan-Am Boeing 747 at Lockerbie), making search, rescue, and recovery extremely difficult.

An incident may occur in flight which does not immediately present a problem although there is potential for a catastrophe at any time (such as emergency decompression, hijacking, and cabin fire).

Speed of impact: survival and the risk of injury has been shown to be related to the forces of deceleration on impact. These forces predominantly act in the G_x and G_z axes, but may be rotational when severe disruption of the aircraft occurs.

The capacity to carry large numbers of passengers: the Boeing 747, for example, can carry almost 500 seated passengers. In exceptional circumstances, more may be aboard (as when the Israeli government evacuated thousands of jews from Ethiopia in May 1991, using 747s with the seating removed; up to 1000 refugees were carried in each aircraft). Paradoxically, as newer aircraft become more crashworthy, there is likely to be a higher number of seriously injured survivors and fewer deaths. Obviously, it is the number of seriously and critically injured patients that will burden the emergency and medical services.

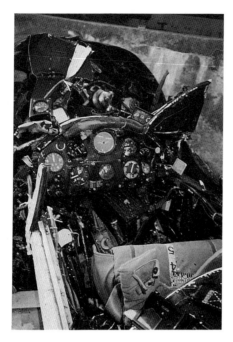

Figure 12.2—Disruption of occupant space after the crash of a light aircraft.

Survivor entrapment: high-speed impacts cause deformity of the aircraft structure with intrusion of flooring and cabin furniture into the vital space around the seat occupant (figure 12.2). The effectiveness of restraint systems is usually compromised and the likelihood of serious injury is vastly increased. Rescue is impeded by the structural disruption, and may be made more difficult by the inversion or rotation of the aircraft cabin into its final resting position. Access to perform lifesaving resuscitation may be limited, especially if the patient is crushed between debris and the bodies of other passengers. Extrication will inevitably be problematic and time consuming, and medical teams working alongside the rescuers must be highly trained and experienced in trauma life support skills. Caution will be needed to avoid further injury to survivors when cutting tools and pneumatic devices are used in the extrication process. Poor handling at this stage can be detrimental to the patient's outcome, especially if airway problems have been experienced, for those in shock and those with spinal damage.

Post-impact fire risk: in a series of 1086 accidents studied between 1960 and 1970, it was shown that the occurrence of fire is associated with an increased mortality rate from 14% to 34%.[1] Likewise, the percentage of serious injuries increased from 3% to 8%. Fire obviously hinders escape, and can be even more catastrophic if it starts whilst the aircraft is in mid-flight.

Hazards to rescuers: the rescuers themselves may be at considerable risk from the dangers of the tangled debris and wreckage and from the threat of fire from ruptured fuel tanks, spillages of oils, hydraulic fluids, and from oxygen sources. The terrain or environmental conditions may also be hazardous, especially since many accidents occur during severe weather. If a conflagration does occur, noxious gases will be produced by the combination of plastics and other materials used in aircraft construction. Hydrogen cyanide and carbon monoxide are probably the most dangerous, and medical teams will need 100% oxygen and specific therapies such as sodium thiosulphate to treat those who collapse.

Multiplicity of interested governments and agencies: confusion may be caused by different national governments and agencies having interests in various aspects of the flight. For instance, the countries of ownership, registration, aircraft manufacture, flight origin, flight destination, location of the crash site, and nationalities of the passengers may all be different.

Risks of aviation accidents

Statistical evidence[1] has shown that the numbers of seriously injured survivors after any aircraft accident is unlikely to exceed 25% of the number of occupants. This may not now be so, especially as new aircraft are designed to meet more stringent crashworthy specifications. The Boeing 737 accident at Kegworth in 1989 resulted in 87 survivors with multiple injuries on an aircraft carrying only 126 occupants.[2]

A study of 473 aircraft accidents between 1977 and 1986 showed that most (68%) occurred in and around airfields—that is, during the take off or approach phases of flight.[3] In 32 of these accidents, injuries were also caused to people on the ground; the largest number being 49.

The problems

In the planning and management of major incidents, it is appropriate to discuss the major recurrent problems that have been clearly identified in recent years. Many are relevant to all disaster scenarios, but particular attention will be paid to the issues that are specific to aviation incidents.

The chaos

All disasters are sudden and unexpected, and their occurrence will bring confusion and chaos. An area which was previously serene and peaceful may be turned into a scene of conflagration, carnage, wreckage, and havoc within seconds. Aircraft accidents may involve overwhelming numbers of casualties who will have suffered a wide range of injuries and who may well be in dispersed groups. In the early minutes there will be no obvious leader and control will be difficult if not impossible. Many people may congregate at the site and it will be vital to identify key personnel from the emergency services. Panic will abound and, during a major incident, one cannot assume that members of the rescue services would be immune from it.

Communications, command, and control

In any disaster, no one will appear to be in overall control during those first vital minutes when decisions need to be made and conveyed to the growing army of helpers. Without effective dissemination of information, leadership is difficult, coordination is impossible, and valuable time is wasted. Communication is vital and there is no place for coded messages. Plain language is essential to avoid confusion. Medical teams need radiotelephone equipment with dedicated frequencies available. Furthermore, if they are to be safe for use around the wreckage, they must be non-spark generating. Alternative methods of communication may also be necessary, such as tannoy, handheld loud hailers, telephone landlines, intercoms, satellite communications, cellular telephones, facsimile, electronic mail, couriers, and messenger runners.

It can not be overemphasised that effective command, control, and coordination depend heavily on efficient communications. Clearly, good communications must exist between the personnel of the rescue and medical services, but there is also a vital need to talk directly to the receiving hospitals in an effort to establish or update information on their capabilities and to convey information on the number of casualties, their injury categories, and an estimate of their times of arrival.

Identification of key personnel

With no obvious leader and so many helpers it is important to identify personnel from the emergency services. If doctors, nurses, and paramedics are indistinguishable from non-trained personnel, instructions given to volunteers and laypeople will go unheeded. It is vitally important that personnel with valuable skills are instantly recognisable by those who need to communicate with them. Similarly, key personnel must be easy to identify. Essentially, these are the incident commanders of the emergency services. Nevertheless, every member of the medical and rescue services should, ideally, have his own personal item of clothing that annotates the wearer's profession or skills, such as a reflective jacket, tabard, brassard, or protective helmet saying "DOCTOR", "NURSE", "PARAMEDIC",

"CHAPLAIN", etc. If all else fails, a simple pin-on badge would help. For military personnel, these items should supplement, not replace, Red Cross armbands.

Medical resources

Personnel

In large incidents it will be essential for a doctor experienced and trained in disaster medicine to take command of the medical services at the site. This doctor will become the medical incident officer (MIO), and will work alongside the ambulance service, giving guidance whenever necessary. The requirements for such an individual are laid out in the DHSS Health Circular HC(90)25,[4] in which it is stated that the MIO should be supplied by a listed hospital or health authority and should not be a membr of a mobile medical team. In reality, he is likely to be on a list of doctors known to the chief ambulance officer, and will be called out by the ambulance service when the extent of the incident becomes known. On arrival, his first duty is to identify himself to the incident officers of the other emergency services[5] and establish the current situation. He should set up his control point in or alongside ambulance control, and then decide on whether a medical/nursing team is required. He must retain an organisational role, and should avoid being drawn into the care of individual patients. Rather, he should delegate, if necessary, by the call up of medical reinforcements.

The MIO must be suitably dressed in protective identifiable clothing and should carry personal communications and some form of identification, such as that provided by the British Association of Immediate Care Schemes (BASICS) (figure 12.3). His personal radio must be compatible with the systems in use by the other emergency services. He must be the communications conduit linking the disaster site, the medical authorities, receiving hospitals, and voluntary agencies.

Once established, there will be a need to decide on the requirement for a casualty clearing station (CCS), so that a suitable balance of holding and evacuation of patients can be achieved (figure 12.4). The MIO will need to ensure that triage is being undertaken and that patients are correctly identified and suitably documented prior to their departure from the site. There may well be a need to arrange for extra medical supplies, fluids, blood products, stretchers, blankets, and so on. If the incident is prolonged, it will also be necessary to ensure food, shelter, water, and latrine facilities for the medical teams will be available. There may even be a need to organise replacement personnel, and the MIO should be alert to the signs of fatigue. In the same light, he would be wise to nominate his own deputy and arrange suitable rest and refreshments after no more than 4 hours on the site.

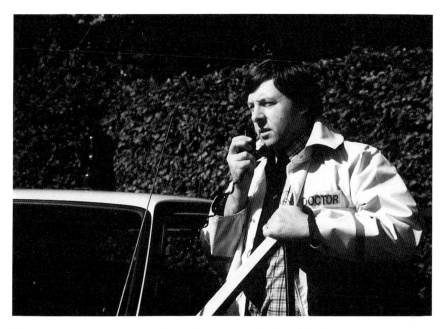

Figure 12.3—The medical incident officer communicating with other emergency services.

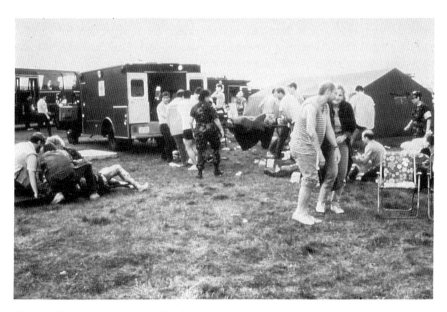

Figure 12.4—One of the collection points for treatment of casualties during the Ramstein air disaster.

Although some authors advocate the importance of dedicated trauma surgical teams, which are moved, intact and with equipment, to the disaster site,[6] this is generally agreed to be useful only when there is likely to be a significant delay in transportation of patients away from the site or when the evacuation chain is long. Such situations are unusual, and it is true to say that hospital staff generally perform better on familiar tasks, with familiar equipment, in a familiar environment, than they do when moved into an alien situation.

Nevertheless, the MIO must decide if or when medical reinforcement will be necessary. Reinforcement might come from nearby NHS hospitals (but not to the detriment of their capabilities if they expect to receive casualties from the incident), military establishments or, alternatively, from voluntary organisations such as BASICS, the Red Cross, and the St John Ambulance Brigade. It is the MIO's responsibility to ensure that all the medical, nursing, and paramedical personnel working under his supervision are logged onto the site, and that they are suitably qualified, dressed, and equipped for the job in hand. He also has the difficult task of trying to integrate the services of these different agencies and volunteers who may well be unfamiliar with each other and even less familiar with the chaos of a major incident.

In consideration of the road congestion that is bound to occur, any medical personnel arriving at the incident in an independent vehicle must be sure to park considerately, so as not to obstruct access to the site. It is worth leaving vehicle keys with the police control centre so that cars can be moved if required. Only one vehicle (marking the control centre) should have an illuminated rotating emergency beacon. All other beacons should be extinguished when vehicles are parked.

Summary of the medical incident officer's role

- Remains an organiser and does not become involved in individual patient care
- Calls up relevant medical personnel and resources and supervises their activities
- Liaises between the site, medical authorities, hospitals, and voluntary organisations
- Organises the casualty clearing station and decides on its function—whether initial treatment followed by rapid evacuation or whether patients are held for later evacuation
- Ensures triage is undertaken
- Decides whether medical reinforcements are needed and which sources to call on, and arranges for replacement personnel if the incident is protracted

---

When all the survivors have been triaged and moved from the immediate area of the wreckage, at least one doctor must be nominated to accompany members of the police force in an effort to identify and certify the dead. Furthermore, there is still a responsibility for the medical services to provide cover for those personnel who must remain at the site and continue their hazardous tasks.

Aid from the military

Aid from the armed forces can provide essential services and important reserves during a major emergency. Guidelines about the assistance that can be requested by local authorities are contained in a pamphlet issued by the United Kingdom Ministry Of Defence.[7]

Ambulance authorities usually develop close ties with military units based within their operational area, and mutual assistance can often be obtained quickly when needed. In addition, Police authorities may request helicopter or fixed wing aircraft support direct from either of the RAF rescue coordination centres—that is, Pitreavie Castle in Edinburgh and Mount Wise at Plymouth (although the latter is due to close in 1994). In addition, RAF mountain rescue teams are available at 1 hour readiness and have the training and expertise to deal with aircraft crash rescue. Requests for other forms of assistance must originate from local authorities themselves, although such requests are usually passed through the police to the district military coordinator.

There are a few tasks that can only be done by the military, such as explosive ordnance disposal. Nevertheless, there is a much larger number of tasks that can perhaps be undertaken more easily by the armed forces than by civilian authorities. These include search and rescue, aerial reconnaissance, aeromedical evacuation, and the provision of specialist signals. Further down the line perhaps, but of equal importance, are those tasks that can easily and quickly be undertaken by the sheer numbers of personnel and ease of availability that only the armed forces can provide. In this context, not only should medical resources be considered but also other supporting assets, such as search/cordon parties, transport, and catering and engineering personnel and equipment.

For civilian authorities, there are many possible advantages to the use of military assets, including the availability of a potentially large pool of personnel, most of whom will be familiar with working in hostile environments. Not only will their individual skills be befitting, but they will be familiar with working in a disciplined manner and will be conversant with communications procedures and a command structure. Many will be used to working long shifts and will not baulk at the prospect of camping out if called upon to do so. Nevertheless, to realise these advantages, there must be an infrastructure already in existence and call outs should be practised whenever possible.

Medical equipment

A dilemma faces the planners—where to place the medical assets? Although it might be considered that some locations may be more prone to the likelihood of an accident (for example, the surrounds of an airport), it is generally impossible to predict where an accident will occur and what might be its effect on surface transport.

Equipment suitable for a mass casualty situation should therefore always be readily available and mobile. Time taken to collect and load such equipment is time wasted. A suitable vehicle or trailer should preferably be permanently loaded and labelled as disaster response medical supplies (DRMS). Obviously, these supplies must be frequently checked and kept up to date. Reserve stocks must also remain easily accessible. As dedicated resources, they should always be tagged ready for rapid augmentation of dwindling supplies. A small number of paramedical personnel should be responsible for updating and packing the supplies so that, in a call out, at least one member of the team is thoroughly familiar with the location and listing of available equipment. The context and compatability of the supplies must be given very careful consideration and in the light of recent experiences, the essential equipment needed should be reviewed frequently.

The DRMS should carry plentiful casualty identification/triage/treatment cards and pencils or chinagraphs. Also, in view of the precautions necessary to prevent the dissemination of HIV virus, the DRMS should contain enough disposable gloves for the entire medical team. Extra gloves will be needed for helpers and volunteers. Consideration must also be given to tentage, generators for light and heating, blankets, stretchers/beds, food, water, and specialised equipment. Close liaison with the other emergency services may be needed to locate all that is required.

Triage

It is difficult to apply the concept of triage in peacetime, since it is unlikely that civilian medical teams will have had the past experience to sort large numbers of seriously and critically injured casualties effectively. Experience during the aftermath of the Ramstein disaster proved that untrained helpers will always try to evacuate those that look worse, often at the expense of more treatable casualties who then suffer the consequences of delayed medical care.[8] Medical teams may be equally reluctant to forsake the moribund in favour of seriously injured survivors who may well be

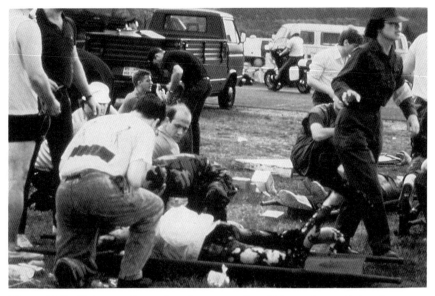

Figure 12.5—Triage at Ramstein, where more than 500 people were injured.

conscious, talking and even mobile, yet who are in urgent need of definitive care.

In a mass casualty situation, results are counted by the number of survivors and are not, unfortunately, reflected by heroic efforts to treat a few individuals. It has been said that the guiding principle is to do as little as possible, as quickly as possible, for as many as possible.[9] The corollary must be that the "little as possible" must, of course, include all that is necessary to sustain life. Medical personnel must triage in such a situation (figure 12.5). It is always preferable that the most experienced member(s) of the team should take on this responsibility, but the injuries that occur are often beyond routine experience, and decisions made in such chaos and confusion, especially in the face of fear, are not always wise ones. It follows, then, that all medical and paramedical personnel who are likely to be required to respond to a disaster scenario need the relevant depth of training and knowledge in advanced resuscitation and life support techniques.

On the subject of the categorisation of casualties sorted by injury severity, there is, unfortunately, still no nationally agreed triage labelling system. However, a recent review of those labels available at the present time advocates labels that are clear, concise, weatherproof, and easily allow change of triange category if the patient deteriorates or improves.[10] There may even be a place for brightly coloured tags or pegs that can be attached to the patient and are distinguishable from a distance.[11]

Training for pre-hospital treatment

Training for medical personnel should follow the lines of the American advanced cardiac (ACLS) and trauma (ATLS) life support courses, or similar courses devised by the Royal College of Surgeons, the Royal Army Medical Corps and BASICS. Doctors must be able to insert intravenous lines peripherally, centrally, or by cutdown if necessary. They must also be skilled in airway management, including the procedures of cricothyroidotomy and both nasolaryngeal and orolaryngeal intubation. Other skills, such as the ability to perform tube thoracostomy and the competence to manage hypovolaemic shock, burns, and cardiac arrest are equally essential. Paramedical personnel can also be trained to insert intravenous lines and should be competent in advanced first aid, including cardiopulmonary resuscitation and the recognition and treatment of shock. The individual's knowledge and proficiency should be tested at every suitable opportunity, but especially during disaster exercises.

Casualty clearing station

At the disaster site the primary objective is to provide life sustaining first aid treatment. Once extricated from the wreckage, survivors must be evacuated to an area at least 200 metres upwind of the aircraft, where triage and initial treatment can begin. This area should be protected both from the elements and from the public (and press). It may be a pre-prepared building on an airport, or it may be a large tent or marquee specially requisitioned for the task.[12,13] Once established, it should be called the casualty clearing station (CCS), and its location should be made known to the emergency services incident officers. By this time, the MIO will have decided on its function—that is, on whether it will simply be an area for initial triage and resucitation, or whether patients will be held before controlled evacuation takes place. If the latter is to be the case, the decision must also be taken as to whether the minimally wounded or the seriously injured should be held. These decisions must be taken in the light of the number of casualties, the assets and resources at the incident site, the availability of transport, the length of the evacuation chain, and the capabilities of the receiving hospitals.

The CCS should be easily approachable by road. A one-way system should be implemented to prevent congestion of arriving and departing ambulances (figure 12.6). The police should be asked to control the entry and exit points, and administrative staff will be needed to help with the documentation of those survivors that are brought in. In addition, consideration must be given to the location of a helicopter landing site if air evacuation is to be required, and the CCS will need to be equipped with

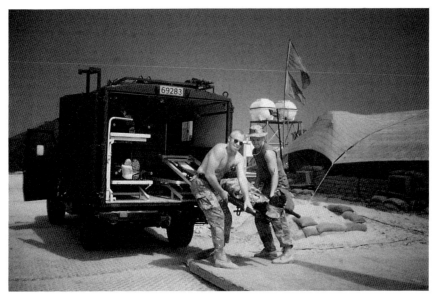

Figure 12.6—Ambulance crew practising movement of patients into a casualty clearing section during the Gulf War.

makeshift beds (or stretchers on stanchions) and suitable blankets, medical equipment, lighting, and heating.

Extra volunteers will be needed to carry stretchers, but they should not be left to wander around the CCS when not busy. A central pool of manpower is preferable, and stretcher bearers can be called forward as required. Similarly, medical personnel should not roam unsupervised around the dangerous environment of the wreckage but should wait until called forward by the rescue services and, when there, should follow all instructions diligently.

Recording the incident

To aid in the after-action report and debriefing, a photographic and video record of events is suggested. A video film is ideal for three-dimensional description of the site and to aid in the identification of victims, especially if they are filmed in situ. Notwithstanding the use of photographic documentation, it is essential to descriptively record the incident in an occurrence log (which should be weatherproof and small enough to put in a coat pocket) or verbally, on a dictaphone. All entries should be prefixed with the time (local—to avoid confusion later) and, if the incident is prolonged, the date.

Transportation of the injured

Since the Vietnam war, much debate has taken place over the use of the scoop and run concept of patient evacuation; the principle being that patients are moved as soon as possible to the nearest medical facility. This method can be used with advantage when the facility is close by and when transport is readily available, though there is an equally vociferous body of support for the opinion that medical resources should be transported directly to the patient. The plan is then to stabilise the patient before evacuating him to his final hospital destination (thereby preventing the need for a possible secondary evacuation later).

The timing and method of medical evacuation remain contentious issues and it is well known that unstabilised traumatised patients travel poorly over long distances. The old adage that evacuation can wait but resuscitation can not is very true, but there is no doubt that early definitive medical intervention saves lives. The average time from injury to definitive treatment was 12–18 hours in the first world war compared with 65–80 minutes in the Vietnam war.[14] The mortality rate of those reaching medical care was 8.5% in the former and only 1.7% in the latter. Clearly, there are many reasons for the decreased mortality rate, but the speed of evacuation is probably of major importance. Also, in a study comparing the mortality of 150 helicopter transported patients with 150 patients (matched by age, sex, and trauma score) who were transported by road, the airlifted group of patients suffered 52% fewer fatalities.[15] Some authors argue that helicopters are best used to deploy medical personnel and equipment to the casualties in a short time and provide for early resuscitative treatment at or near the site of injury, especially when the incident site is isolated or surrounding areas are likely to be congested by heavy traffic (figure 12.7).[16–18]

The speed with which all the casualties are triaged, treated, and evacuated may cause problems further down the medical chain of evacuation. Hospitals may become inundated if casualties begin arriving in large numbers. Delay in treatment is then simply shifted from one location to the next. This will be compounded if evacuation has been so rapid that patients arrive with no pre-hospital care and little or no clinical documentation. Furthermore, if the staff at the hospitals have little idea of how many more casualties to expect, they are likely to fill their casualty unit and acute beds with the first wave of patients, who may in fact not be those in most need.

There is no doubt that some casualties will have to be evacuated early, in order that the medical personnel at the disaster site can concentrate on the resuscitation of those left behind. The problem appears to be one of identifying the casualty chain "bottleneck" so that sensible decisions to hold or release casualties can be made. In this way they can be seen and treated, either on scene or at a nearby hospital, with minimal waiting time.

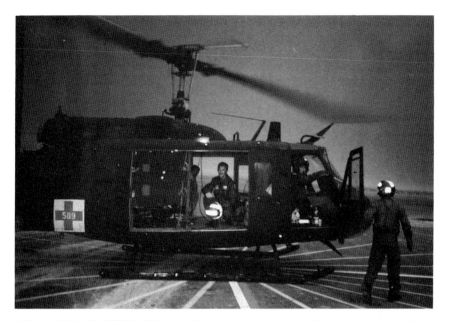

Figure 12.7—Bell UH1 (Huey) helicopter commonly used for casualty evacuation.

Inevitably, this means that a sensible mixture of scoop and run evacuation and on-site stabilisation must be applied in each case. The correct balance of both can only be reached by the MIO at the scene of the disaster.

In a mass casualty situation there are likely to be many distressed and confused survivors who are otherwise uninjured. It is important that they are not sent directly to hospital, at least not in the early phase. They should be transported to a private area where they can be counselled, interviewed, and eventually reunited with relatives or friends. This area must be dedicated for this sole purpose and must be located distant from the bustle of the rescue activities. Members of the press should be excluded from the area, if necessary with the help of the police.

The role of aeromedical evacuation has already been discussed, and there can be no doubt of the value of helicopter support when patients need to be moved quickly and the surrounding roads are blocked or the distances are great. However, consideration may also be given to the use of fixed wing transport aircraft or air ambulances for long distances when airfields are conveniently located near to the destination medical facilities. In general, though, fixed wing aircraft are more appropriate for secondary evacuation at a later stage.

Road transport (coaches in preference to trucks) is equally valuable and should be readily identifiable as suitable for "re-rolling" in stretcher fit, in case of urgent need. In some situations it may also be appropriate to consider the use of trains.[19]

Casualty identification and tracking

In the chaos and confusion of the scene of a major incident, many family members and friends travelling together will be separated. As described above, those who are uninjured should not be allowed to wander around but should be persuaded to return to a central point where they can rejoin their missing travelling companions or their "meeters and greeters". At such a place, telephone lines should be installed to allow the survivors to call out, and computers will be necessary to help with the compilation of a list of identified survivors and another of those who are missing.

Untrained volunteers, thinking only of the benefits of rapid evacuation, may attempt to move patients from the scene without belongings or clothing, which may be useful for identification purposes later. Some of these patients may lose consciousness or subsequently die, and will prove difficult to identify. This will cause great distress to the relatives of the missing, and a great deal of confusion amongst the team who must try to keep track of all the evacuated patients. Nevertheless, the collection of effects from the disaster site is a controversial issue, since some see it as tampering with potential evidence. However, it is preferable that all survivors are identified before being transported away from the disaster site or CCS; ideally, they should be photographed.

It is feasible that victims of an air disaster may have travelled from anywhere in the world, and language problems should not be underestimated. It will be essential to identify a number of interpreters at the earliest opportunity and, at the very least, medical planners should have access to the International Red Cross medical translation booklet which gives 43 commonly used medical questions in 28 languages.[20]

Significant numbers of casualties may need to be transported to a large number of hospitals. After initial treatment and identification of remaining major problems, some patients will be evacuated to a second or even third echelon of medical care. This may serve to compound the problem of tracking patients, and every effort must be made to update the police casualty bureau of the final destinations of all patients.

Disaster planning

Disasters are always unexpected and are usually unpredictable. Anticipation and specific planning is therefore difficult. Nevertheless, a sound working framework is essential, whilst flexibility remains crucial. Disaster exercises need to be practised frequently so that each member of the team knows his or her exact role and location in the system. In the United

Kingdom there is, at present, no national body that coordinates disaster planning and reponse. Department of Health policy dictates that contingency planning is a regional responsibility, but a national civil emergencies adviser, responsible for overseeing emergency operations, has been recently appointed by the Home Office. His main responsibility will be the development and dissemination of "good practice and information". He will liaise with all emergency services, local authorities, government departments, and voluntary bodies that have a direct interest in the management of major incidents. In addition to advising on disaster exercises and training, he will ensure that the lessons of past incidents are learned and applied. To assist with this task, the Civil Defence College at Easingwold (now known as the Emergency Planning College) has been given a wider remit to act as a centre for the study of the broader issues involved in peacetime emergency planning.

It is essential that planners have a working liaison with the local emergency services and hospital staffs. It is vital to know where mass casualties are to be sent, especially if they are to be transported to burns or other specialist centres, or to other hospitals distant from the disaster site. Planners should not forget the voluntary organisations. They should be included in all disaster exercises, since their help will be invaluable on the day.

Airport disaster planning is a special case, since many international airports have their own medical personnel and resources. These are central to the plan, because they will inevitably be the first attenders at airfield incidents. In the design of emergency contingency plans for airports, it is useful to have an assessment of the number of seriously injured casualties that may be anticipated. As discussed previously, it has been estimated that no more than 25% of occupants will survive with major injuries in most (95%) of aircraft crashes.[1] For the largest of modern transport aircraft, this effectively means no more than 140 serious casualties. The International Civil Aviation Organisation (ICAO) has produced guidelines towards airport emergency planning[21] and excellent examples of contingency plans have been published,[6,13,20] but planning must differ for each individual site to cater for a multiplicity of variables such as aircraft type and size, traffic density (air and ground), airport layout, climate, surrounding geography, and proximity of local emergency services and medical facilities.

Format of the plan

It is important to be able to rapidly read the essential details of any plan, and to be able to extract relevant orders precisely and quickly. The ideal method is to have an indexed checklist format. There should be an introductory narrative which reads clearly, and contains concise and vital information necessary to understand the organisation of the plan. Putting

163

the orders in a checklist type layout is the ideal approach to ensure that vital actions are not omitted. Nevertheless, even the most carefully conceived plan will be of minimal value if it is not regularly put to the test, reviewed, and critiqued.

Major incident exercises

The importance of the frequent practise of good disaster plans can not be overstated. In fact, a condition for the Civil Aviation Authority licence to operate public services at an airport is that the management should satisfy certain stringent safety requirements, including the capability to respond to a disaster. As part of this requirement, it is mandatory that an annual full scale disaster exercise is performed.

It is important that the "incident" and subsequent scenarios are made to be as realistic as possible. To this end, moulaged casualties, actual aircraft, and the true assets available on the day should be used. Every member of the emergency services and disaster response team should be thoroughly familiar with his role in the plan and should be confident that he can play his part.

It is not enough simply to practise the major incident scenario on airfields. Medical teams, especially, need to exercise with the other emergency services. In addition, doctors need to be aware that disaster medicine is unlike any other form of medicine and that it requires a distinct approach. Doctors who are likely to be used as MIOs will benefit greatly by liaising and coordinating with other emergency workers, and by understanding more of the organisational and communications roles of their counterparts from the police, fire, and ambulance services.

Tabletop exercises also have their place. They are less expensive in terms of both manpower and finance, and take less organisation to set up. The participants will include only the senior staffs of the emergency services and other interested parties, such as airport and/or airline management, hospital administrators, and voluntary agencies. Scenarios should be played with the true assets that are available on the day of the exercise, and actions decided as the play unfolds. Although not a substitute for full scale exercises, they have proved most useful and cost effective additions.

After the evacuation of survivors

For many, the work will continue long after the casualties are cleared from the site. These include the fire and rescue personnel who must ensure that there is no further risk of conflagration, police and special investigators (from the Air Accidents Investigation Branch and the aircraft manufacturer), and environmental health personnel who must ensure the complete and correct disposal of all potentially infective or soiled medical waste and

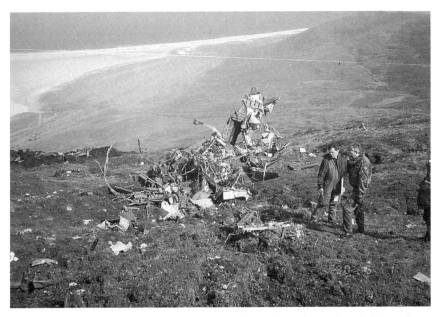

Figure 12.8—Air accident investigators after the crash of a large aircraft in Scotland.

who also have the task of collecting soil samples at the sites of fuel and chemical spillage (figure 12.8). There may also be a need for specialist teams such as military explosive ordnance experts who may have the task of disarming ejector seats, and RAF recovery personnel who will eventually clear the site and transport the wreckage to Farnborough for further examination.

Planners should also consider that there will be many victims who are not physically injured. Post-traumatic stress disorder is now well recognised,[22] and experience gained at Ramstein and other recent catastrophes has shown that we should anticipate psychiatric casualties amongst the personnel of the emergency services as well as amongst the survivors and their relatives. Mental health services therefore need to be available in sufficient numbers to deal urgently with the many cases that are bound to occur. Crisis intervention will be needed at the disaster site and at all stages down the chain of medical evacuation where chaplains, social workers, and psychiatrists will all be required in the long task of counselling the survivors, relatives, and health and rescue workers alike. In the ensuing days, open support groups may well be needed, preferably on a "walk in" basis. Many sufferers may require more formal treatment, perhaps lasting many months, before they can eventually come to terms with their exceptional experiences.

Summary

- The objective of any disaster plan must be to ensure the best quality of triage and treatment of the survivors in an effort to minimise the risks of mortality and increased morbidity

- In the real event, success will depend on prior planning, thorough training, medical reinforcement, co-operation with other agencies, and availability of suitable medical assets and transportation

- Clear and efficient communications will be fundamental to successful command and the effective coordination of rescue efforts

- A favourable outcome will be the result of the intelligent interpretation of a simple yet flexible plan that has been rehearsed and frequently reviewed.

1 Lane JC, Brown TC. Probability of casualties in an airport disaster. *Aviat Space Environ Med* 1975; **46**: 958–61.
2 Rowles JM, Kirsh G, Learmonth DJA, Martindale JP. The NDLB aircraft accident study: the injuries and consequences of the M1 aircraft accident [Abstract]. Sixth World Congress Emergency and Disaster Medicine, 1989.
3 Rutherford WH. An analysis of civil aircrash statistics 1977–86 for the purposes of planning disaster exercises. *Injury* 1988; **19**: 384–8.
4 Department of Health. *Emergency Planning in the NHS: health service arrangements for dealing with major accidents.* London: HMSO, 1990. (HC(90)25).
5 Robertson B, ed. *Guide to major incident management.* British Association for Immediate Care, 1985.
6 Dove DB, Del Guercio LRL, Stahl WM, Star LD, Abelson LC. A metropolitan airport disaster plan—coordination of a multihospital response to provide on-site resuscitation and stabilisation before evacuation. *J Trauma* 1982; **22**: 550–9.
7 Defence Council Instruction (General) Order No 17, 1969.
8 Martin TE. The Ramstein Airshow disaster. *J Br Assoc Immed Care* 1990; **13**: 2–8.
9 Grollmes EE. Aviation emergency management/disaster response: the getting ready. *Proc Int Aviat Emerg Manage Conf* 1989; **I(1)**: 1–13.
10 Robertson B. Medical management at the scene of the accident. *Proc Int Aviat Emerg Manage Conf* 1989; **I(3)**: 31–42.
11 Martin TE. Al Jubail—an aeromedical staging facility during the Gulf conflict. *J R Soc Med* 1992; **85**: 32–6.
12 Abelson LC, Star LD, Goldner AS. Twenty years of medical support in aircraft disasters at Kennedy airport. *Aerospace Med* 1973; **44**: 560–6.
13 Bergot GP. Disaster planning at major airports. *Aerospace Med* 1971; **42**: 449–55.
14 Trunkey D. Towards optimal trauma care. *Arch Emerg Med* 1985; **2**: 181–95.
15 Baxt WG, Moody P. The impact of a rotorcraft aeromedical emergency care service on trauma mortality. *JAMA* 1983; **249**: 3047–51.
16 Perry IC. The helicopter as a civilian emergency vehicle. *Injury* 1972; **3**: 254–6.
17 Bock KH, Lampl L, Helm M. Management of mass casualties by the emergency physician. *Med Corps Int* 1988; **3**: 17–20.
18 Wilson A, Cross F. Helicopters. *J R Soc Med* 1992; **85**: 1–3.
19 Coe LG. Heathrow evacuation plan. *Proc Int Aviat Emerg Manage Conf* 1989; **I(3)**: 43–59.
20 *Emergency multi-lingual phrasebook.* London: British Red Cross, undated.
21 Secretary General. *Airport Emergency planning in the NHS: health service arrangements for dealing with major incidents.* London International Civil Aviation Organisation, 1980. (Doc 9137-AN/898 Part 7.)
22 Raphael B, Middleton W. After the horror. *BMJ* 1988; **296**: 1142–3.

13
Management of abdominal trauma in the multiply injured patient

NIGEL WILLIAMS, MILES IRVING

EDITORS' INTRODUCTION

The general surgical injuries in the survivors of the M1/Kegworth aircrash were reported in the *Annals of the Royal College of Surgeons* 1990; **72**: 378–81. In the M1 aircrash there were remarkably few abdominal injuries. Of the 87 initial survivors of the accident only five had suspected intra-abdominal injuries that required a laparotomy. In two patients the laparotomy was carried out because of a fall in blood pressure and revealed no significant intra-abdominal problem. Both patients died as a consequence of their multiple injuries. In one patient a laparotomy carried out because of a fall in blood pressure and a rigid abdomen revealed a liver haematoma, another patient had a fall in blood pressure, a tense abdomen, and at laparotomy was found to have a ruptured spleen and perinepheric haematoma, and a fifth patient with abdominal tenderness and a positive diagnostic peritoneal lavage was found to have a ruptured bladder and a tear of the serosan of the sigmoid colon.

Despite abdominal injuries being uncommonly associated with major disasters, when they do occur they usually are life threatening. For this reason we have invited Mr Nigel Williams and Professor Miles Irving to write this chapter, which focuses on the modern views about management of abdominal injuries. There has been a considerable change in emphasis, with a much more conservative approach to abdominal injuries being adopted in the 1990s compared with the 1970s, and we feel that this contribution will allow those who may be presented with major disasters to make up to date management decisions on their patients.

Introduction

Trauma may be categorised according to the mechanism of injury—that is, blunt or penetrating. In mainland Britain blunt trauma accounts for the vast majority of cases of abdominal injury admitted to accident and

167

Mechanism of injuries

Blunt: High velocity—high energy
      Low velocity—low energy

Penetrating: Gunshot
      Shotgun
      Stab
      Explosive
      Missile/projectile/shrapnel

---

emergency departments, and nearly all of these are the result of road traffic accidents. In many trauma centres, such as those in the USA, penetrating injuries account for a greater proportion of injuries encountered. Although this classification is arbitrary it has practical and predictive advantages. Blunt and penetrating abdominal injury are usually distinguishable at the time of presentation and these two categories usually have different management patterns. Blunt and penetrating injuries can be further subdivided according to the magnitude of energy of the injurious agent (see box). Whereas penetrating injuries (other than high velocity bullet wounds) usually divide anatomical structures directly in their path, blunt injuries cause crushing and tearing of solid viscera because of the sudden rapid deceleration that occurs inside the body. Blunt injuries are more often associated with multiple skeletal injuries. As a result, blunt abdominal trauma has a higher mortality than penetrating injury.

In the past, all penetrating injuries to the abdomen were explored. However, as the incidence of visceral injury from a stab wound has now been shown to be only 30–40%, mandatory laparotomy is no longer necessary. In contrast, visceral injury occurs in more than 90% of gunshot wounds to the abdomen, and therefore these nearly always have to be explored.

After severe multiple injuries (such as those sustained in an aircraft accident), abdominal trauma is often part of a wider spectrum of injury, and it is probably inappropriate to consider thoracic and abdominal trauma separately. Indeed, it is easier to divide the torso into three coronal zones (figure 13.1a), one mid-zone and two lateral zones. Blunt or penetrating injury to structures in the mid-zone, such as the heart and great vessels, has a higher mortality because of the vital function of the heart and the high risk of haemorrhage. Conversely, injuries to structures in the lateral zones have a lower mortality. The torso can also be divided into three sagittal zones; zone I from the nipples and above, zone II between the nipple and the umbilicus, and zone III from the umbilicus downwards (figure 13.1b). Injuries to zones II and III are more likely to require operative treatment and will be discussed in detail later.

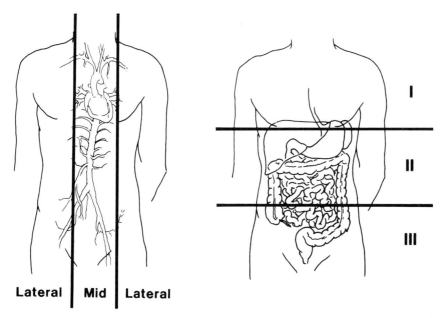

Lateral | **Mid** | **Lateral**

Figure 13.1—The torso can be thought of as three coronal zones, two lateral zones, and a medial zone (left), and three sagittal zones, I, II, and III (right).

Assessment

The first hour after injury is now recognised as being the most critical period. This is the "golden hour", when resuscitation and formal assessment of all injuries should be carried out and a management strategy should be clearly defined. The most widely accepted schema of trauma management is that used in the advanced trauma life support (ATLS) approach of the American College of Surgeons. The sequence of assessment and priority is:

A—airway and cervical spine control
B—breathing and ventilation
C—circulation and control of haemorrhage.

This is followed by a brief neurological examination and the complete undressing of the patient to avoid missing injuries hidden by clothing.

History and examination

Of necessity, the initial history and examination is brief and will be performed concurrently with resuscitation. During this primary survey those conditions that present an immediate threat to the patient's life are identified and dealt with in an expeditious manner. Of paramount import-

169

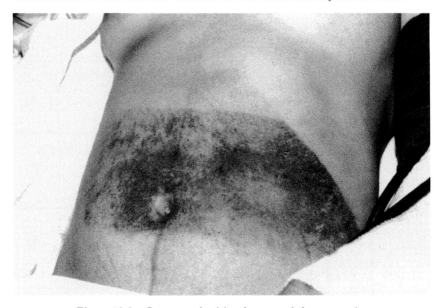

Figure 13.2—Cutaneous bruising from seat belt compression.

ance in the history is the time and mechanism of trauma, as this will allow an assessment of the likely possible injuries.

On abdominal inspection the presence of ecchymoses and abrasions may be an indication of underlying organ damage. The location of bruising may or may not fit with the presumed mechanism of injury and a clinical suspicion of possible underlying injuries should always be considered. Seat belt bruising should be sought as it may declare an underlying visceral and abdominal wall injury (figure 13.2). The site(s) of penetrating injuries should be noted. Foreign bodies embedded in the abdominal wall or other objects penetrating the abdomen should be left undisturbed as their removal may result in sudden and significant intra-abdominal haemorrhage. Such foreign bodies should only be removed at laparotomy, when control of bleeding can be obtained if the object has penetrated a major vessel. Although the contour of the abdomen should be noted, it must be remembered that abdominal distension is not a reliable sign of intraperitoneal haemorrhage. Guarding and peritonism are significant signs suggesting intraperitoneal bleeding or contamination with bowel contents. Auscultation of the abdomen offers little useful information in the acute situation. If the patient with surgical shock does not respond to fluid resuscitation, the highest priority should be given to the rapid localisation of bleeding site(s) and the control of bleeding. The patient who becomes stable following fluid resuscitation can be more formally assessed within the framework of the secondary survey.

Diagnostic peritoneal lavage

Death from the consequences of internal haemorrhage used to be quite common in cases of blunt abdominal trauma managed in the days before modern diagnostic techniques were available. In an attempt to increase diagnostic accuracy, methods of aspirating fluid from the abdominal cavity, such as paracentesis, culdocentesis, and four quadrant taps, were developed. However, these techniques were not demonstrated to have a significant greater diagnostic accuracy than physical examination alone. In 1965, Root et al[1] introduced the method of diagnostic peritoneal lavage (DPL) which had an accuracy of 100% in their first 28 patients. Since then, DPL has become the standard method for evaluating blunt abdominal trauma because it is considered to be quick and sensitive in detecting the presence of intra-abdominal blood. It is used to detect the presence of intraperitoneal free blood, bacteria, vegetable matter, or amylase. It is not specific for type or extent of organ injury. It can resolve the question as to whether exploratory laparotomy is indicated with an accuracy of greater than 97%. Diagnostic peritoneal lavage comes close to fulfilling all the criteria recognised for the ideal test for blunt abdominal trauma—high sensitivity, high specificity, expediency, ease of use, and low morbidity—and it is currently considered the gold standard for the diagnosis of intra-abdominal injury after blunt abdominal trauma. It is of particular value when there is a severe concomitant closed head injury, when no history is available and findings on physical examination are equivocal.[2] In a series of 2586 patients managed over a 14 year period, Fischer et al found DPL to have a 1.2% false negative rate and a 0.2% false positive rate.[3]

Computed tomography

Computed tomography (CT) has been evaluated as a diagnostic tool for abdominal injuries in patients who are haemodynamically stable and therefore do not warrant urgent laparotomy. Used in this way it is valuable for the diagnosis of haematomas and non-bleeding parenchymal injuries and for the detection of intraperitoneal free gas and blood. Although the diagnostic specificity of CT is superior to DPL, it is not as sensitive. Also, CT does not reliably exclude the presence of a hollow viscus injury. Thus, the opportunity to prevent significant intraperitoneal infection at an early stage may be lost. This is of importance in adults, who are more likely to sustain hollow viscus injuries from blunt trauma than are children.[4] Computed tomography is particularly useful in identifying splenic, hepatic and renal parenchymal, and subcapsular haematomas, and in these situations may permit further conservative management. Indeed, the increasing use of CT has uncovered many more of these injuries than were previously suspected. The presence of a large splenic or hepatic parenchymal haematoma with an intact capsule could have easily produced a negative result with DPL, whereas the same injury can now be visualised by CT.

In assessing hepatic trauma, recent studies have found little agreement between the degree of injury seen on CT with that seen at laparotomy. None the less, CT has had a positive impact in trauma management, as many patients with subcapsular or intraparenchymal haematomas who may have previously undergone laparotomy based on abdominal pain and tenderness can now be observed with sequential CT assessment and repeated clinical examination. In such instances, not only is laparotomy unnecessary but it may lead to inappropriate and sometimes dangerous surgical intervention. Therefore the main impact of CT has been in promoting non-operative management.

More recently, CT has been used to guide non-operative management of selected stable patients with right-sided penetrating thoracoabdominal wounds in several trauma centres in the USA.

Ultrasonography

Although operator dependent and at times limited by excessive bowel gas or open wounds, ultrasound scanning is non-invasive and may be performed rapidly at the bedside. The latter is an important advantage over CT in the patient who has some cardiovascular instability as monitoring and resuscitation of patients in the radiology department during CT investigations is often less than optimal. Because ultrasound investigation is non-invasive it may be used in instances where DPL may be contraindicated—for example, pregnancy, coagulopathy, and previous laparotomy.

Ultrasonography can reveal subcapsular intraparenchymal haematomas and other contained injuries, and information can be obtained about both extraperitoneal and intraperitoneal structures. It relies heavily on detecting the presence of free abdominal fluid to indicate the presence of an abdominal injury, and correspondingly the sensitivity of ultrasonography in detecting intra-abdominal injury is greatly reduced in the absence of free peritoneal fluid. This explains the low sensitivity of ultrasonography (approximately 70%) in detecting the less severe parenchymal and retroperitoneal injuries.[5] Therefore a negative ultrasound scan does not exclude the presence of injury to an abdominal organ, and ultrasound has been found to have poor precision in the assessment of pancreatic or hollow viscus injuries. Ultrasonography has, however, established itself in the subsequent management of patients with abdominal injury, for both the follow up of renal or splenic injuries that are managed conservatively and the detection of abdominal collections that may require surgical drainage. The role of ultrasonography in the acute situation when assessing blunt abdominal trauma continues to evolve, but for the present its use should normally be supplemented by other diagnostic techniques.[6]

Arteriography

Arteriography has a very selective role in the diagnosis and treatment of abdominal trauma. In the presence of haematuria it is mandatory for the demonstration of a non-visualised kidney following intravenous urography. It is of value in the assessment of retroperitoneal haematomas and pelvic fractures and can be followed by embolisation to control bleeding in patients with pelvic fractures.

Intravenous urography

Intravenous pyelography (IVP) is the initial imaging study in the staging of renal injuries and should be considered in all cases of haematuria.[7] If the IVP is abnormal or indeterminate, then CT or arteriography is indicated.

Laparoscopy

Increasingly, laparoscopy is being used to assess the abdominal contents following blunt or penetrating abdominal injury.[8] With developing skills and technique, one can foresee treatment of visceral injuries by this technique, using materials such as fibrin glue.

Immediate operative management of abdominal injuries

The midline incision is preferred for emergency laparotomy, because the abdomen can be entered in minutes and virtually the whole abdominal viscera can be exposed, as the incision may be extended cranially or caudally. In the emergency situation, the incision is associated with minimal blood loss from the divided midline tissues. On entering the abdominal cavity, free blood and clots are rapidly scooped out, but only enough to allow for a rapid assessment of the sites and extent of injuries. Immediate management priorities are to control haemorrhage and to repair visceral injury. If bleeding is still profuse after entering the abdomen, the bowel is eviscerated and the quadrants of the abdomen packed separately to control bleeding while replacement of the circulating blood volume is carried out rapidly. Venous bleeding is usually amenable to packing. If bleeding is arterial, then manual compression of the abdominal aorta below the oesophageal hiatus may be sufficient to temporarily control major haemorrhage while the bleeding site(s) are located and controlled. Repair can then proceed under more favourable conditions. Complete abdominal exploration should be undertaken to determine whether multiple sites of haemorrhage are present. Manual assessment of the spleen will usually reveal the extent of the damage and will also allow the surgeon to decide whether splenorrhaphy or splenectomy should be performed. The liver should be palpated next, making sure that all surfaces are examined. In the presence of multiple solid visceral injuries, bleeding sites are packed and attention should be directed to major vascular injuries, the spleen, and the liver. Once haemorrhage is controlled and physiological stability restored, priority should be given to containment of faecal spillage and repair of visceral injury.

Splenic injuries

The spleen is the most commonly injured organ in blunt abdominal trauma and is also frequently involved in penetrating wounds of the left lower chest and abdomen. In children, blunt trauma is responsible for the great majority (>90%) of splenic injury.[9] Although splenic injury may be isolated, associated abdominal injuries are seen in 30–70% of patients and extra-abdominal injuries in up to 90%. Penetrating injuries to the spleen are associated with other serious abdominal injuries in up to 94% of cases.[10]

Anatomy

Located below the left hemidiaphragm, the spleen is bounded by the fundus of the stomach medially, the splenic flexure of the colon anteriorly, and it is attached to the retroperitoneum by the lienorenal ligament. The splenic artery courses over the superior border of the pancreas and bifurcates into two branches to supply the superior and inferior poles, delivering approximately 5% of the cardiac output. Polar vessels either from the splenic artery or from the coeliac axis are not uncommon and variation in splenic arterial anatomy is often seen.

Classification

Many classifications of splenic injuries exist. Because of these different classifications, comparisons between institutions treating such injuries using differing management techniques has often not been possible. In an attempt to remedy this problem the organ injury scaling committee of the American Association for the Surgery of Trauma (AAST) devised a new classification in 1987, which is now used in most centres. This splenic injury scale is based on an assessment of the macroscopic damage sustained by the organ (see box).

The mechanism of injury should normally alert the clinician to have a high index of suspicion of there being a splenic injury. Patients with an underlying splenic abnormality or with splenomegaly as a result of a haematological diathesis are much more susceptible to splenic injury. Recognition of such disorders also has implications for the patient's preoperative and postoperative care. The clinical manifestations of splenic injury are due either to the irritant effect of blood in the peritoneal cavity, causing abdominal pain, or under the diaphragm, producing local and left shoulder tip pain and tenderness, or the significant blood loss that occurs,

The splenic injury scale of the American Association for the Surgery of Trauma

Grade		Injury description
I	Haematoma	Subcapsular, non-expanding; <10% surface area
	Laceration	Capsular tear, non-bleeding; <1 cm deep
II	Haematoma	Subcapsular, non-expanding, 10–50% surface area
		Intraparenchymal non-expanding, <2 cm diameter
III	Haematoma	Subcapsular, >50% surface area or expanding
		Ruptured subcapsular haematoma with active bleeding
		Intraparenchymal haematoma, >2 cm or expanding
	Laceration	>3 cm deep or involving trabecular vessels
IV	Haematoma	Ruptured intraparenchymal haematoma with active bleeding
	Laceration	Laceration involving segmental or hilar vessels, producing major devascularisation (>25% of spleen)
V	Laceration	Completely shattered spleen
	Vascular	Hilar vascular injury devascularising the spleen

which presents as hypotension, tachycardia, and circulatory shock. Circulatory shock is present on admission in approximately 30% of all splenic injuries.

Management

During the early decades of the twentieth century splenectomy for trauma was carried out frequently but mortality remained at between 30% and 40%. Removal of the spleen was regarded as of little consequence. Indeed, it was Kocher who said that, "injuries of the spleen demand excision of the gland, no evil effects will follow its removal while danger of haemorrhage is effectively stopped." The practice of splenectomy for trauma therefore continued unchallenged until 1952, when King and Shumaker reported five cases of overwhelming postsplenectomy infection (OPSI) in infants who had previously had splenectomy for haemolytic anaemia. As well as the risk of OPSI, which has a reported incidence of 1–2% in adults following splenectomy for trauma, many other immunological changes occur.[11] From the currently available information, it is recommended that splenectomy should be avoided in infants and children younger than 2 years old because of the much higher documented risk of OPSI. In adolescents and adults, the risk is significantly less; however, the multiple immunological deficits that have now been recorded suggest that splenectomy should be avoided whenever possible. These data have resulted in enthusiastic interest in splenic preservation (splenorrhaphy) after splenic injury. Successful reports of suture splenorrhaphy and partial splenectomy by William Mayo date back to 1910, and interest in these techniques has now been rekindled. Clearly, if a patient is haemodynamically unstable and splenic injury is suspected then emergency laparotomy is appropriate. The majority of patients (approximately 70%) with acute blunt splenic trauma will be haemodynamically stable or will be rapidly stabilised by crystalloid infusion, thus allowing for DPL. If the injury was sustained by low velocity trauma, management may be adjusted, depending on patient's age. In the child in whom haemodynamic stability is rapidly restored and the mechanism of injury is "low energy" there is clearly a role for a non-operative approach. The following criteria must be satisfied in order to select patients suitable for non-operative managment:

- The patient must be haemodynamically stable following fluid resuscitation

- There should be no other serious associated abdominal injury

- There should be no extra-abdominal injuries that could prevent or alter abdominal assessment—for example, severe closed head injury.

Using these criteria, 40–70% of children can be managed without operative intervention. However, if lavage indices suggest other visceral injury, such as increased white cell count or amylase or the presence of enteric stained effluent, then immediate laparotomy is indicated. This concept has been practised successfully in the management of paediatric trauma for over two decades now and is beginning to influence adult trauma management. However, not all surgeons agree that this is the best method of splenic preservation; some suggest that early laparotomy and splenorrhaphy can preserve more spleens. A non-operative management strategy should only be adopted if there are facilities available for repeated regular clinical assessment and haemodynamic monitoring and access to a fully staffed operating theatre for emergency splenectomy should the patient become unstable. Such conservative management is probably inappropriate in those aged over 60 years. In children, laparotomy should be contemplated when estimated blood loss exceeds 40 ml/kg.

After laparotomy has been performed and the degree of splenic injury ascertained, a decision must be made whether to remove the spleen or attempt salvage. It must not be forgotten that splenorrhaphy requires greater expertise and is more time consuming than splenectomy, therefore it is not for the inexperienced surgeon or an unstable patient.[12] Splenorrhaphy also requires special sutures and other materials, such as vicryl mesh, and there is a recognised incidence of rebleeding requiring subsequent splenectomy. Splenorrhaphy is contraindicated in patients with peritoneal contamination due to gastrointestinal injuries and rupture of diseased spleens. Therefore although splenic preservation is desirable, it should certainly not be done if it causes extra risk to the patient.

Splenectomy: emergency splenectomy should be performed briskly and boldly. The surgeon's left hand is placed over the body of the spleen and the organ is retracted anteromedially and out into the wound. If the lienorenal ligament is not torn by this manoeuvre then it is incised under direct vision while a retractor is used to the left of the wound to improve access and vision. Superiorly the phrenicolienal ligament and inferiorly the lienocolic ligament may also need to be divided. The spleen is now completely visible in the wound and safe removal of the organ can now proceed. The main splenic vessels are isolated at the hilum of the gland and are doubly ligated, taking care not to incorporate the tail of the pancreas. The short gastric vessels also require ligation, and care should be taken to preserve the gastroepiploic vessels and not to include the stomach wall in these ties. Nasogastric intubation is mandatory to avoid acute gastric dilatation and subsequent haemorrhage from a slipped short gastric artery ligature. The splenic bed should be packed and a systematic and thorough laparotomy repeated. At the end of the procedure the splenic bed should be inspected again to ensure there is no continued bleeding. The surgeon can only be certain there is adequate haemostasis once the patient's blood pressure has returned to a normal level. Prior to abdominal closure, low-pressure suction drains should be placed in the splenic bed.

Splenorrhaphy: once the spleen has been adequately delivered into the wound all surfaces may be visualised. In cases of small non-bleeding lacerations or capsular avulsions (grade I), when there is little or no blood in the perisplenic area, then it may not be necessary to fully mobilise the spleen. In such instances intraoperative packing of the spleen, with removal of the pack to verify haemostasis (in a normotensive patient) before the abdomen is closed, may be justified. In all other instances the spleen must be fully mobilised and brought out into the wound for a full assessment of the severity of injury. After inspection the splenic injury score can be ascertained and should be recorded. Options for splenic preservation may be divided into the following groups:

- Application of topical agents—for example, Gelfoam or Surgicel

- Electrocautery

- Suture splenorrhaphy (with or without collagen or Teflon buttresses)

- Meshes—for example Teflon or Vicryl

- Partial resection.

Simple capsular avulsions and superficial parenchymal fractures (grade I and II) are usually managed by topical haemostatic agents applied to the bleeding sites combined with pressure. For grade II injuries suture splenorrhaphy is the most commonly used technique, employing absorbable sutures in much the same manner as hepatic or renal parenchymal repairs. Diffuse bleeding requires interlocking mattress sutures approximating the parenchyma. The relatively thick splenic capsule in a child will permit direct suturing but in the adult buttresses are usually necessary. Grade III–V injuries require exposure of the hilar vessels in order to obtain complete haemostasis. Complex splenic fractures with deep parenchymal involvement require anatomic resection and surgical management is based on the same principles as those for hepatic resection. However, if the spleen is pulverised or haemostasis cannot be achieved by splenorrhaphy, splenectomy remains the safest option.

Complications and outcome

Many of the complications encountered following emergency splenectomy are similar to those seen following elective surgery—for example, acute gastric dilatation, greater curve necrosis, recurrent bleeding, subphrenic abscess, pancreatitis, and pancreatic fistula. Following splenorrhaphy delayed haemorrhage has been observed as late as 45 days after splenic repair. Patients should therefore be advised to avoid contact sports for at least 3 months. They should be made aware that they have had a splenectomy and should be advised to have pneumococcal vaccine and to seek medical attention promptly should they develop symptoms of nonspecific "flu like" illness. It is important that the parents of children who have had splenectomy are made aware of this.

Hepatic injuries

As with splenic injury, in mainland Britain blunt abdominal trauma remains the commonest cause of hepatic injury, in contrast to the USA where penetrating injury is more common. Although it sits under the diaphragm, protected by the lower ribs, the liver remains particularly vulnerable to compressive injury because of its relatively thin capsule. Because it is the largest solid organ in the abdomen it is injured in 20–45% of patients sustaining severe blunt trauma and in up to 45% of cases of penetrating injuries. Associated injuries to other viscera are very common, and penetrating injuries are associated with a greater number of injuries than are blunt injuries (in a 2.7:2.0 ratio).[13] Splenic, pulmonary, and head

---

The liver injury scale of the American Association for the Surgery of Trauma

Grade		Injury description
I	Haematoma	Subcapsular, non-expanding, <10% of surface area
	Laceration	Capsular tear, non-bleeding, <1 cm deep
II	Haematoma	Subcapsular, non-expanding, 10–50% surface area
		Intraparechymal non-expanding, <2 cm diameter
	Laceration	Capsular tear, active bleeding, 1–3 cm deep, <10 cm long
III	Haematoma	Subcapsular, >50% surface area or expanding
		Ruptured subcapsular haematoma with active bleeding
		Intraparenchymal haematoma >2 cm or expanding
	Laceration	>3 cm deep
IV	Haematoma	Ruptured intraparenchymal haematoma with active bleeding
	Laceration	Parenchymal disruption involving 25–50% of hepatic lobe
V	Haematoma	Parenchymal disruption involving 50% of hepatic lobe
	Vascular	Juxtahepatic venous injuries (retrohepatic vena) cava/major hepatic veins
VI	Vascular	Hepatic avulsion

---

injury occur commonly in association with blunt trauma, whereas vascular, gastrointestinal, and adjacent solid visceral injuries are seen more frequently in association with penetrating injury.

Classification

Although a variety of classifications exist, the most accepted in current practice is that devised by the AAST (see box).

Diagnosis

The diagnosis of a severe liver injury may be immediately obvious from the mechanism of injury and the patient's physiological status. Unstable patients with penetrating abdominal injuries require immediate laparotomy to control intra-abdominal haemorrhage, and in this situation diagnositic procedures merely delay appropriate management. Although there may be co-existing injuries requiring attention, few will or should take precedence. With haemodynamic instability in patients sustaining blunt trauma it is more difficult to ascertain from which body cavity blood is being lost. However, if there are strong physical signs—for example, distended abdomen or cutaneous abdominal bruising—then urgent laparotomy is indicated. Patients who are stable require formal evaluation of the nature and degree of injuries sustained, as there is no immediate risk of exsanguination or threat to life. Diagnostic peritoneal lavage remains the initial diagnostic procedure of choice in most cases and is very sensitive (>98%) for diagnosing hepatic injury after blunt trauma.

There is currently a resurgence of interest in the non-operative management of liver injuries, and CT is the cornerstone of this mode of management. There are conflicting reports as to the efficacy of CT in the assessment of abdominal trauma. This discrepancy is almost certainly related to observer expertise, and therefore if CT is to be used to guide management then good quality scans and an experienced radiologist are essential. Assessment of the use of ultrasound in this situation thus far has indicated that it does not have the diagnostic sensitivity of DPL. Radioisotope scanning and arteriography do not offer any advantage over DPL or CT in the acute situation but may be of value in the evaluation of complications arising from hepatic injuries. Arteriography gives the additional option of embolisation for the control of bleeding.

Management

The management of liver trauma has seen a full swing of the pendulum back to a more conservative approach, as practised at the beginning of the century and during the first world war, and away from the aggressive approach of resectional surgery. In part, this has been prompted by the recent prominent role of CT in identifying lesions that may be managed non-operatively (figure 13.3).

In those unstable patients in whom laparotomy is mandatory, methods of controlling haemorrhage short of resection are now employed. The techniques used are suture hepatorrhaphy, hepatotomy with selective vessel ligation, resectional debridement, resection, selective hepatic artery ligation, and perihepatic packing. Major hepatic resection in trauma is associated with an unacceptably high mortality rate (>50%) even in very experienced hands and is losing favour as a treatment option in trauma surgery.[14] This is reflected in its decreasing use. Resection is used only when haemorrhage has been controlled and a necrotic piece of liver would be left in place were it not resected. In experienced hands, liver lacerations are extended to explore the bleeding vessels and selective vessel ligation is employed. Topical haemostatic agents are often quite helpful in patients with grade I and grade II injuries, where parenchymal oozing from the surface of the liver is the predominant problem.

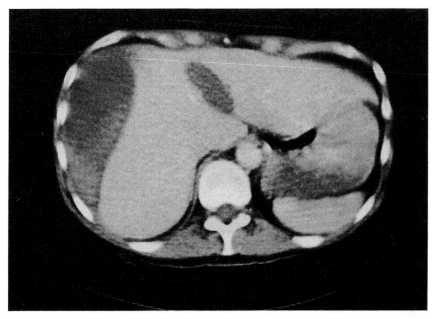

Figure 13.3—Intrahepatic haematoma seen on CT.

The use of viable omentum as a pack or filler continues to be a useful technique. Although its efficacy has not been validated by controlled studies there is adequate documentation of its positive benefits. It is presumed that this method works because the omentum is able to tamponade deep intrahepatic venous bleeding, local oozing from hepatotomy sites, and biliary leaks. More recently, temporary packing has re-emerged as an acceptable technique in managing liver injuries after the failure of other resectional techniques in controlling haemorrhage. The renewed interest in perihepatic packing was precipitated by the poor results obtained in patients who had hepatic injuries associated with intraoperative hypothermia, metabolic acidosis, and coagulopathy. Packing allows for a quick exit from the abdomen in these critically ill patients and is a valuable technique for the surgeon encountering a hepatic injury that is beyond his surgical capability. It is also of benefit in patients who will require hospital transfer to a more experienced unit because of continued bleeding following the performance of routine measures for hepatic haemostasis. Indeed, there now appears to be a more positive approach to the general use of intra-abdominal packing as a first measure in the exsanguinating patient. Under the label of "damage control", packing a temporary abdominal closure is advocated as the initial procedure to enable physiological stability to be restored prior to conducting definitive procedures on a stable patient.

Debate continues as to whether perihepatic packing is associated with a greater incidence of intra-abdominal sepsis (IAS) in comparison with resectional surgery. Large series show the infection rates to be similar (approximately 10–15%). It is probable that one of the main contributing factors in the development of IAS is the magnitude of the original injury and the extent of tissue that has been devitalised.[15]

Mesh hepatorrhaphy: this technique of compressive haemorrhagic control employs a synthetic absorbable mesh of polyglycolic acid or polyglactin which is wrapped around the liver to obtain haemostasis. This is similar to the method used for splenic preservation and a more detailed account of the technique can be found in a recent paper by Reed *et al.*[16] Because the liver has two points of vascular fixation (the portal triad and the inferior vena cava) the two lobes of the liver have to be wrapped separately. It is important that the compression provided is tight enough to achieve haemostasis but not so tight as to cause ischaemia. The technique appears to be most useful in patients with gaping lacerations, hepatotomy sites, or several large viable hepatic fragments still attached to the hilum, or when decapsulation has occurred. Mesh hepatorrhaphy appears to control haemorrhage in patients without retrohepatic venous injuries and has the major advantage of avoiding re-operation. However, the main criticism of this technique is the amount of time that it takes, and some would argue that the patient may be better served by the rapid insertion of perihepatic packs.

Retrohepatic injuries: injury to the hepatic veins and inferior vena cava are fortunately rare but are more common with blunt than penetrating trauma. Management of this type of injury requires greater surgical expertise and even in the best hands mortality is high (50–90%). Recent evidence appears to justify the use of perihepatic packing in some cases. However, if this fails then the use of an atriocaval shunt prior to haemostasis and repair may be necessary. These techniques have been described in more detail by Reed *et al*[16] and Wilson and Moorhead.[10]

Complications

Sepsis and haemorrhage are the major complications encountered. The latter may be exacerbated by the development of a coagulopathy. Hyperpyrexia (moderate—temperature $> 38°C$ for > 3 days; severe—temperature $> 39°C$ for > 3 days) occurs in up to two thirds of patients though its cause remains unknown. Biliary fistulae or haemobilia may also develop, the latter often requiring angiographic embolisation in severe cases.

Intestinal injuries

The management of small bowel and colon injuries is very different. In general, injuries to the small intestine can nearly always be managed by primary reanastomosis regardless of the mechanism of injury, severity of devitalised tissue, and presence of associated injuries.

Blunt injury

Blunt trauma is a recognised cause of intestinal injury and is typically associated with abdominal compression by seat belts in motor vehicles. The mechanism of injury is either by direct compression or by rapid deceleration. Compression may cause a spectrum of injuries to the bowel, ranging from simple serosal tears to complete transection and contusion as the bowel is forcibly compressed. Rapid deceleration is usually the cause of mesenteric tears, which may result in intestinal ischaemia.

Penetrating injuries

Penetrating injuries encountered in combat are different from those seen in civilians. The use of high velocity firearms in war results in extensive tissue destruction around the path of the missile. The time from injury to hospital transfer and surgery may also be greater, and under these circumstances colonic injuries are nearly always managed by the formation of a colostomy. In contrast, in civilians these injuries are nearly always due to knife and gunshot wounds and can therefore be managed differently.

Management of colonic injuries

The traditional management of colon wounds by exteriorisation or proximal colostomy was influenced by the wartime experience that these injuries resulted in a high complication rate. Unacceptably high morbidity and mortality rates associated with colon wounds and primary repair in the early months of the second world war led military surgeons to establish exteriorisation of the colon proximal to the site of the injury as the appropriate method of management. The goal of early colostomy was to establish an alternative pathway for the faecal stream and to prevent intra-abdominal sepsis as a result of peritoneal soiling. Despite this background, however, the management of civilian colonic injuries has undergone significant changes in the last two decades, with many surgeons questioning the validity of the practice of exteriorisation.[17] Citing the facts that civilian wounds are generally less destructive than those of high velocity missiles and shrapnel encountered during combat and that there have been major advances in fluid resuscitation, antibiotic treatment, and prompt trauma management, surgeons began to consider primary closure of colonic injuries.

Generally speaking, right-sided colonic injuries can be managed either by primary repair or by hemicolectomy. The problems of management tend to be associated with injury to the left colon. In a prospective randomised trial comparing obligatory colostomy and primary repair,

---

Factors influencing the need to fashion a colostomy

Absolute indications: Rectal injury
Open pelvic fracture
Blunt colonic injury

Relative indications: Rectal impalement
Penetrating trauma
Delayed/missed diagnosis
Military wounds
Civilian injury

Contraindications: Open abdomen
Massive transfusion
Coagulopathy
Acidosis
Hypothermia
Staged repair

---

where one of seven high risk factors were present, Stone and Fabian found that patients with primary closure fared better overall.[18] Additionally, colostomy patients required more hospital resources than those with primary repair, both during the initial hospital stay and subsequently for colostomy closure. There are now generally accepted guidelines that may help to decide whether to perform primary repair. Factors that have been considered to be adverse for primary repair include:

- Preoperative shock; systolic blood pressure less than 80 mm Hg

- More than 1 litre of intraperitoneal blood

- More than two intra-abdominal organs injured

- Significant faecal peritoneal contamination

- A delay of greater than 6 hours from injury to laparotomy

- Colonic injuries requiring major resection

- Major loss of tissue from the abdominal wall.

Indications for colostomy (see box): injuries sustained from high velocity missiles, blast injury, and other combat wounds should all be managed by repair and proximal defunctioning colostomy, or by resection and end colostomy. For colonic injuries encountered in civilians the indications for colostomy can be divided into absolute and relative. Absolute indications include open pelvic fractures, extensive rectal injury, and extensive colonic injury due to blunt trauma.[19] Relative indications include most types of blunt trauma, rectal impalement, and injuries that are associated with a delay in treatment as a result of a misdiagnosis or triage error. There are relatively few contraindications to the use of a colostomy in the management of colonic injuries.

It is the general conclusion from the many studies on the subject that most penetrating colonic injuries can be repaired regardless of the presence of most of the risk factors previously described.[20] Colostomy is recommended only for those with a significant delay to definitive surgery or in those in whom there is a coagulopathy as a result of major blood loss. Suture repair of the colon is associated with a much higher success rate than when resection and primary anastomosis are employed. Current practice in trauma centres suggests that greater than 75% of those with penetrating colonic injuries may be candidates for primary repair, with surgical judgment regarding associated risk factors relegating the remainder of the patients to a diverting colostomy.

Vascular injuries

In the USA abdominal vascular injuries are seen much more frequently in civilians than in a military combat situation.[21] This is more a reflection of the modest wounding capacity of the many handguns in the public domain in comparison with high velocity firearms and also the much shorter transit time from the incident to arrival in hospital. Blunt trauma is associated with a much lower incidence of vascular injuries (5–10%) than that observed with penetrating injuries (10–20%). Blunt injuries cause vascular impairment either through an avulsion injury or as a result of an intimal tear with subsequent thrombosis of the vessel, and they are much more likely in the upper abdomen (zone II).

Management

Clearly, initial management will depend on the patient's condition. Those with contained retroperitoneal haematomas are likely to be rapidly stabilised with intravenous fluids. Conversely, those with a distended abdomen due to free intraperitoneal haemorrhage are likely to be difficult if not impossible to stabilise. In such circumstances emergency thoracotomy with cross clamping of the descending thoracic aorta may be necessary to maintain cerebral and coronary blood flow during the period of transit to the operating theatre. Although the use of this technique remains controversial,[22] it is the only available technique that attempts to prevent the irreversible ischaemic changes to the oxygen starved brain. Active haemorrhage requires prompt control by proximal and distal isolation of the artery concerned. In contrast, injuries to major veins may not be amenable to vascular clamping because of size and location of the vessel and in these circumstances direct compression with packs may be more appropriate.

Once vascular control has been obtained attention should focus on the gastrointestinal tract in order to prevent further enteric contamination of the peritoneal cavity. Vascular repair or reconstruction can then proceed and may range from simple suture repair to prosthetic graft reconstruction. The decision whether to open and explore a retroperitoneal haematoma is clearly very difficult and should only be made by an experienced surgeon, often after consultation with his orthopaedic colleagues if a pelvic fracture is present. In general, upper abdominal retroperitoneal haematomas should be explored, whereas most pelvic retroperitoneal haematomas are now managed non-operatively. In the mid-abdomen it is generally wise to explore such haematomata.[22]

Pancreatic and duodenal injuries

The low incidence of pancreatic and duodenal injury is a reflection of their deep seated position in the retroperitoneum where they are shielded posteriorly by the bony vertebrae and by the paravertebral musculature. Injury to these organs therefore implies high energy blunt injury or a deep penetrating injury. The incidence of pancreatic and duodenal injuries has increased over the last two decades as the speed of motor vehicles has increased. Because of their location and proximity to so many surrounding structures, multiple abdominal injuries are the rule rather than the exception, the liver being the other structure most frequently involved.

Diagnosis and management

With blunt injuries of the pancreas and duodenum concomitant vascular injury is seen in 10% of cases. The key to diagnosis in these cases rests on a high index of suspicion. The serum amylase is raised in approximately 80% of patients with pancreatic injury due to blunt trauma, but in only 25% when injury is penetrating in nature. Computed tomography has not been demonstrated to be useful in the assessment and diagnosis of pancreatic injury.

The diagnosis of pancreatic and duodenal injury is more often than not made at laparotomy. However, injuries of the pancreas and duodenal loop are the most commonly missed of all abdominal injuries. Thus in all cases of upper abdominal trauma a thorough and careful exploration of this area of the abdomen is mandatory. This will include opening the lesser sac to inspect the pancreatic body and kocherising the duodenum to inspect the second and third parts of the duodenum and pancreatic head. If necessary, the peritoneum at the inferior border of the pancreas may be incised to allow elevation of the body and tail of the pancreas to inspect the posterior surface. If bile staining is present and no cause is found with the above procedures then the ligament of Treitz should be divided, allowing mobilisation and full circumferential inspection of the fourth part of the duodenum.

Most duodenal injuries are minor tears on the anterior surface. Although simple suture repair is effective in these cases it is essential that the posterior wall of the duodenum is also examined. In cases of duodenal wall loss, repair may be by side to side duodenojejunostomy or by a jejunal serosal patch. When there has been gross tissue destruction management should aim to exclude the duodenal loop from the pylorus. This is effectively achieved by cross stapling the pylorus and constructing a gastrojejunostomy. Duct transection or transection of the gland itself and contusion of the pancreatic head are the main types of pancreatic injury encountered. Management of these injuries is either by repair and drainage or by resection with reconstruction and drainage.

Outcome

Despite many improvements in the management of such injuries the mortality remains high and, as might be anticipated, the highest mortality rates are in patients requiring pancreatic resection, with fatality rates approaching 25%. The majority of deaths in patients sustaining pancreaticoduodenal injury result from haemorrhage and shock, and most die within 24–48 hours. Late death is usually due to pulmonary and systemic septic complications, specific pancreatic complications being the cause of death in only a small proportion of cases.

Urological injuries

Genitourinary injuries occur in 10–15% of cases of abdominal trauma with blunt injuries accounting for 80% of cases of renal trauma.

Renal injuries

Although the kidney appears to be relatively well protected by the vertebral bodies and postvertebral muscles, renal injuries are not as rare as one would expect. The kidneys receive approximately 20% of the cardiac output. Therefore major parenchymal or vascular injuries rapidly result in major blood loss and hypovolaemic shock. Most blunt injuries are minor and a subcapsular haematoma is the only finding. However, the degree of haematuria does not correlate with the degree of injury. Arterial injury is usually the result of rapid deceleration. As the renal artery is stretched on deceleration, the intimal layer ruptures and separates from the media. This is followed by thrombosis and renal ischaemia. In 85% of cases the renal artery is a solitary end artery and the small amount of collateral circulation is insufficient to support renal viability. Early diagnosis and treatment of a renal vascular injury is therefore mandatory. Similar arterial injuries may be seen in the segmental branches of the renal artery. Blunt trauma affecting the renal parenchyma results in transection of the organ in the transverse plane, beginning at the border of the cortex and spreading into the medulla and collecting systems. The deeper the parenchymal laceration the greater the likelihood of significant blood loss as a result.

Classification: minor injuries account for up to 90% of all blunt renal injuries and include parenchymal contusions and superficial lacerations that extend only into the renal cortex. Lacerations extending into the deep medullary portion of the kidney are classed as major injuries. Vascular injuries, regardless of degree, are also classed as major injuries.

Management: approximately 95% of blunt renal injuries can be managed conservatively. All patients with minor trauma and a few with major injuries may be managed conservatively. Patients with gross haematuria should be placed on strict bed rest with ambulation commencing when gross bleeding has stopped. Bleeding from small calibre renal arteries can be controlled by selective embolisation at angiography. Penetrating injuries require surgical exploration unless staging information suggests that non-operative management may be sufficient.

There are no clear or universally accepted guidelines which can be used as an indication for renal exploration. The following, however, are suggested: vascular injury, pulsatile haematoma, extensive extravasation, expanding retroperitoneal haematoma, and non-viable tissue in more than 20% of the kidney. Operative intervention should aim to achieve early vascular control by isolating the renal arteries at the aorta. Gerota's fascia can then be opened and the kidney exposed. After careful inspection all non-viable tissue is debrided. Haemostatic sutures should be placed and the renal capsule held in approximation. Absorbable sutures should always be used. If the capsule has been destroyed, coverage with omentum or peritoneum may aid in preventing delayed bleeding or urinary extravasation. Nephrostomy is rarely required because internal stents may be placed if required. Closed system drainage of the perirenal space may be necessary for several days until all extravasations cease. In the face of continued drainage of urine, distal ureteric obstruction must be excluded.

A full discussion of the management of renal vascular injuries is beyond the scope of this chapter.[23]

Outcome: renal salvage can be expected in more than 90% of cases and late hypertension is uncommon, occurring in less than 5% of patients. However, the outcome following primary repair of major renal pedicle injury appears to be poor and some suggest that autotransplantation is a better procedure to deal with this problem.

Other genitourinary injuries

The rest of the urinary tract will only be briefly considered. For a more detailed account of ureteric, vesical, and urethral injuries a more specialist text should be consulted.

Ureteric injuries: ureteric injury following blunt trauma is rare and when seen is usually an avulsion injury. Gun shot and stab wounds are more common causes of ureteral injury. Diagnosis of such injuries is usually made by IVP or surgical exploration. The principles of ureteric repair are adequate debridement, tension free repair, adopting a spatulated anastomosis, the use of ureteral stenting in selected cases, and retroperitoneal drainage. Fistulas are unusual after ureteric repair but may occur if a stricture or obstruction develops, although most cases will close spontaneously with adequate drainage.

Bladder injuries: these are often seen in association with pelvic fractures. Rarely is bladder rupture seen without an associated pelvic fracture, and in these cases rupture is due to a direct blow to the full bladder. Non-operative management by prolonged catheter drainage (about 14 days) may be adopted if the rupture is extraperitoneal and the urine is sterile at the time of injury. If low pressure cystography demonstrates continued leakage then catheter drainage can continue until spontaneous closure occurs. The main risk from this approach is the potential for infection within any associated retroperitoneal haematoma. Intraperitoneal rupture usually requires a multilayer repair of the bladder wall. Extraperitoneal lacerations are repaired from within the bladder. Severe venous bleeding from pelvic fractures should be initially managed by application of an external fixator to the pelvic ring, but continued bleeding can be managed by packing and re-exploration. Arterial bleeding can respond dramatically to arterial embolisation. Cystostomy drainage should be maintained for 7–10 days. Fortunately, vesical injuries nearly always heal uneventfully without any complications.

Uretheral injuries: these are nearly always associated with pelvic fractures. The major cause of urethral rupture is blunt trauma at the level of the urogenital diaphragm. Blood at the external urinary meatus is the single most important physical sign in the diagnosis of urethral trauma. Rectal examination in these cases is mandatory to exclude a major bladder neck or prostatic injury. The decision whether to attempt urethral catheterisation in this situation remains contentious, as in doing so an incomplete laceration may be converted into a complete laceration. Many would agree that the absence of blood at the external urethral meatus and the presence of a palpable prostate on rectal examination are sufficient evidence to allow careful and gentle passage of a narrow urethral catheter by an experienced surgeon. Alternatively, if the bladder is palpable, the insertion of a suprapubic catheter is relatively simple and safe. In cases of doubt, a

189

retrograde urethrogram will establish the diagnosis. If a urethral tear is confirmed then a suprapubic catheter is generally thought to be the treatment of choice. Subsequent management should be by an experienced urological surgeon.

1 Root HD, Hauser CW, McKinley CR, *et al*. Diagnostic peritoneal lavage. *Surgery* 1965; **57**: 633–7.
2 Day AC, Rankin N, Charlesworth P. Diagnostic peritoneal lavage: integration with clinical information to improve diagnostic performance. *J Trauma* 1992; **32**: 52–7.
3 Fischer RP, Beverlin BC, Engrav LH, *et al*. Diagnostic peritoneal lavage: fourteen years and 2586 patients later. *Am J Surg* 1978; **136**: 701–4.
4 Fischer RP, Miller-Crotchett P, Reed RL. Gastrointestinal disruption: the hazard of nonoperative management in adults with blunt abdominal injury. *J Trauma* 1988; **28**: 1445–9.
5 Tso P, Rodriguez A, Cooper C, *et al*. Sonography in blunt abdominal trauma: a preliminary progress report. *J Trauma* 1992; **32**: 39–44.
6 Bode PJ, Niezen RA, van Vugt AB, Schipper J. Abdominal ultrasound as a reliable indicator for conclusive laparotomy in blunt abdominal trauma. *J Trauma* 1993; **34**: 27–31.
7 Eastham JA, Wilson TG, Ahlering TE. Radiographic assessment of blunt renal trauma. *J Trauma* 1991; **31**: 1527–8.
8 Ivatury RR, Simon RJ, Weksler B. Laparoscopy in the evaluation of the intrathoracic abdomen after penetrating injury. *J Trauma* 1992; **32**: 101–9.
9 Koury HI, Peschiera JL, Welling RE. Non-operative management of blunt splenic trauma: a 10 year experience. *Injury* 1991; **22**: 349–52.
10 Wilson RH, Moorehead RJ. Management of splenic trauma. *Injury* 1992; **23**: 5–9.
11 Feliciano DV, Spjut-Patrinley V, Burch JM, *et al*. Splenorrhaphy. The alternative. *Ann Surg* 1990; **211**: 569–82.
12 Feliciano DV, Bitondo CG, Mattox KL, *et al*. A four-year experience with splenectomy versus splenorrhaphy. *Ann Surg* 1985; **201**: 568–75.
13 Wilson RH, Moorhead RJ. Hepatic trauma and its management. *Injury* 1991; **22**: 439–45.
14 Cogbill TH, Moore EE, Jurkovich GJ, *et al*. Severe hepatic trauma: a multi-center experience with 1335 liver injuries. *J Trauma* 1988; **28**: 1433–8.
15 Croce MA, Fabian TC, Stewart RM, *et al*. Correlation of abdominal trauma index and injury severity score with abdominal septic complications in penetrating and blunt trauma. *J Trauma* 1992; **32**: 380–8.
16 Reed RL, Merrell RC, Meyers WC, *et al*. Continuing evolution in the management of severe hepatic trauma. *Ann Surg* 1992; **216**: 524–38.
17 George SM, Fabian TC, Voeller GR, *et al*. Primary repair of colon wounds; a prospective trial in nonselected patients. *Ann Surg* 1989; **209**: 728–34.
18 Stone H, Fabian T. Management of penetrating colon trauma. *Ann Surg* 1979; **190**: 430–6.
19 Fallon WF. The present role of colostomy in the management of trauma. *Dis Colon Rectum* 1992; **35**: 1094–102.
20 Demetriades D, Pantanowitz, Charalambides D. Gunshot wounds of the colon: role of primary repair. *Ann R Coll Surg* 1992; **74**: 381–4.
21 Rignault DP. Abdominal trauma in war. *World J Surg* 1992; **16**: 940–6.
22 Feliciano DV. Management of traumatic retroperitoneal haematoma. *Ann Surg* 1990; **211**: 109–23.
23 McAnich JW. Renal injuries. In: Mattox KL, Moore EE, Feliciano DV, eds. *Trauma*. East Norwalk: Appleton and Lange, 1988: 537–52.

14

Handling of casualties by the fire service, with experiences from the Manchester air disaster

ROBERT W DOCHERTY

Introduction

This chapter deals with aircraft accidents where firefighters from the airport fire service and the local authority fire service have to deal effectively with a potentially hazardous situation. Tasks to be considered by firefighters will include extinguishing or suppressing an already burning fire, eliminating the danger of ignition where fire is not present, and rescuing casualties.

In all cases the main aim is the saving of life, but in order to achieve this aim it is essential to control any fire, eliminate the danger of ignition, and secure the scene for rescue personnel. All initial firefighting techniques are therefore designed to allow evacuation and assist survival.

No one aircraft accident is the same as another and so different types of aircraft fires can be expected. It is therefore difficult to employ any fixed strategy or tactic without first adapting it to the particular incident. Fires can be external or internal and may not involve fuel. However, the risk of a fire is a constant threat. The plan, tactics, and techniques for fighting aircraft fires must therefore form a framework of reference for firefighters and this framework must be flexible enough to fit any situation that is encountered.

An aircraft fire can intensify quickly and bring with it a situation that rapidly deteriorates. The skill of firefighters in the use of their equipment, with the correct techniques, is essential and can only be accomplished by having the correct selection of personnel who are highly trained and practised in all fire and rescue techniques.

Firefighting techniques

When an aircraft accident occurs, large numbers of people become involved. These range from rescue and firefighting personnel to other groups, including the press, government officials, airline officials, public sightseers, etc. The latter groups all add to complicate the firefighter's role and need to be effectively controlled. The use of tabards—brightly coloured tunics, preferably with identification marks—by rescuers aids the identification of key personnel, and the policing of others is important. Control of the accident site is best achieved by classifying zones of control.

Zones of control

Incident zone (Bronze control):

- The actual incident site and fire area immediately surrounding the aircraft, including the major sections of wreckage

- In this zone, rescue workers and firefighters can operate to establish control and can act to coordinate for both the rescue and firefighting operations

Assisting services zone (Silver control):

- An area preferably selected upwind and uphill from the incident zone

- This zone functions as a triage (casualty handling) point together with ambulance loading, forward incident control points, and parking for other emergency vehicles

- Part of this area may be designated for the collection and removal of the uninjured and a separate area may also be used as a temporary mortuary

Outer zone (Gold control):

- Houses all the other assisting services such as emergency hospitals, "permanent" mortuaries, and airline offices

- In specific instances, this area may be used for the casualty loading area so that ambulances can get to the accident site without going over rough terrain

---

Aircrashes at airports

When approaching an accident on an airport site the route chosen will usually be the one that provides the quickest transportation for firefighting vehicles. This may not be the most direct route: it should avoid going over rough ground that may result in more delay than a more conventional but longer route.

When there is a rapid intervention vehicle provided, this will normally be the first to reach the scene. The aim of this vehicle and its crew is to prevent an outbreak of fire and assist in the rescue phase. Where fire has broken out an attempt should be made to extinguish the fire and clear an evacuation path. The officer in charge of this vehicle should assess the situation and determine the best positioning for the major vehicles when they arrive.

Airport rescue and firefighting vehicles will normally be the first to arrive at the scene and the officer in charge will deploy his resources in a manner which does not obstruct escaping passengers or crew and ensures that doorways and escape slides are kept usable.

As a general rule, firefighting vehicles should be kept upwind and uphill of the incident, but wind direction may not always be the most important factor in dictating the direction of approach and positioning of appliances. Indeed it may play a part in keeping parts of the fuselage free of flame. All parts of the fuselage are highly vulnerable to fire, and a careful watch must be maintained on the integrity and stability of the aircraft structure at all times. One of the main considerations of vehicle positioning is that the vehicles themselves are not threatened by fire, heat, or the terrain that they are working on.

If the aircrash happens off the runway and in soft terrain, all rescue and firefighting vehicles may have to be kept on the hard standing surfaces. This will result in the need to use hand lines for firefighting. Free flowing fuel may surround firefighters and it should always be covered by an extinguishing agent to reduce the risk of ignition that would engulf the firefighters in fire.

The correct positioning of all gear is vital if the operational rescue and firefighting response is to be successful.

The primary aim of firefighters will be to keep the fire away from the escape routes and the escaping occupants. This must be done without hindering or obstructing the rescue operation. It should always be borne in mind that foam or water on surfaces that escaping occupants have to cross or use, such as the aircraft wings, will make them slippery and therefore more dangerous.

Foam has to be applied in sufficient quantities to achieve rapid flame knockdown and prevent re-ignition. Firefighting will normally be initially directed to the fuselage and then outwards, care being taken not to disturb fuel with too direct an application of foam, which may in some circumstances drive fuel under the fuselage.

As soon as possible, a crew of firefighting personnel will enter the fuselage to give warning of any fire penetration of the fuselage. If this occurs, then water fog or fine spray jets should be used to cool the area involved and extinguish any fire that has entered the fuselage.

If fire does penetrate the fuselage, there can be a rapid build up of heat and smoke and the cabin will become quickly filled with smoke. If this occurs, firefighting crews may find it necessary to ventilate the fuselage to allow the heat and smoke to dissipate and thus reduce the atmosphere to tolerable levels.

Aircrashes away from airports

Where an aircraft is forced to make an emergency landing away from an airport, the location of the accident site will dictate the direction of access to the incident that the emergency services should make. Firefighting vehicles will not normally be able to cross rough terrain and crews may therefore have to proceed to the incident on foot. When this happens care will have to be taken with regard to the parking of firefighting vehicles so that they do not block or hinder the movement of other vehicles that need to approach the crash site. Vigilance is essential when approaching the area of the crash site in case survivors have been thrown clear or have crawled or walked away from the aircraft.

If the crash has happened within an urban area, then firefighting will be carried out in a similar manner to a crash at an airport, although there may have to be firefighting crews deployed in a conventional role using water sprays and jets on fires in any buildings that have become involved.

Crashes that occur in remote areas may be hampered by fires in fields, woodland, etc. that may have been burning for some time and delays in attending the scene may result because of the distance that the firefighting vehicles and crews may have to travel. Other problems such as a lack of water supplies and poor access may be encountered and the officer in charge will need to assess such priorities as:

- Tackling the main body of the fire with the resources available

- Using extinguishing agents or water to prevent the spread of fire that might hamper further resources from attending the scene

- Looking for survivors while waiting for adequate reinforcements before tackling any fire

- Looking for additional supplies of water and starting to relay them to the site.

Handling of casualties

An early systemic and careful search will be made of the whole of the crash area and beyond, including the flight path that the aircraft has taken prior to its final resting position. Survivors must always be considered a possibility even in the most serious crashes; they may wander from the immediate vicinity of the crash and may collapse in places where they are obscured from view, such as ditches or under hedges. Injured survivors may also have been thrown clear and be lying around the wreckage, while others may still be in or under the debris.

Handling casualties will be an important consideration in any off-airport incident, as the injured may be placed in an area demarcated for casualty handling and clearance (a triage post). In this area, first aid can be given and the injuries assessed. Documentation of the personal details of the casualties and identification of their location when rescued should be made if practicable before transfer to ambulances. The casualty handling and clearance area should be sited in a position that is clear of any risk of fire and is near to the ambulance loading area.

Some casualties may be so badly injured that it may be best to treat them initially where they are found, providing there is no further risk to them, until medical treatment can be administered. The closest cooperation and liaison is required between the medical services and firefighting crews to ensure that this part of the rescue operation is coordinated correctly.

Rescue

For effective evacuation and rescue, firefighters need to protect the normal aircraft escape routes and the other routes that the survivors may take in order to escape. The evacuation and rescue must proceed at the greatest possible speed, the initial emphasis being on the safety of the rescuers, the safety of the occupants, the maintenance of escape routes, and the protection of the fuselage.

Other activities frequently expected of firefighters are involvement in improving the efficiency and effectiveness of the rescue by coping with and resolving the problems of areas around an aircraft soaked in fuel and covered with foam, the provision of lighting for the accident if it occurs at night, and the movement of occupants away from the hazardous area.

During the period when occupants are escaping from the aircraft, no entry should be made by rescuers through any of the routes being used by the escaping occupants. There may be some occupants who cannot make their own way via escape routes without help, and their rescue can be a long, arduous, and harrowing task. Their rescue may involve the use of a variety of rescue equipment and rescue personnel—for example, firefighters, aircraft engineers, medical teams—all of whom have different jobs to do and tasks to perform: although these may seem to conflict at times, the efforts of all have to be coordinated in order to achieve the fastest and safest extrication and evacuation of the casualties without aggravating their injuries.

During this time, firefighting operations and protection will be maintained both inside and outside the aircraft, including the maintenance of any foam blanket that has been laid.

Firefighters have three main tasks to perform once the fire is under control. These are:

- To make an entry into the cabin to assist any occupants who are still inside. Entry may only be possible for firefighters wearing breathing apparatus; they should take with them sufficient equipment to help free any occupants who are trapped and give first aid treatment where necessary

- To ensure that firefighting equipment is taken into the cabin upon entry

- To ensure adequate lighting equipment is provided and adequate ventilation is obtained within the cabin.

It should always be remembered that for some accidents—and the M1 accident was such a case—entry to the cabin can be obtained not only through the normal doors and emergency exits but also through artificially created access holes in the fuselage.

Once entry has been made, firefighters may be confronted with tangled wreckage, loose luggage and debris, seats torn from mountings, and interior lining ripped away. Any internal fire should be tackled immediately, although one of the first priorities must be to clear a working space. It may then be necessary to make the aircraft safe, and the movement of any switches or controls will be noted, so that such information can be passed on to the accident investigating authority.

Where passengers and crew are found inside the aircraft, it should be assumed that they will be either dazed, injured, trapped, or dead. An assessment of the situation is carried out quickly and a system for prioritising the first aid treatment and the release and rescue of the survivors is set up. Firefighters should then consult any medical teams available on site as to the medical state of casualties and to the prioritising of their rescue. All firefighting crews must work carefully and in unison, applying a common sense approach.

Lessons from the Manchester air disaster

Each aircraft accident is unique. The Manchester air disaster highlighted the effects of smoke and the great difficulty occupants have in exiting from an aircraft that is on fire. The result of this accident was the introduction of illuminated strips that lead to aircraft exits. The introduction of smoke hoods remains controversial, but the increasing use of less flammable materials will improve fire safety.

In the M1 aircrash one of the problems was obtaining access to the different parts of the plane, and an artificially created access point in the fuselage might have made a big difference to the speed of the rescue operation.

Summary

- Successful firefighting, rescue, and casualty handling in aircraft accidents are dependent upon the skills, abilities, and competence of the first crews to arrive at the crash

- Their efforts and endeavours allow precious time to be gained so that rescue and medical teams can maximise their efforts in saving life

- The firefighters' role combines preventing and extinguishing fire with evacuation and rescue

- Their efforts must be coordinated with those of other rescue workers

- To ensure the maximum benefit from all rescue workers, there is a need to pre-plan for such disasters and to train and practice the plan regularly

- By training and practice, not only is the effectiveness of the rescue workers maximised but also there follows a greater understanding between the disciplines involved and greater cooperation can be developed

- Plans must be flexible—no two aircraft accidents are the same

15

Management of burns in trauma victims, with experiences from the UK and the USA

CHARLES M MALATA, JC FITZPATRICK,
BA PRUITT JR, DAVID T SHARPE

Introduction

Aircraft accidents, although infrequent, have a fearsome reputation for producing fatalities and a large number of critically injured subjects. Those injured can be the crew, passengers, or spectators, as occurred at the Ramstein Airshow in 1985.[1] Aircraft accidents are often accompanied by fire, thus adding thermal injury to the wide range of mechanical injuries. The United States National Transportation Safety Board (NTSB) has estimated that between 1965 and 1974 15% of all fatal US air carrier accidents were attributable to the effects of fire.[2] Fire, as compared with impact trauma, drowning, or blast injury, was involved in at least 65% of the deaths in US airline accidents between 1965 and 1982.[3] In recent years the percentage of airline deaths in which fire was involved has not decreased.[4] Smoke inhalation is also common in these accidents, adding to the morbidity and mortality of the victims. Burns and their complications stand out as the most frequent cause of death among passengers in survivable aircraft accidents.[5]

Although important, the management of burns in multiply injured patients takes second priority to the management of immediately life threatening injuries, the maxim being to "first forget all about the burns" (DM Heimbach, personal communication). Only after treatment of the immediately life threatening injuries should attention be turned to the cutaneous burns. With few exceptions, the subsequent management of the

198

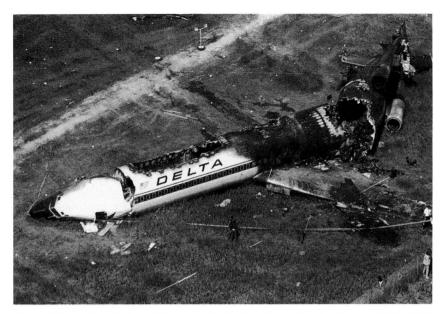

Figure 15.1—The Delta Airlines crash, Dallas-Fort Worth, Texas, 1988. With permission of the Dallas Morning News *and Juan Garcia.*

aircraft burns victim is along similar lines to that of burns patients with multiple injuries due to other forms of trauma. The purpose of this chapter is to provide a review of aircraft fires and to discuss the proper triage and care of burns victims following survivable aircraft accidents.

Aircraft fires

General points

Fires and explosions are a common occurrence in aircraft accidents for three primary reasons: large quantities of fuel are present; aircraft interiors are lined and furnished with combustible materials; and the high impact velocities of aircraft increase the likelihood of igniting a fire in the event of an accident. The materials that may burn are petroleum products, interior furnishings, baggage, cargo, and finally the metallic frame of the aircraft. The two main hazards of an aircraft fire are cutaneous burns resulting from heat and "flashover", and inhalation injury resulting from smoke and toxic fumes.

Aircraft fires may occur post-crash, in flight, and on the ground. Post-crash fires (see figure 15.1) are the most common by a large margin, followed by in-flight, and lastly the rare (and least dangerous) on-ground

199

fires. In-flight fires may begin in the cabin interior, engines, or baggage compartment. Full-blown fires are nearly impossible to escape from and claim many lives, but most in-flight fires occur in accessible areas, such as toilets or galleys, where the fire is discovered early and extinguished.[6,7] Most commonly, post-crash fires result from fuel ignition. In post-crash fires there is only a short escape period after impact before fire and toxic fumes occur. These periods average 135 seconds in airplanes and 16 seconds in helicopters, and are important because at least 12% of the fire associated deaths in US airline accidents are believed to be due to the release of carbon monoxide (CO) or cyanogen gases.[3] Victims of the crash should be evacuated quickly—not forgetting that they may have associated spinal fractures that must be stabilised before movement—both for their welfare and for the safety of the rescue teams. Even if fires do not occur immediately post-crash, ruptured fuel tanks may release flammable vapours that can collect near the cabin ceiling and "flashover" within 60–90 seconds after the exits are opened.[3] These flashover fires can spread throughout the length of the fuselage, instantaneously consuming the remaining oxygen. Mortality from post-crash fires is 2.4 times greater than from in-flight fires.[4] The initiation, extension, and propagation of post-crash fires was reviewed by Hill[4] and Galea and Markatos,[6] and interested readers are referred to their excellent discussions of the sequential events occurring in aircraft fires.[4,6]

Thermal injuries are not universal in air accidents; they appear to be directly related to impact velocity and the quantities of flammable substances present. Notable examples are the M1 aircrash at Kegworth, in which the low velocity (100 miles/h) at impact was found to be an important factor in the lack of fire,[8] and the Avianca 052 air crash in New York in which little jet fuel (6% of its capacity) remained as the aircraft was about to land.[9] Despite such exceptions, fire is still a serious cause of mortality and morbidity in aircraft accidents.[10] A useful classification of aviation accidents is that of Dudani,[11] which relates injury characteristics to the presence, alone or in combination, of impact, fire, explosion, and hazardous cargo. Determination of which of these components are present on arrival at the scene of the accident promotes effective and informed patient triage, ensures appropriate initial care, and identifies rescuer safety needs.[9]

Factors that increase the risk of burn injury

Factors that impede escape from the fuselage of a burning aircraft increase the risk of burn injury. These factors include the degree of structural damage, the number of passengers on board, the trauma sustained by the passengers during the crash, and the thermotoxic environment present in a fire. The specific problems that escaping passengers are faced with include the following.

Visibility problems

Smoke is opaque, and smoke, gases, and toxic fumes are all highly irritating to the eyes and cause profuse lacrimation. Decreased visibility resulting from atmospheric opacification and lacrimation makes it difficult to identify exit signs and operate emergency exits.

Structural problems

At least 50% of exits are unusable after a crash,[12] due to twisting of the fuselage or blockage due to the position of the exit relative to the ground, water, or other wreckage. The exits and aisles may also be blocked with victims incapacitated by crash associated injuries or the thermotoxic environment.

The degree of mental and physical incapacitation

Injuries, especially concussions and limb fractures, make escape from a disorienting, structurally damaged, irritating, and low visibility environment difficult. Even seat belts may be hard for survivors to release. Pre-existing cardiac and respiratory diseases or sedating drugs may also contribute to the inability of the victims to escape.

Chemical incapacitation

Toxic effects from carbon monoxide (CO) inhalation and respiratory irritation from fumes and smoke particles can lead to hypoxia, laryngospasm, bronchospasm, and inhalation injury. These effects may be of sufficient severity to be lethal on their own. Hydrogen cyanide (HCN) inhalation contributes its lethal effect by impairing cellular respiration through its crippling effect on the oxidative phosphorylation pathway, preventing ATP generation. Experimental studies[13] show that CO and HCN in the cabin quickly rise to physiologically intolerable levels. Laboratory studies[13] indicate that a combination of CO and CN have a synergistic pharmacological effect causing incapacitation.

Emotional factors

Rational thought processes are impaired in the face of the above problems and by the intense fear and panic experienced by the victims of mechanical trauma. Passenger ignorance regarding the operation of exit doors and emergency escape windows, especially when coupled with crew incapacitation, compounds the fear and panic of the situation.

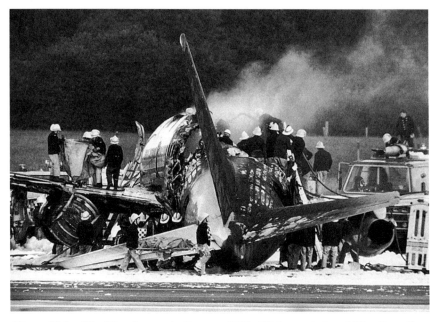

Figure 15.2—The Manchester air disaster, 1985. With permission of The Guardian.

These variables constitute the primary determinants affecting morbidity and mortality of burns following a survivable aircraft accident.

Injury pattern in aircraft accidents

General points

The burns victims of air crashes often have multiple trauma. The variety of injuries encountered depends upon the causative mechanisms involved— usually impact, fuel explosion, or escape from the aircraft.[14] In the 1988 Delta Airlines crash in Dallas, Texas, most of the passengers died immediately but the six burned survivors had also sustained multiple fractures, head injuries, and intra-abdominal injuries, two of which required laparotomies (JL Hunt, personal communication). All but one of these survivors eventually died. Mechanical trauma does not always occur, in particular when the accident is an on-ground fire such as the Manchester air disaster (figure 15.2).[15,16] These fires are usually associated with improved survival compared with in-flight and post-crash fires.

Differences exist between injuries sustained in fatal and non-fatal air accidents. The nature and severity of injuries reported from forensic postmortem examinations[4,14,17] contrast sharply with the experience of the

Box 15.1
Aircraft accident burns treated at the US Army Institute of
Surgical Research (1987–92)

	Patients
Aircraft type	
Helicopter	30
Fixed wing	10
Total	40
Types of associated injuries in aircraft crashes	
Transmetacarpal fractures, multiple lacerations, mandible fractures, humeral head fractures, radial head dislocations, Le Fort I fractures, L5 spine fractures, pneumothorax	
Inhalation injury	
Yes	20
No	20
Outcome*	
Alive	37
Died	3 (all had inhalation injury)

*p = 0.12 by Fisher's exact test

US Army Institute of Surgical Research (USAISR) burn unit (WF McManus, personal communication), and demonstrate that those who present to burns units for treatment tend to be those who have escaped with lesser injuries (Box 15.1). It is important to know the trauma pattern following fatal air crashes[14] to anticipate the likely injuries present in the seriously injured patients presenting to the accident and emergency department. Common occult injuries include basilar skull fracture, cerebral contusion, vertebral fracture, myocardial contusion, aortic transection, and intra-abdominal and extremity trauma. The importance of cerebral injuries is underscored by their occurrence in at least two thirds of air accident fatalities,[4,9,18] highlighting the susceptibility of the brain to impact trauma. In reviewing aircraft accidents between 1955 and 1979, Hill stated that there has been no change in the incidence of head injuries.[4] It is vitally important to seek and rule out associated injuries following standard trauma protocols to prevent morbidity and mortality secondary to missed injuries.

Types of burns and notable injuries in aircraft accidents

A wide spectrum of thermal injuries occurs in aircraft fires. Besides cutaneous thermal burns, the notable features of aircraft fires are an increased incidence of smoke inhalation injury, conjunctivitis and pronounced psychological problems. Cutaneous thermal burns do not seem to differ from burn injuries sustained in other circumstances. In the experience of the USAISR burn unit staff there is nothing unique about them. The various burns sustained by victims are related to certain causative factors (box 15.2).

Box 15.2
Types of burn injury and their causes

- *Radiant burns* result from proximity to the high temperatures (> 400°C) generated by the fire.[4] The radiant heat may ignite passengers' clothing, causing direct flame burns

- *Flash burns* are usually superficial, as occurred in the Ramstein Airshow disaster in which hundreds of spectators received partial thickness burns[1]

- *Chemical burns* may result from contact with aviation fuel or hydraulic fluid[14]

- *Contact burns* are caused by plastic interior fixtures that can melt and drip when ignited; hot plastic is very adherent to skin and has a high heat capacity, causing deep burns

- *Hypothermic injury* is also possible. In a recent accident in Denver, Colorado, an aircraft overturned on the runway, and it took rescue workers hours to free the passengers. A number of victims became hypothermic and some sustained cold thermal injuries. Similar problems were experienced in a recent Alaskan aircrash

- *Inhalation injury* is common in burns patients from aircraft accidents. A 6 year survey of the deaths from burns in army aircraft showed that respiratory complications were the main cause of delayed death in 80%.[19] The USAISR has the world's greatest experience of managing burns patients from aircraft accidents (see Box 15.1): of the 40 patients treated over the last 5 years 50% sustained inhalation injury. In the 1988 Delta Airlines crash in Dallas, Texas, 33% (2/6) of the burns survivors had inhalation injury (JL Hunt, personal communication)

- *Conjunctivitis* is caused by the rapid generation of dense and highly irritating fumes and particulate matter

- *Thermal injury* to the cornea, resulting in corneal opacification, is rare but has been reported

- *Psychological problems* are common in survivors of aircraft burns. All patients from the Manchester air disaster had nightmares, guilt feelings, and phobias about travel, crowds, and smoky rooms. Rod Watts, an Australian social worker who sustained severe burns following an aircraft accident, gives a vivid description of the short attention span, cloudiness of thinking, and sleeping difficulties he experienced in its aftermath[20]

Triage and general care of burns patients

Triage and first aid

Following an aircraft accident the prompt arrival of the rescue services, their efficient action, and the availability of appropriate medical help may enable those who survived the impact of an aircraft crash to live. The fire must be extinguished and controlled and the passengers evacuated or retrieved from the burning wreckage.

The general principles of burn patient evacuation and triage and hospital response employed in civil emergencies also apply to burns following air craft disasters.[21-25] Efficient triage will result in the greatest good being done for the greatest number of patients. Initial triage is frequently performed by the first paramedic or emergency medical technician arriving at the scene but should be taken over by the medical incident officer (accident site physician) when he or she arrives at the scene. After initial triage is performed and the magnitude of the injuries assessed, additional personnel may be requested as needed by the medical incident officer. A second person should assume responsibility for communication with area hospitals, relaying pertinent patient information, and distributing casualties among hospitals, with consideration of transport time to and capacity for patient treatment in each facility. A third person should organise specific areas outside the danger zone surrounding the site of the accident for triage, treatment of casualities, and evacuation of patients. A fourth person should collect information from the victims and ensure that all victims' destinations are recorded and that they can be accounted for at all times. Rescue personnel may then be directed to patients by the medical incident officer at the accident site by priority for treatment. Additional personnel should be assigned to crowd control and management of the site hazards to prevent additional casualties, under the supervision of law enforcement officers, rescue personnel, and fire department personnel.

Patients should be quickly examined and assigned to a treatment category. A typical system might contain four categories, in order of priority:

(1) Those who are in immediate danger of asphyxiation or exsanguination, and those already in shock—immediate treatment, advanced life support and transfer
(2) Patients who are at risk of developing shock—initial treatment and transfer within 1 hour
(3) Patients with minor injuries—transfer within 3 hours
(4) Patients who are dead or have sustained such overwhelming injuries that survival is very unlikely (for example, decapitation, severed trunk, unwitnessed cardiac arrest following blunt trauma, incineration).

205

The highest priority of treatment should be assigned to patients with airway obstruction or respiratory failure, witnessed cardiac arrest, uncontrolled external bleeding, tension pneumothorax, pericardial tamponade, open thoracic or abdominal wounds, severe closed head injuries, and severe burns (especially when complicated by inhalation injury). Second priority patients usually consist of patients with open or multiple fractures, spinal injuries, smaller burns, eye injuries, and hand injuries. Third priority patients usually have simple fractures, sprains, simple lacerations, and other minor injuries.

On receiving news of an aircraft accident the hospital should declare a major incident and activate its major accident plan. The specific cascade of subsequent events depends on the hospital's major accident plan, which must be rehearsed regularly in conjunction with the emergency services and neighbouring airports. A control centre (called a command post in the USA) is established by the medical, nursing, and administrative co-ordinators. They mobilise and prepare for reception of casualties in the accident and emergency department, operating theatre, and intensive care facilities. They should establish a triage point in the hospital emergency department. A separate burns ward should be opened if significant numbers of burns casualties are present.

The care of the aircraft accident victim, although frequently complicated by the additional thermal and inhalation injuries sustained as the result of post-crash fires, is not significantly different from the non-burned multiply injured patient and is still governed by the encompassing principles of good trauma care. Lifesaving first aid procedures must be carried out before the transfer of the patients by the paramedics or mobile medical team. The primary care giver must be certain that the burning process has been stopped. Thereafter any burning clothing is removed and suspected chemical burns irrigated with copious amounts of water before and during transfer to the hospital.

A clear airway and adequate breathing are secured. Cervical spine stabilisation is applied before moving the patient. One hundred per cent oxygen by facemask is administered to all aircraft burns patients because of the frequency of inhalation injury. At the crash site the burnt areas are covered with clean dry sheets and the patients kept warm by wrapping them in blankets before transfer to the hospital. If it does not delay transport of the patient, an intravenous line may be established and resuscitation begun. The victims of aircraft accidents are triaged with consideration given to all their injuries. For the burns victims, first priority goes to those with pulmonary distress, or serious associated mechanical trauma followed by severe isolated cutaneous burns.

Box 15.3
An outline for the management of burns patients

- Check the airway and ventilation (intubate if necessary)
- Support systemic perfusion via intravenous fluid administration (Muir and Barclay, Parkland, or modified Brooke formula)
- Provide emergency treatment of inhalation injury
- Diagnose and treat concomitant life threatening injuries
- Obtain a full medical history
- Perform a complete systemic (clinical) examination and map the burn wound
- Catheterise the bladder (after ruling out urethral injury)
- Perform an ophthalmological examination, including use of fluorescein drops
- Obtain pertinent laboratory and radiological tests
- Provide analgesia—small doses of intravenous narcotics as needed
- Provide tetanus prophylaxis
- Re-evaluate the burn wound and perform "second" triage
- Transfer to burns unit after stabilisation

Emergency department

The management of burns after aircraft accidents is similar to that of burns sustained in other circumstances and broadly follows the principles utilised in managing mass burn disasters.[21-26] The burn injury, although frequently the most spectacular injury sustained by the patient, is not the injury that is immediately life threatening. The associated mechanical trauma is very important and takes precedence over the burns treatment. A clear plan of action to be followed in the emergency department and on the ward is essential. A simple outline is offered in box 15.3 (after Settle).[27]

Emergency measures related to the care, resuscitation, and triage of the multiply injured burn patient should follow the guidelines established by the American College of Surgeons Advanced Trauma Life Support (ATLS) Course. Briefly, the ABCs (airway with cervical spine control, breathing and ventilation with supplemental 100% oxygen, and circulation with haemorrhage control) are treated as necessary and secured, and the gross neurological status of the patient is documented. Several criteria for endotracheal intubation are listed in box 15.4. The threshold for endotracheal intubation must be low to avoid later difficult intubation secondary to oedematous swelling of the upper airway. The presence of

---

Box 15.4
Emergency room indications for endotracheal intubation

Absolute indications
- Posterior pharyngeal swelling or burns of the tongue and pharynx

- Stridor and hoarseness

- Inhalation injury with coma or respiratory depression

Relative indications
- Deep burns of the face and neck

- Soot in nostrils

- Singed nasal vibrissae

- Carbonaceous sputum

---

carbonaceous sputum, singed nasal vibrissae, or nasopharyngeal soot should also prompt careful observation for clinical indications for intubation. The patient's respiratory rate and mental status must be followed carefully, with oxygen saturation and arterial blood gas determinations as needed. Tachypnoea, vocal changes, and disorientation are sufficient clinical indications for urgent intubation, before respiratory arrest occurs. If respiratory obstruction has already occurred or endotracheal intubation is unsuccessful, a cricothyroidotomy (minitracheostomy in the UK) is required, to be followed later by a formal tracheostomy.

The patient is completely undressed so that no injury is overlooked. Wide bore intravenous lines are established and blood taken for pertinent laboratory tests (box 15.5). Urinary catheters and nasogastric tubes are

---

Box 15.5
Initial laboratory and radiological studies for major burns (adapted from Robertson and Fenton)[29]

- Full blood count and haematocrit

- Serum electrolytes, creatinine, glucose

- Blood group and cross match

- Arterial blood gases

- Carboxyhaemoglobin concentration

- 12 lead electrocardiogram

- Chest *x* ray

---

inserted unless their use is contraindicated (suspicion of urethral injury or basilar skull fracture, respectively). A thorough secondary survey is performed to look for occult life threatening intracranial, spinal, thoracic, abdominal, pelvic, and extremity trauma. A rapid estimation of the extent of the burn injury (percentage total body surface area (TBSA) involved with second or third degree burns) utilising Wallace's rule of nines[28] may be made at this time, and an appropriate resuscitation fluid rate calculated and initiated (see later). After initiation, fluid rates are titrated to urine output. A complete neurological examination should be performed expeditiously. All appropriate diagnostic, laboratory, and radiological assessments may be performed at this time, to complete the secondary survey.

All intravenous fluids should be warmed before administration, and the patient should be covered with a clean dry sheet and kept warm to minimise hypothermia. The patient's list of injuries and response to therapy up to this point may now be reassessed, and adjusted to return the patient to homeostasis.

Of particular concern in the burns patient, once immediately life threatening injuries are treated, is the need to identify the presence of specific burn-related injuries and to initiate therapy to minimise the potential morbidity. In particular, inhalation injuries need to be carefully looked for and treated if found. Ocular injuries are also common, and prompt flushing of the eyes with copious amounts of water or saline is necessary to remove the irritant chemicals or particles and reduce the inflammation. Fluorescein drops are useful in searching for corneal abrasions and must be part of the routine physical examination of the burns patient. Ophthalmological consultation for more specialised examinations and for the removal of embedded particles is also necessary. Evidence of vascular compromise, as defined by loss of palmar arch or pedal Doppler signals or peripheral neurological deterioration, requires the performance of an escharotomy or fasciotomy (see later).

Fluid resuscitation

Since the pathophysiological hallmark of burns injury is the loss of isotonic fluid from the intravascular compartment into the injured tissue secondary to impaired microvascular integrity, fluid resuscitation is of the utmost importance in the acute treatment of the burns patient. Additionally there is loss of protein rich fluid from the plasma at the site of the burn and elsewhere, and the resulting hypoproteinaemia contributes to the fluid loss from the intravascular compartment into the non-burned tissues. Hypovolaemia and shock ensue if the burn is large enough and the fluid is not replaced. Patients with inhalation injury need increased volumes of resuscitation fluid compared to those without.[30] A reduction in the total number of red blood cells, caused by their direct destruction by heat (haemolysis) and by their decreased life span (abnormal fragility), results in the loss of up to 10% of the circulating red cell mass in the first day post-burn and up to 9% per day for the next 3–4 days in patients with large burns, especially deep burns.[31] If this haemolysis is significant enough it may manifest as obvious haemoglobinuria.

The aim of fluid management in the first 24–48 hours is to restore and maintain adequate tissue perfusion and oxygenation, thus avoiding organ ischaemia and preserving injured but viable soft tissue while minimising any iatrogenic contribution to the generalised oedema. It should be noted that microvascular instability in burn patients is short lived, with a new transcapillary equilibrium reached in 12–24 hours; therefore the resuscitation must carry the patient through this period with the minimum iatrogenic morbidity.[32]

Resuscitation formulae

These vary greatly from country to country. They are all effective if monitored with care[33] and modified according to the patient's clinical response. The fluid need is independent of burn depth, but is directly proportional to the size of the burn and the pre-burn weight of the patient.

Isotonic crystalloid: in the USA the most widely used regimen is the Parkland (or Baxter) formula using Ringer's lactate during the first 24 hours followed by 5% dextrose in water (D-5-W) and colloid in the second 24 hours. It estimates the initial Ringer's lactate needs at:

4 ml/kg per %TBSA burned

Half is administered over the first 8 hours and the remaining half over the next 16 hours, with the rate being adjusted to maintain an adequate urine output (30–50 ml/hour). The modified Brooke formula is similar, but bases the initial resuscitation rate, for the first 24 hours, on:

2 ml/kg per %TBSA burned

with the same time considerations for administration. Apart from their simplicity, the main advantage of isotonic crystalloid solutions stems from the fact that clinical and laboratory investigations have shown that colloid given in the first 24 hours post-burn is no more effective than crystalloid in restoring plasma volume and maintaining cardiac output,[33] and may have deleterious pulmonary effects secondary to trapping in the pulmonary extravascular space.[34] Colloid is, however, more efficacious than crystalloid in maintaining intravascular volume in the second 24 hours and minimises the salt and volume load that the patient will eventually need to excrete. The 24 hour volume of 5% albumin to be administered is calculated by the following formulae:

0.3 ml/kg per %TBSA burned for burns of 30–50% TBSA burned
0.4 ml/kg per %TBSA burned for burns of 50–70% TBSA burned
0.5 ml/kg per %TBSA burned for burns of over 70% TBSA burned.

This volume is administered as a 5% solution of albumin in lactated Ringer's at a constant rate over the second 24 hours. During the second 24 hours, D-5-W is administered to maintain the urine output between 30 and 50 ml/hour. Care must be taken when the required rate of fluid administration results in a dextrose administration rate greater than 5 mg/kg/min, as glucosuria and the associated osmotic diuresis may cause some degree of hypovolaemia.

Hypertonic saline: the mechanism of hypertonic saline resuscitation is that the sodium ion—the key element in crystalloid resuscitation—osmotically draws intracellular fluid into the extracellular fluid compartment to fill the deficit induced by the burn injury. Less fluid is required initially, although the exact amount needed remains unclear. It finds marginal use in the elderly with cardiovascular disease. Contrary to popular belief there is no evidence that inhalation injury is made worse by administration of appropriate resuscitation volumes; thus inhalation injury is not an indication for hypertonic saline. On the contrary, under-resuscitation may be worse for patients with inhalation injury and their volume requirements for adequate resuscitation are often higher than predicted. The mechanism(s) by which inhalation injury increases the fluid requirements are not clear but may be related to the release of vasoactive mediators from the injured lung and the increase in the amount of tissue injured when there is significant lower respiratory injury.

Colloid: Plasma proteins exert a colloid osmotic pressure that counteracts the outward hydrostatic pressure in the capillaries, thus decreasing or reversing the fluid shift into the interstitial space and thereby decreasing oedema in non-burned tissue. By this action they increase haemodynamic stability and maintain blood volume better than crystalloid alone, provided there is no capillary leak of colloid into the interstitial space, a phenomenon that is present for the initial 12–24 hours post-burn. A continuous infusion of protein is more efficacious than pulsed administration. The protein preparations used are human albumin solution, fresh frozen plasma, freeze dried plasma, plasma protein fraction (PPF), and various heat fixed proteins. Albumin is the most oncotically active plasma protein and does not transmit disease. Fresh frozen plasma carries the entire osmotic load of plasma and all the normal clotting factors but can transmit disease, such as hepatitis or HIV. *In the UK the most popular intravenous resuscitation regimen uses the Muir and Barclay formula[31] and PPF.* The likely colloid requirement for 24 hours is 2.5 ml/kg/%TBSA. It is given according to designated time periods, the estimated colloid volume (ml) for each period being:

0.5 to 0.65 ml × kg body weight × %TBSA burned.

The first 12 hours from the time of burn (not arrival in hospital) is divided into *three* time periods of *4 hours* each, while the next 12 hours is divided into *two* periods each of *6 hours*. Thereafter, the periods are *12 hours* long. Increased protein requirements are found in patients with more than 50% burns, older patients, and those with significant inhalation injuries.[33]

Non-protein colloid: the mechanism of action of non-protein colloid is identical to that of protein. However, it does not decrease burn tissue oedema or hypoproteinaemia. Examples used occasionally for burns resuscitation are dextran (Dextran 40 (USA) and Dextran 70 (Europe)) and hetastarch (Hespan).

Monitoring

This is a critical part of patient care because resuscitation is a dynamic process and formulae are only guidelines for the initiation of care; adjustments need to be made regularly according to the response of the patient to optimise the result. Regular checks and recordings of the following must be made. In our opinion, urine output and arterial blood gases are fundamentally important in monitoring burned patients.

Urine output: this is an excellent guide to the adequacy of resuscitation with the use of crystalloids. This is because the urine so produced is not due to an osmotic diuresis as produced by dextran or hypertonic saline. The target is an output of 30–50 ml/hour for adults, or 0.5–1.0 ml/kg/hour (for children of less than 30 kg).

Pulse rate: this is a helpful indicator of the adequacy of resuscitation in young patients. However, it is affected by the degree of pain control and catecholamine levels, and is not reliable in the elderly due to blunted physiological responses, pre-existing heart disease, and medication use (for example, β blockers). The trend in the pulse rate is frequently of greater significance than the absolute value itself in assessing the response to resuscitation.

Blood pressure: due to difficulties in obtaining accurate and reproducible pressures without invasive techniques, blood pressure is an insensitive monitor. The difficulties are related to the relative hypovolaemia and lack of suitable sites for non-invasive monitoring in burns patients, as well as the neuroendocrine response to stress. Stress-induced catecholamine release can maintain blood pressure spuriously in the face of hypovolaemia, especially in the young patient. Even if invasive techniques are used, pressure measurements are still not as sensitive to small changes in perfusion as urine output.

Indices of peripheral perfusion: these include surface temperature, transcutaneous oxygen measurements, laser Doppler flow metering, capillary refill, etc. All these methods have poor reproducibility and thus are rarely used.

Blood gases: preferably from an indwelling arterial line to avoid multiple painful arterial punctures. These are useful for assessing the degree of metabolic acidosis, which reflects tissue perfusion. Persistent metabolic acidosis is a good indicator of inadequate perfusion and therefore the need for increased fluids, except in CO poisoning, in which the metabolic acidosis represents lactic acidosis secondary to hypoxic crippling of the oxidative phosphorylation pathway. An arterial line also gives a constant recording of the arterial blood pressure.

Serial haematocrit determinations: generally, these are insensitive to the adequacy of resuscitation, but they are useful in that a dropping haematocrit may indicate an occult source of blood loss (such as an undiagnosed abdominal injury) and thus prompt a careful reassessment of the patient to locate such an injury.

Invasive monitoring: Swan-Ganz catheter monitoring of pulmonary artery wedge pressures (PAWP) and cardiac output may be necessary in elderly patients with cardiovascular disease or in patients requiring unusually large resuscitation volumes (> 6 ml/kg/%TBSA). The interpretation of Swan-Ganz data is difficult in many burn patients and must be done with consideration of other parameters (urine output, base deficit, and arterial pH). Central venous pressure measurements by themselves are of limited use and Swan-Ganz monitoring is preferred if central monitoring is necessary to guide resuscitative efforts.

Reassessment and transfer to burns unit

Only after all the above measures are carried out is the final destination of the patient determined. This depends on the total number of casualties, the extent of their injuries, ages, presence or absence of inhalation injury, and available local and regional resources. In an aircraft accident many of the burns will be life threatening and may be complicated by inhalation injury or significant non-burn trauma and will therefore require admission.

Minor burns in non-critical sites (<10% TBSA in children under 10 and adults over 50, and <20% TBSA in those aged 10-50) may not need admission. In contrast, minor burns occurring in critical sites (hands, face, feet, and perineum) warrant admission, but may not need to be sent to a burns centre if resources are being overwhelmed and if the burns can be adequately managed by a local general or plastic surgeon in consultation with a burns centre.

Topical antimicrobial therapy

This constitutes the single most important method of minimising septic complications in those patients in whom wound closure is not achieved promptly.[35] It has decreased burns patient mortality by 50%.[32] The rationale for its use is that (a) systemic antibiotics do not penetrate the eschar that forms on partial thickness and full thickness burns, and (b) topical agents are at the greatest concentration on the wound surface, where the risk of exogenous contamination is greatest. Although the burn wound is initially sparsely colonised, the bacteria proliferate with time. If untreated the initially predominant Gram positive flora are progressively replaced so that within 5–7 days Gram negative aerobes from the patient's own GI tract and the environment predominate. These organisms can invade healthy tissue from the burn wound; therefore topical therapy must be instituted promptly. A number of agents may be used.

1% silver sulphadiazine

Applied once or twice a day with or without dressings, silver sulphadiazine is active against Gram positive and Gram negative bacteria, *Candida albicans* and possibly herpes virus. It is non-staining and most patients find it soothing. The problems associated with its use are the lack of penetration of the burn eschar (allowing subeschar suppuration to occur in large full thickness wounds when it is used as single agent topical therapy), formation of a thin pseudoeschar, occasional leucopenia, and rare instances of haemolytic anaemia, Stevens–Johnson syndrome, and induction of resistant enterobacteriaceae and *Pseudomonas aeruginosa*.

0.5% silver nitrate solution

A virtually non-toxic, painless broad spectrum agent, silver nitrate solution is applied by soaking bulky wet dressings every 2 hours. Its drawbacks include lack of penetration of burn eschar, staining of linen and equipment, hypochloraemia, and hyponatraemia (because of chloride precipitation and hypotonicity), necessitating prophylactic electrolyte supplementation, and the rare induction of methaemoglobinaemia. Its minimal eschar penetration precludes its use for established wound sepsis.

11.1% mafenide acetate

The broad antibacterial spectrum of mafenide acetate and its outstanding ability to penetrate eschar make it the agent of choice for prevention of burn wound infection on full thickness burns, and for the topical treatment of areas of burn wound infection after operative debridement of all infected tissue. Side effects include some pain on application to areas of partial thickness burn and (rarely) hyperchloraemic metabolic acidosis secondary to carbonic anhydrase inhibition when used on extensive burns.[32] The use of mafenide acetate is not recommended in patients with glucose-6-phosphate dehydrogenase deficiency, due to the possibility of haemolytic anaemia and diffuse intravascular coagulation.

A suitable dressing regimen would be twice daily dressing changes with silver sulfadiazine for burns of $< 40\%$, and twice daily dressings with alternate silver sulfadiazine and mafenide acetate for burns of $> 40\%$ TBSA. Straight mafenide acetate is used on burnt ears and noses to prevent septic chondritis and resulting disfigurement. At the time of dressing changes the wounds are thoroughly cleansed and inspected to ensure that there are no areas of fluctuance or tinctoral change in the eschar, which may indicate the presence of an occult wound infection, and to check for evidence of healing in the wound bed.

Inhalation injury

The significance of inhalation injury in burn patients as a comorbidity factor is well documented, and is particularly apparent in aircraft accidents in which escape is delayed. Toxic fumes may cause an inhalation injury without the presence of facial burns or carbonaceous secretions. With the advances in the treatment of burns, shock and sepsis, respiratory complications have emerged as the dominant killer of individuals with major thermal injury. Pulmonary pathology, primarily as a result of inhalation injury, in various reports accounts for 20–84% of burn mortality.[36] Inhalation injury increases mortality by a maximum of approximately 20% over that predicted by standard formulae using age and extent of injury alone, making it "the single most important comorbid factor in severely burned patients today".[37] It is not surprising that inhalation injury is a major cause of death after aircraft fires. Pulmonary complications were responsible for 80% of delayed deaths in Braunohler and McMeekin's (1974) series.[19] It is interesting that of the 40 aircraft burns victims treated at the USAISR burn unit over the last 5 years, 20 had concomitant inhalation injuries; the three patients who died (out of the group of 40) all had inhalation injury, although this is statistically not a significantly greater mortality than that of the patients without inhalation injury (p = 0.12 by Fisher's exact test).

Pathogenesis

Inhalation injury in aircraft fires can occur even with a short exposure time to fumes (within 2 minutes in the 1985 Manchester air disaster)[15] because of the enclosed space and extremely rapid generation of large amounts of smoke and toxic fumes. The most serious pathological changes are due to the smoke particles and fumes causing a chemical tracheobronchitis and pneumonitis, while the direct effect of heat is a relatively unimportant mechanism.[17,38–40]

A large number of highly toxic materials are inhaled during an aircraft fire. The interior fabrics are made of a number of flammable materials, such as polyvinyl chloride (PVC), polyvinyl fluoride, chlorinated acrylics, urethane, isocyanates, polyacrylonitrile, and polyurethane to name a few. Their combustion generates a highly toxic combination of HCN, hydrochloric acid (HCl), hydrogen fluoride, hydrogen sulphide (H_2S), phosgene, nitrogen dioxide, isocyanates, chlorine, and CO. The last of these (CO) is a product of incomplete combustion, resulting from a lack of sufficient oxygen for complete combustion. Cyanide gases can come from polyurethane (in seat cushions, carpet pads, hat racks, etc.), wool (seat upholstery), modacrylics (dust panes), and acrylonitrilebutadienestyrene (plastic windows).[40] Burning PVC releases HCl, chlorine gas, and phosgene. The toxicological effects of these gases allow them to be divided into two groups: those with primarily systemic toxicity and those with primarily local (pulmonary) toxicity.

Systemic toxicity: CO is responsible for causing hypoxia by occupying oxygen binding sites on the haemoglobin molecule, thus decreasing the oxygen carrying capacity of blood. Its levels are usually higher than normal in patients with inhalation injury.[41,42] Cyanide is a highly toxic gas that uncouples the electron transport chain of oxidative phosphorylation. It causes unconsciousness and death rapidly. Lethal levels of CO, CN, and fluorine (F) are found in the victims' blood after aircrash accidents.[7]

Local toxicity: short chain aldehydes can produce pulmonary oedema. The toxic gases (H_2S, HCl) cause local irritation to both upper and lower airways and act systemically as direct cellular poisons. The strong acids and alkalis produced by water soluble chemicals cause irritation, laryngospasm, bronchospasm, ulceration of mucous membranes, and oedema. Gases such as HCl can be transported on carbon particles to the lower airways, causing bronchiolitis, and alveolitis.

Pathophysiology and complications

There are a number of excellent reviews of this subject.[30,36-38,43-45] The effects of smoke inhalation can be local to the airway and pulmonary parenchyma (related to the irritant particles and gases) or systemic, especially to the myocardium and systemic vasculature (related to CO). Currently, a great deal of research is being focused on the effects of cellular inflammatory mediators (cytokines, leukotrienes, and interleukins) on the pathophysiological response by the lung to smoke inhalation.

The symptoms and signs of inhalation injury are not very specific, requiring the clinician to have a high index of suspicion in order for the diagnosis to be made. A history of being burned in a closed space, such as an aircraft cabin, is classic. This was present in 82% of 66 consecutive inhalation injury patients in one series.[46] Seventy per cent of patients with inhalation injury have facial burns or singed nasal vibrissae but 70% of patients with facial burns do not have significant respiratory tract injury.[47] In Braunohler and McMeekin's (1974) series 10% of aircraft burn deaths had nasopharyngeal burns clinically or on autopsy and 92% of these had flame burns about the face and neck.[19] Cough, hoarseness, bronchorrhoea, dyspnoea, and wheezing are often delayed in onset. Wheezing is frequently absent for the first 24–48 hours after injury. The presence of carbonaceous material in the airway secretions is usually a reliable indicator of inhalation injury when present but may be the result of soot trapped in the nasal passages only. Additionally carbonaceous material can be rapidly cleared and may not be evident on admission to the burns centre.

Respiratory failure usually presents as three different clinical entities at various times in the post-burn course, all associated with 50% mortality rates.[36] Severe inhalation injury may present as acute pulmonary insufficiency with inability to clear CO_2 as well as difficulty oxygenating, generally occurring within the first 36 hours in the most severely burned patients. Pulmonary oedema with difficulty oxygenating but free clearance of CO_2 usually manifests between post-burn days 3 and 6 while resuscitation fluids are being mobilised and excreted, and may be a consequence of either underlying inhalation injury or fluid loading during resuscitation. All burns patients are at risk for the latter mechanism, but those with a history of congestive heart failure are most likely to develop this complication. Lastly, tracheal mucosal sloughing and bronchopneumonia, as complications related to underlying inhalation injury, may appear between post-burn days 7 and 14.

Diagnosis and evaluation

The respiratory status of the acutely burned patient must be accurately assessed. The specific tests available to evaluate the three major sites of inhalation injury are carboxyhaemoglobin determinants (for CO toxicity), fibreoptic bronchoscopy (for upper respiratory tract damage) and xenon-133 pulmonary scintigraphy (for parenchymal damage). The non-specific tests that provide useful baselines are arterial blood gases and chest radiographs.

The diagnosis of inhalation injury rests on traditional clinical signs supplemented by fibreoptic bronchoscopy[37,48,49] and xenon-133 scanning.[50] A combination of fibreoptic bronchoscopy and xenon-133 scintigraphy diagnoses the presence of inhalation injury with a 93% accuracy.[46] Bronchoscopy remains the most sensitive and specific method of documenting the presence of an inhalation injury, and is also therapeutically important, allowing careful examination of the upper airways and removal of inspissated mucus plugs and carbonaceous debris that promote atelectasis and can coalesce and cause obstruction. Early accurate diagnosis is important because of the increased incidence of respiratory failure and bronchopneumonia. It permits the timely application of high frequency ventilation, which appears to decrease the incidence of pneumonia and to reduce mortality.[37,51] At present, however, there is no diagnostic modality that can quantify the severity of inhalation injury or the volume of lung tissue involved.[37,51]

Treatment

The treatment of inhalation injury begins before confirmation of the diagnosis. The subsequent management depends on whether the patient is stable or has a complication. The treatment of patients with parenchymal inhalation injury is largely supportive.[47] They should be managed in an intensive care unit or a burns unit and should be closely monitored because of the possible rapid development of airway obstruction. Initially, patients suffering from smoke inhalation may seem relatively well, but lung function may deteriorate rapidly in the first 24 hours. Among the 85 survivors at Manchester only one patient required ventilation at the time of admission, but within 12 hours another five had deteriorated to such an extent as to require ventilation.[15]

Emergency management:
(1) Humidified high flow oxygen (F_iO_2 of 100%) through a facemask or endotracheal tube is administered depending on the patient's degree of respiratory distress. One hundred per cent oxygen, initiated at the scene of the crash, is the single most effective treatment of CO toxicity. It decreases the half life for elimination of CO from the blood from almost 4 hours to approximately 45 minutes. Treatment should continue until the carboxyhaemoglobin level is less than 15%
(2) Protection of the compromised airway by tracheal intubation. The threshold for intubation should be low. Early endotracheal intubation is needed to prevent the development of respiratory distress during

transfer and to obviate a cricothyroidotomy for emergency airway access

(3) Bronchodilators delivered through an oxygen-powered nebuliser (β_2 agonists, such as salbutamol) or intravenously (aminophylline) are given for those patients who present with or develop wheezing. If the bronchospasm is intractable and severe, intravenous steroids (hydrocortisone or prednisolone) may be considered. However, steroids increase sepsis related mortality and are best avoided if possible.

Early management: this focuses on keeping the upper airways open to reduce the risk of small airway occlusion and resultant alveolar collapse (atelectasis) which contribute to ventilation–perfusion mismatching, hypoxaemia, and the development of pneumonia. This is achieved by:

(1) Cough exercises and incentive spirometry—regular physiotherapy hourly, for at least 48 hours

(2) Tracheal suctioning (nasotracheal, orotracheal, or bronchoscopic) frequently (every 2 hours and as needed) is very important to help clear the profuse secretions present secondary to the impaired mucociliary clearance mechanism and stimulation of bronchial glands. Sputum production in the order of 300–400 ml/day was commonplace in the victims of the Manchester aircraft fire[15]

(3) Mechanical ventilation (either conventional or high frequency) may be necessary if the patient cannot maintain an adequate minute ventilation. Recent data from Cioffi[52] and Pruitt[37] demonstrate that high frequency pressure controlled ventilation allows adequate ventilation to be maintained at lower peak and mean airway pressures and with lower inspired oxygen concentrations than can be achieved with conventional volume ventilation. A lower incidence of pneumonia was noted in the high frequency ventilation group, possibly related to better clearance of secretions and decreased barotrauma. A significant reduction in the expected mortality of these patients was found.

Prophylactic antibiotics (parenterally or aerosolised) should be avoided because (a) clinical trials have shown them to be of no value in preventing later pulmonary infection, as documented by radiological findings, the need for mechanical ventilation, sepsis rate, and mortality,[53] and (b) they promote the emergence of later infections with multiply resistant organisms. Prophylactic steroids have no effect on the course of inhalation injury, they increase the infectious complications, and may even lead to increased mortality.[54,55]

Complications and their treatments

The complications of inhalation injury are related to infection, oedema, and mechanical obstruction. Although they are usually not preventable, early diagnosis and treatment is important to minimise the considerable additive effect they have on morbidity and mortality.

Tracheobronchitis and pneumonia (38% incidence):[37] specific antibiotics are administered on the basis of identification of the offending organism and the culture and sensitivity results, in patients with clinical evidence of infection (fever $> 102.5°F$; sputum Gram stain with $> 20–25$ white blood cells per high power field, few squamous epithelial cells, and a preponderant organism; evidence of an infiltrate on chest radiograph). Before the culture and sensitivity results are available, empirical antibiotic therapy should be started with coverage of the preponderant organism noted on sputum Gram stain, usually penicillinase-producing *Staphylococcus aureus* in the initial post-burn days and Gram negative rods, especially *Pseudomonas aeruginosa*, later in the hospital course. At the US Army Institute of Surgical Research vancomycin has been used successfully for many years both for empirical and specific staphylococcal therapy without emergence of in vitro resistance. Regular chest physiotherapy with meticulous pulmonary toilet is also important.

Pulmonary oedema (5–30% incidence):[37] the aetiological factors are inhalation injury, fluid overload during the resuscitation phase, and/or cardiac failure. Meticulous fluid management assisted by Swan-Ganz haemodynamic monitoring (as needed) and ventilatory support is the mainstay of its treatment. Diuretics are avoided if possible, due to the risk of causing hypernatraemia and hypovolaemia,[44] but are necessary if the degree of fluid overload results in hypoxia, hypotension, or atrial fibrillation. Patients requiring mechanical respiratory support respond well to positive end-expiratory pressure (PEEP). Patients with a previous history of congestive heart failure frequently require inotropic support (digoxin and/or dopamine) in addition to careful haemodynamic monitoring and ventilatory support to proceed through resuscitation successfully.

Mucosal sloughing: this complication usually occurs during the second post-burn week as the damaged tracheobronchial mucosa separates from the tracheal wall. Increased amounts of bleeding occur during this time, resulting in the formation of haemorrhagic casts of dried blood and necrotic tracheal mucosa. The cornerstones of therapy are:

(1) Minimising barotrauma to the injured tracheobronchial epithelium by careful adjustment of mechanical ventilation to the minimum mean airway pressure consistent with adequate minute ventilation and oxygenation
(2) Appropriate clearance of sloughing airway mucosa to prevent accumulation of occlusive tissue plugs
(3) Maintenance of optimal humidification in the ventilator circuit to

prevent desiccation of the injured mucosa or of the haemorrhagic casts, which can make their removal more difficult.

Rigid bronchoscopy may be necessary to extract the occluding debris. Pulmonary insufficiency and continued sloughing of the tracheal mucosa in patients with severe inhalation injury is sometimes associated with a need for assisted ventilation beyond 2 weeks. The endotracheal tube should then be replaced by a formal tracheostomy for patient comfort and continued simple access to the central airways for pulmonary toilet.

Nutritional therapy

A comprehensive review of the many and far reaching metabolic effects of thermal injury is beyond the scope of this chapter and the reader is referred to the excellent review of this subject by Tredget and Yu,[56] who said "Major thermal injury is associated with extreme hypermetabolism and catabolism as the principal metabolic manifestations encountered following successful resuscitation from the shock phase of the burn injury." This hypermetabolic response to stress induced by the burn is of greater magnitude and duration than that due to sepsis or non-burn trauma and lasts until the wound is closed.

The aim of nutritional supplementation is to prevent the loss of greater than 10% (moderate sized burns) to 20% (large burns) of the pre-resuscitation lean body weight. Significant systemic complications (morbidity or mortality) may occur with losses of more than 20% of the lean body mass, and smaller losses may make the rehabilitation phase of burn recovery more difficult and prolonged. It is indicated in any patient who does not meet their estimated or measured nutritional needs, which is common in patients with burns greater than 20% TBSA. The nasojejunal enteral route, available for use in the vast majority of burns patients, is preferable to the parenteral route because central vein catheters are associated with catheter-related septicaemia and iatrogenic thoracic injuries. Jejunal rather than gastric feedings are preferred to minimise the risk of aspiration pneumonia in these critically ill patients. Continuous nasojejunal enteral feeds should be started on post-burn day 2 or 3, as soon as bowel function returns.

There are many formulae for determining caloric and protein requirements, but what is most important is the monitoring of the patient's clinical response to the particular formula used and adjusting the intake accordingly, through routine measurement of body weight, calorie counts, nitrogen balance, cholesterol and triglyceride levels, liver function tests, urinary glucose and ketones, electrolytes, calcium, magnesium, and phosphate, and by use of indirect calorimetry.

TABLE 15.1 Formulae for estimating calorie requirements of burn patients (results in calories per day)†

Harris-Benedict

Male: $[66 + (13.7 \times W) + (5 \times H) - (6.8 \times A)] \times 2$ (stress factor)

Female: $[655 + (9.6 \times W) + (1.8 \times H) - (4.7 \times A)] \times 2$ (stress factor)

Curreri

Adult: $(25 \times W) + (40 \times \%\text{TBSA burned})$

Junior:
  age 0, 1 years: $(\text{BC} \times W) + (15 \times \%\text{TBSA burned})$
  age 2, 3 years: $(\text{BC} \times W) + (25 \times \%\text{TBSA burned})$
  age 4–18 years: $(\text{BC} \times W) + (40 \times \%\text{TBSA burned})$

Basal calories (BC) by age (years) for Curreri Junior formulae:

Age	BC	Age	BC	Age	BC
0	60	7	48	14	36
1	59	8	47	15	35
2	55	9	46	16	32
3	53	10	45	17	31
4	52	11	44	18	30
5	51	12	40		
6	50	13	38		

Galveston

Children: $[1800 \times \text{BSA}] + [2200 \times \text{burn(m}^2)]$

USAISR

$\text{BMR} \times [0.89 + (0.013 \times \%\text{TBSA burned})] \times \text{BSA} \times 24 \times 1.25$

BMR male: $54.34 - (1.2 \times A) + (0.025 \times A^2) - (0.0002 \times A^3)$
BMR female: $54.75 - (1.5 \times A) + (0.036 \times A^2) - (0.0003 \times A^3)$

---

† W = weight (kg), H = height (cm), A = age (years), BSA = body surface area (m²), TBSA = total BSA.

Calories

Formulae estimating requirements are predicated on age and burn size (and some on gender). Commonly used formulae include the Harris-Benedict formulae for males and females, the Curreri and Curreri Junior formulae for adults and children, the Galveston formulae for children, and the USAISR formula. These formulae are given in table 15.1.

Carbohydrates

Carbohydrates are an important substrate following injury, providing glucose for peripheral glycolysis. The maximum tolerated rate of administration of dextrose in most patients is approximately 5 mg/kg/min from all sources. Rates of administration in excess of 5 mg/kg/min usually result in hyperglycaemia and glycosuria, and may result in fatty infiltration of the liver; if rates of administration must exceed this limit, exogenous insulin via continuous infusion should be provided as needed to maintain normo-glycaemia and prevent osmotic diuresis.

Proteins

These are necessary to provide substrate for wound healing, gluconeo-genesis, maintenance of visceral and skeletal protein stores, and for preservation of immunological function. Although there are some animal data that suggest a beneficial (protein sparing) effect from the administration of protein with increased proportions of branched chain amino acids, there are no compelling human data to support their use at this time. The goal of supplementation is to achieve a normal nitrogen balance (between -2 and $+2$). The recommended calorie to nitrogen ratio is between 100 k cals to 1g nitrogen and 150 k cals to 1g nitrogen, with the lower ratio (100:1) closest to optimal for the more severely stressed patients.

Fats

These should comprise no more than 30% of the dietary caloric intake to prevent sequestration of fat in the reticuloendothelial system. Much less fat is necessary to prevent fatty acid deficiency (1–4% of the total caloric intake) and no clear benefit has been demonstrated for the preferential supply of calories in the form of fat. A satisfactory programme is to provide essential fatty acids once or twice a week, and to provide additional calories in the form of fat only if the amount of carbohydrate necessary to meet the estimated or measured caloric need exceeds the carbohydrate tolerance of the patient.

Definitive burn wound care

Expectant (conservative) therapy

After treatment of immediately life threatening injuries, smoke inhalation, and occult mechanical trauma has occurred and resuscitation has been initiated with haemodynamic stability attained, burn wound care becomes a priority in the care of the patient.

The initial wound debridement and dressing must be performed in a warm room under adequate analgesia (see later) and constant monitoring of vital signs and core temperature. Medical photographs (for records and medicolegal purposes) should be taken at this time.

The burns should be gently washed with warm saline or water and a surgical detergent disinfectant to remove soot and debris. Loose skin and any blisters larger than 1 cm should be debrided. After careful inspection of the wounds and final mapping of the burn extent, topical antimicrobial agents may be applied to the wound and the patient returned to bed to continue resuscitation. Burned extremities are placed in splints to maintain joints in a position of function and to prevent early contractures from interfering with physical and occupational therapy. Active and passive range of motion and exercises to maintain muscle strength are also initiated immediately to preserve as much function as possible.

The daily debridement of non-adherent eschar is important because it allows maximal penetration of topical antibiotic into the wound surface, hastens the healing of partial thickness burns, and makes full thickness burns suitable for skin grafting more quickly. Suitable analgesia, such as morphine or another narcotic, must be provided. Dosages are larger than those commonly used; frequently, for adequate pain control, the average sized adult patient will need 10–20 mg of morphine sulphate intravenously. For patients in whom tolerance to narcotics develops, short acting intravenous anaesthesia (ketamine or propofol) may be necessary. Occasionally, anxiety regarding wound care will require the administration of anxiolytics such as midazolam or diazepam. Debridement has classically been performed in an immersion facility (for example a Hubbard tank) but cross infection with resistant organisms can occur if such tanks are not adequately cleansed between patients. Therefore the use of a showering cart or the patient's own bed may be preferable. The dressings should be changed at least twice a day to maintain an adequate concentration gradient of antibiotic in the cream over the wound.

Surgical management (surgical excision and closure)

The surgical care of the burn wound involves the use of skin grafts to provide wound cover. The timing of the skin grafting can either be late or early. "Late" skin grafting entails waiting for spontaneous eschar separation, usually occurring at 3 weeks (due to autolysis) aided by bedside eschar debridement, and then grafting the remaining granulation tissue bed. Postoperative graft care and rehabilitation are identical to that described for early burn wound excision and grafting (see later).

At present, the excision of deep burns relatively soon after injury is common and has become routine practice in many centres. This process is usually started during the first post-burn week, after the patient has begun to mobilise his or her resuscitative fluid load and approach pre-burn weight, and as soon as it has become clear which areas will not heal spontaneously. First described in 1970 by Janzekovic, the practice of early excision and grafting provides excellent graft take and results in a clean closed wound.[57] The techniques, operative and postoperative management of burns by early excision and skin grafting, have been reviewed in the excellent work of Heimbach and Engrav[58] and Heimbach.[59] Guidelines for early excision and debridement are:

- An experienced surgeon is required because inadequate excision leads to skin graft loss

- Associated medical problems must be controlled before surgery to decrease mortality and morbidity

- The degree of intraoperative blood loss requires that an adequate quantity of blood be crossmatched and available in the operating theatre

- Burns of the foot and hand should be excised as soon as possible to assist progress in physical and occupational therapy.

There is unanimity that small full thickness burns can be easily excised and grafted with excellent results and that the technique is an ideal treatment for hand burns.[59,60] In a prospective randomised trial, Engrav *et al*[61] showed that early excision and grafting of indeterminate burns of less than 20% TBSA resulted in decreased hospital stay, reduced costs, and less need for reconstruction. What is more important, these patients returned to work twice as fast as the traditionally treated group, and Heimbach[59] concluded that this method decreases the number of painful wound debridements required by all patients and stated that there is suggestive, but not definitive, evidence that it also decreases scarring and mortality from infections and other burn complications. Curreri *et al*[62] found no difference in mortality between early and late excision and grafting. Clearly, due to its emergence at a time when there were marked improvements in all aspects of burn care, it remains unproven whether prompt wound excision confers a survival advantage (or functional and cosmetic benefits) and, if so, to what extent.[63] Controversy also exists as to whether patients with major burns are best managed by (a) a series of staged excision and grafting procedures governed by availability of donor sites, or (b) by excision of all the deep burns within a few days post-burn in one or two extensive operative procedures with cutaneous allograft wound coverage at the time of the procedure followed by replacement of the cutaneous allograft with autograft skin as donor sites become available.

The timing of surgery is crucial. For haemodynamically stable patients without complications of smoke inhalation precluding general anaesthesia, the "golden period" is between days 3 and 9.[58] Before 48 hours, resuscitation and stabilisation take priority. Surgery before post-burn days 7–9 is preferable due to the lesser degree of bacterial colonisation in the burn wound. A number of different excisional techniques are used in different circumstances, as detailed below.

225

Tangential excision

Using an electric dermatome (suitable for large planar surfaces) or a hand dermatome (ideal for small irregular surfaces such as the hands or feet), excision of the burn wound is continued until uniform brisk capillary bleeding is seen in the recipient dermis. Full thickness burns will require excision into the subcutaneous fat and may have poorer graft take in comparison to an intradermal excision. Blood loss may be reduced by the use of a tourniquet and the use of topical thrombin (or adrenaline) for haemostasis. Hypotension may be avoided by limiting the area of excision, effecting rapid meticulous haemostasis, and ensuring that the pace of the excision does not exceed the capacity of the anaesthetist to provide volume replacement.

Excision at the level of the investing fascia

This method can easily be performed with a tourniquet and requires less experience to obtain a reliable bed for grafting. Minimal blood loss may be achieved with this method, and this is occasionally the most important consideration, especially in patients with poor physiological reserve. It can, however, produce a significant cosmetic deformity and risks distal oedema (if circumferential) and damage to superficial nerves and tendons. It is reserved for burns extending deep into the subcutaneous fat, large life threatening full thickness burns, and for patients with small full thickness burns and multiple medical problems complicating anaesthetic management.

Excision with primary closure

Some burns are sufficiently small that they can be excised and primarily closed without tension, giving an optimal cosmetic and functional result. This approach may also be used to eliminate small donor sites after the graft has been taken.

Skin harvest and application

The skin is harvested using a hand knife or dermatome (powered or manual). It is applied as sheet grafts in areas of cosmetic or functional importance (face, hands, and feet) or grafts meshed for expansion from 1.5:1 to 9:1 depending on the size of the burn, available donor sites, and number of times the donor sites have been used. The grafts are secured with staples or sutures. Sheet grafts are not dressed so that they may be inspected periodically and gently rolled as needed to prevent accumulation of serum or blood beneath the graft, which can cause graft loss. Meshed grafts are covered with fine mesh gauze and bulky dressings kept continuously moistened to prevent desiccation of the interstices. The dressings are fastened in place with elastic net or cotton gauze to prevent shearing of the graft. Extremities are placed in splints to prevent rotational shearing, with immobilisation of joints above and below the grafted area required for adequate results. In extensive burns where adequate donor sites are not available for immediate autografting, temporary coverage may be achieved using fresh frozen, or lyophilised cadaver (allograft) or porcine (xenograft) skin. Rarely, human placental membranes (amnion) or synthetic tissue derivatives have been used.

Postoperative care and rehabilitation

Postoperative graft immobilisation and elevation of the extremities are crucial for graft take. Expert nursing care is required for patient monitoring, feeding, and local care of the burn dressings. The dressings are changed and the grafts inspected on post-graft day 5 (day 3 for hand grafts) for initial assessment of graft take and every 24–48 hours subsequently. Adequate narcotic premedication should be administered to maintain patient comfort. Occasionally, small children may require a general anaesthetic for dressing changes. Moistened dressings are kept on the grafts until the interstices heal. Following interstitial closure, the grafts may be left open or in dry protective dressings. Hand splints on sheet grafted hands are generally removed on postoperative day 3 to allow quicker mobilisation and prevent loss of joint range of motion.

Physiotherapy to maintain joint mobility is very important. Physical and occuaptional therapy play crucial roles in the rehabilitation of the patient beginning in the immediate post-burn period, while joint mobility and conditioning are maintained, and throughout the remainder of the hospital stay, when prevention of scar formation and improvement of fine motor movements needed for functional rehabilitation become important considerations. Social workers and psychologists provide much needed family support and psychological counselling, respectively, and are vital in arranging postoperative placement in appropriate rehabilitation units.

Complications of burns

Monitoring for complications of the thermal injury and their therapy is important to minimise their effect on morbidity and mortality. These complications primarily affect the immunological, renal, pulmonary, gastrointestinal, and cardiac systems.

Infection

The most frequent cause of mortality in burn patients is infection. The most common sites of infection are the respiratory tract, urinary tract,

---

Box 15.6
Tests for infection in burns patients

- Temperature or haemodynamic instability, ileus, oliguria, or glucose intolerance

- Serial chest *x* rays, sputum Gram stains, and urinalyses

- Cultures of blood, urine, sputum, surface swabs, intravenous catheter tips, etc.

- Biopsy of the wound, including the eschar and adjacent viable tissue, for visualisation of invading microorganisms—allows distinction of colonisation of the burn wound from microbial invasion into viable tissue

---

blood, and the burn wound, in decreasing order of frequency. Other potential problems include sinusitis, prostatitis, soft tissue cellulitis, suppurative thrombophlebitis, endocarditis, peritonitis secondary to visceral perforation, and infection at skeletal pin insertion sites and fractures. Burns patients are susceptible to invasive sepsis for several reasons: the burn constitutes a breach in the body's mechanical barrier to infection and is a good growth medium for bacteria; there is immunosuppression, related to burn size, of the specific and non-specific immune systems; and the myriad of invasive devices that these critically ill patients require, including endotracheal tubes, bladder and vascular catheters, and nasogastric tubes, allow micro-organisms to bypass some of the normal host defence mechanisms.

The dominant pathogens in most burns centres are *Staphylococcus aureus* and *Pseudomonas aeruginosa*. *Candida* species are the most frequently seen yeast and usually appear 2–3 weeks after the burn.

Diagnosis requires a high index of suspicion because often the first indicators of incipient sepsis are subtle changes in the patient's clinical condition. Changes in the burn wound appearance due to the development of sepsis occur in only half of such patients. There is no substitute for serial clinical and laboratory monitoring of the patient in the diagnosis of sepsis (box 15.6).

Treatment of burn patients who have laboratory and clinical evidence of infection involves antibiotic therapy based on Gram stains, biopsy, or initial culture results when available: empirical therapy may be necessary if no clinical information is available. A suitable 'regimen' is a broad spectrum penicillin or cephalosporin with an aminoglycoside. For fungal infections, systemic amphotericin B is administered. Steroids should never be used unless there is evidence of acute adrenal infarction, chronic adrenal insufficiency, or a history of prolonged steroid administration in the past year that could result in adrenal suppression. Subsequent treatment may be adjusted on the basis of culture and sensitivity results. If the burn wound is identified as the source of the infection it is standard practice in the USA to undertake immediate excision (preceded by subeschar clysis for 24–72 hours when there is Gram negative bacterial invasion) to control the septic episode.

Renal failure

Oliguria during resuscitation usually indicates inadequate resuscitation. Appropriate resuscitation of the burn patient has been the single greatest advance in decreasing both mortality and renal failure. With the exception of electrical burns (and the resultant myonecrosis and myoglobinuria) the incidence of renal failure in appropriately resuscitated burn patients is near zero. The subset of patients at greatest risk for renal complications (excepting electrical injuries) is those with limited cardiovascular reserve who cannot mount an appropriate hyperdynamic response and those in whom resuscitation has been inordinately delayed or grossly inadequate. These patients require monitoring with pulmonary artery catheters to ensure adequacy of intravascular volume and to assess the need for inotropic support.

The presence of urinary haemochromogens, usually as a complication following electrical injury, requires an increase in urinary output to approximately 100 ml/h, alkalisation of administered intraveneous fluid to obtain a urine pH above 7.0, and may require administration of an osmotic diuretic to prevent crystallisation of these nephrotoxic agents in the renal tubules, with its resultant acute tubular necrosis. After the haemochromogens have visually cleared from the urine the urine output may be allowed to return to normal levels (30–50 ml/h in adults, 1 ml/kg/h in children).

Renal failure occurring later in the post-burn hospital course is usually the result of sepsis and frequently progresses to multiorgan system failure. Appropriate and rapid treatment of the underlying cause may result in improvement.

Pulmonary failure

The common pulmonary complications of burns include pulmonary oedema, pneumonia, and pneumothorax. Pulmonary oedema usually occurs as the result of resuscitation. As resuscitation volumes rise above 6 ml/kg/%TBSA burned the possibility of pulmonary oedema (usually non-cardiogenic) increases and the utility of PAWP becomes apparent. Non-cardiogenic pulmonary oedema is frequently accompanied by pleural effusions and generalised oedema and may be related to circulating cytokines from the burn, although no specific factor has been identified yet. Cardiogenic pulmonary oedema is rare and occurs almost exclusively in elderly patients with pre-existing congestive cardiac failure. These patients are best managed by early PAWP monitoring and may need inotropic support to allow resuscitation to take place.

Pneumonia (both tracheobronchitis and true bronchopneumonia) is a frequent complication in burn patients. Before the use of topical antimicrobial agents pneumonias were usually secondary to haematogenous seeding, but currently most pneumonias are airborne. Gram positive organisms are somewhat more common than Gram negative organisms as causative agents. The diagnosis of pneumonia or tracheobronchitis depends on the presence of white blood cells (at least 25 per high power field) and organisms on the Gram stain of endobronchial secretions. Radiographs alone are inadequate to make the diagnosis of pneumonia and frequently miss the presence of tracheobronchitis. Treatment is based on the results of culture and sensitivities; empirical therapy while awaiting results is based on Gram stain results.

Pneumothorax is usually an iatrogenic complication of central line placement, occurring in approximately 1% of placement attempts. Positive pressure ventilation and pre-existing pulmonary disease increases the chance of pneumothorax. Other causes are related to blunt or penetrating trauma associated with the burn event and to positive pressure ventilation, especially at high mean airway pressures. Early treatment of pneumothorax is important, especially for patients on positive pressure ventilation to prevent the development of a tension pneumothorax. The diagnosis is suspected when clinical symptoms such as tachypnoea, pain, and air hunger are present. Signs on physical and radiographic examination include hyperresonance, crepitus, absent breath sounds, absence of lung markings on chest radiographs, and elevated airway pressures in patients on positive pressure ventilation. Treatment usually requires insertion of a chest tube to effect drainage, re-expansion, and healing of the injured lung.

Gastrointestinal failure

The gastrointestinal tract is the site of several severe complications in the burn patient. These include problems as mundane as ileus and as dramatic as stress ulceration. Excellent reviews may be found in standard references (such as Pruitt)[64] or standard surgical textbooks and we will limit our discussion to the most commonly seen problems—ileus, stress ulceration, and pancreatitis.

Ileus is the earliest as well as the most frequent gastrointestinal complication experienced by burn patients. The vast majority of patients with burns greater than 20–25% will have the onset of ileus within the first 6 hours of the burn event. The ileus persists throughout the period of haemodynamic instability and resolves spontaneously after the patient is adequately resuscitated. Oral feeding (or feeding via a nasojejunal tube) may be instituted as soon as the ileus has resolved. Ileus occurring at any other time during the post-burn course is usually associated with sepsis and requires investigation to identify the cause of the ileus.

Stress ulceration (Curling's ulcer) usually occurs as multiple small acute ulcers in the gastric or duodenal mucosa, although large solitary ulcers can occur in either location. Within 48 hours of significant burns mucosal lesions appear in the stomach and duodenum. The lesions are punctate, with little inflammatory reaction. In the past, operative intervention was required in approximately 10–15% of patients; recently, however, stress ulceration has become much less of a problem because of the advent of H_2-receptor blockers. Adequate prophylaxis (usually a combination of H_2-receptor blockers and antacids to maintain a gastric pH above 5, or the more recently introduced drug sucralfate) permits the superficial erosions to heal and prevents progression of the lesions to the point of frank bleeding or perforation. Rarely, when operative intervention is required, the procedure of choice is vagotomy and partial gastric resection.

Pancreatitis usually occurs as an additional complication in patients with sepsis or multiorgan system failure. These complications frequently result in alterations of blood flow in the splanchnic bed, resulting in pancreatic ischaemia with subsequent pancreatitis. Pancreatitis of widely varying severity is seen, from clinically insignificant elevations of serum amylase without overt gastrointestinal symptoms to haemorrhagic pancreatitis associated with adult respiratory distress syndrome (ARDS). Treatment is symptomatic and supportive: cessation of feedings, adequate intravenous hydration, nasogastric decompression if nausea or vomiting occurs, a search for a septic focus to rule out occult infection, and respiratory support if indicated.

Cardiac complications

Myocardial complications of burns include congestive cardiac failure (CCF) and myocardial infarction. These events almost always occur in patients with pre-existing cardiac disease. A history of myocardial disease should increase the clinician's index of suspicion, allowing early intervention and preventing (if possible) major cardiac events from occurring through careful cardiodynamic monitoring and pharmacological support.

Congestive cardiac failure occurs most frequently in patients with pre-existing congestive failure or renal failure and is a direct result of the volume of fluid that must be administered to resuscitate the patient. If the patient is known to have a history of CCF, prompt insertion of a pulmonary artery catheter to assist in control of the resuscitation to prevent pulmonary oedema is recommended. These patients may also require inotropic support to obtain an adequate myocardial response to stress.

Myocardial infarcts usually occur in patients with pre-existing atherosclerotic disease. The peak incidence of infarction is toward the end of the first post-burn week, when the hypermetabolic response to stress has reached its peak. Routine measures to provide inotropic support, control afterload, and maintain preload are indicated, but the prognosis is poor.

Conclusions

Aircraft fires and burns constitute a significant danger following aircraft accidents. The majority of aircraft burns follow post-crash fires. In accidents in which fuselage structural integrity renders the crash survivable the main factor affecting mortality and morbidity of passengers is their ability to escape from the fire.

It is important to remember that burns in trauma victims, especially after aircraft accidents, almost invariably form only part of the injuries sustained by the individual victim, who must be evaluated as a whole to determine correctly the treatment priorities. The management of the burns is along well established lines, keeping in mind that first airway, breathing, circulation, and spine stability are achieved; then cranial, thoracic, and intra-abdominal trauma must be ruled out or treated according to standard trauma care. These burns will tend to be severe and inhalation injury is frequent. The latter ranks highly among the immediate threats to life alongside craniothoracic and intra-abdominal trauma. After the immediate life threatening injuries have been treated, the burn becomes the major focus of the patient's care. These victims, most of whom have major burns, are best treated in specialised burn care centres with appropriate specialist surgical input.

The authors would like to thank Dr IL Naylor of the Postgraduate School of Pharmacology at Bradford University, UK, and Dr RD Cooter of the Plastic Surgery Department of Royal Adelaide Hospital, Australia, for their guidance and constructive criticism in the design and preparation of the early drafts of this manuscript.

1 Martin TE. The Ramstein Airshow disaster. *J R Army Med Corps* 1990; **136**: 19–26.
2 National Transportation Safety Board, *US air carrier accidents involving fire, 1965 through 1974, and factors affecting the statistics*. 1977. (Report NTSB-AAS-77-1.) Washington, DC United States Government: 1–60.
3 Gunby P. Fire, gases, smoke lower crash survival chances. *JAMA* 1984; **252**: 3349.
4 Hill IR. The immediate problems of aircraft fires. *Am J Forensic Med Pathol* 1986; 7: 271–7.
5 Berner WH, Sand LD. Deaths in survivable aircraft accidents. *Aerospace Med* 1971; **42**: 1097–100.
6 Galea ER, Markatos NC. Progress in mathematical modelling of aircraft cabin fires. *Disaster Management* 1988; 1: 32–40.
7 Pane GA, Mohler SR, Hamilton GC. The Cincinnati DC-9 experience: lessons in aircraft and airport safety. *Aviat Space Environ Med* 1985; **56**: 457–61.
8 Fulford P. An aircraft accident: How to survive. *J Bone Joint Surg* 1991; 73B: 694–5.
9 Greenberg BM, Brewer BW. Avianca Flight No. 052 accident: a plastic surgical perspective. *Plast Reconstr Surg* 1991; **88**: 529–35.
10 Mimpriss JG. *Fire and smoke in aircraft fuselages*. London: Flight Safety Committee Discussion Group, Royal Aeronautical Society, 1969.

11 Dudani N. Experience in medical coverage of airport disasters at Logan International Airport in Boston. *Aviat Space Environ Med* 1983; **54**: 612–8.

12 Carr JN, Omans LP. The ins and outs of aircraft passenger rescue. *Fire Engineering* 1991; Sept 83–98.

13 Mohler SR. Aircrash survival: injuries and evacuation of toxic hazards. *Aviat Space Environ Med* 1975; **46**: 86–8.

14 Hill IR. Mechanism of injury in aircraft accidents—A theoretical approach. *Aviat Space Environ Med* 1989; **60**(suppl): A18–25.

15 O'Hickey SP, Pickering CAC, Jones PE, Evans JD. Manchester air disaster. *BMJ* 1987; **294**: 1663–7.

16 Samuels A. The Manchester Airport Disaster. *Med Sci Law* 1987; **27**: 118–20.

17 Hill IR. An analysis of factors impeding passenger escape from aircraft fires. *Aviat Space Environ Med* 1990; **61**: 261–5.

18 Mason JK. Injuries sustained in fatal aircraft accidents. *Br J Hosp Med* 1973; 9: 645–54.

19 Braunohler WM, McMeekin RR. Deaths from burns in army aircraft, 1965–1971. *Aerospace Med* 1974; **45**: 939–41.

20 Watts R. Surviving a plane crash. *Med J Aust* 1990; **152**: 547–8.

21 Griffiths RW. Management of multiple casualties with burns. *BMJ* 1985; **291**: 917–8.

22 Mabrouk AW. A plan for the management of burns disasters. *Burn Incl Therm Inj* 1981; **8**: 139–40.

23 Sharpe DT, Roberts AHN, Barclay TL, et al. Treatment of burn casualties after the fire at Bradford City football ground. *BMJ* 1985; **291**: 945–8.

24 Sharpe DT, Foo ITH. Management of burns in major disasters. *Injury* 1990; **21**: 41–4.

25 Sharpe DT, Malata CM. The law and best practice of burns treatment in the 3 phases of a civil emergency. In: Suddards R, ed. *Encyclopaedia of civil emergencies*. Bradford, Sweet and Maxwell. In press.

26 Pegg SP. Burns management in a disaster. *Aust Fam Physician* 1983; **12**: 848–521.

27 Settle JAD. *Burns—the first five days*. Romford: Smith & Nephew Pharmaceuticals Ltd, 1986.

28 Moylan JA. First aid and transportation of burned patients. In: Artz CP, Moncrief JA, Pruitt BA, eds. *Burns: a team approach*. Philadelphia: WB Saunders; 1979: 151–8.

29 Robertson C, Fenton O. Management of severe burns. In: Skinner D, Driscoll P, Earlam R, eds. *ABC of major trauma*. Cambridge: Cambridge University Press, 1991: 83–7.

30 Herndon DN, Barrow RE, Linares HA, et al. Inhalation injury in burned patients: effects and treatment. *Burns Incl Therm Inj* 1988; **14**: 349–56.

31 Muir IFK, Barclay TL, Settle JAD. *Burns and their treatment*. London: Butterworths, 1987.

32 Press B. Thermal and electrical injuries. In: Smith JW, Aston SJ, eds. *Grabb and Smith's plastic surgery*. 4th ed. Boston: Little, Brown; 1991: 675–730.

33 Demling RH. Fluid replacement in burned patients. *Surg Clin North Am* 1987; **67**: 15–30.

34 Goodwin CW, Dorethy J, Lam V, Pruitt BA Jr. Randomized trial of efficacy of crystalloid and colloid resuscitation on hemodynamic response and lung water following thermal injury. *Ann Surg* 1983; **197**: 520–31.

35 Monafo WW, Freedman B. Topical therapy for burns. *Surg Clin North Am* 1987; **67**: 133–45.

36 Herndon DN, Langner F, Thompson P, Linares HA, Stein M, Traber DL. Pulmonary injury in burned patients. *Surg Clin North Am* 1987; **67**: 31–46.

37 Pruitt BA, Cioffi WG, Shimazu T, Ikeuchi H, Mason AD. Evacuation and management of patients with inhalation injury. *J Trauma* 1990; **30**(12 suppl): 63–9.

38 Traber DL, Linares HA, Herndon DN, Prien T. The pathophysiology of inhalation injury—a review. *Burns Incl Therm Inj* 1988; **14**: 357–64.

39 Hill IR. Inhalation injury in fires. *Med Sci Law* 1989; **29**: 91–9.

40 Pane GA. Toxic smoke inhalation and aircraft fires [letter]. *Am J Emerg Med* 1988; **6**: 82.

41 Clark CJ, Campbell D, Reid WH. Blood carboxyhaemoglobin and cyanide levels in fire survivors. *Lancet* 1981; **i**: 1332–5.

42 Clark CJ, Reid WH, Gilmour WH, Campbell D. Mortality probability in victims of fire trauma: revised equation to include inhalation injury. *BMJ* 1986; **292**: 1303–5.

43 Prien T, Traber DL. Toxic smoke compounds and inhalation injury—a review. *Burns Incl Therm Inj* 1988; **14**: 451–60.

44 Madden MR, Finkelstein JL, Goodwin CW. Respiratory care of the burn patient. *Clin Plast Surg* 1986; **13**: 29–38.

45 Fein A, Leff A, Hopewell PC. Pathophysiology and management of the complications resulting from fire and the inhaled products of combustion: review of the literature. *Crit Care Med* 1980; **8**: 94–8.

46 Agee RN, Long JM III, Hunt JL, *et al.* Use of [133]xenon in early diagnosis of inhalation injury. *J Trauma* 1976; **16**: 218–24.

47 Moylan JA. Inhalation injury—a primary determinant of survival. *J Burn Care Rehabil* 1981; **3**: 78–84.

48 Hunt JL, Agee RN, Pruitt BA, Jr. Fibreoptic bronchoscopy in acute inhalation injury. *J Trauma* 1975; **15**: 641–9.

49 Moylan JA, Adib K, Birnbaum M. Fiberoptic bronchoscopy following thermal injury. *Surg Gynaecol Obstet* 1975; **140**: 541–3.

50 Moylan JA Jr, Wilmore DW, Mouton DE, Pruitt BA Jr. Early diagnosis of inhalation injury using [133]xenon lung scan. *Ann Surg* 1972; **176**: 477–84.

51 Cioffi WG, Rue LW, Graves TA, McManus WF, Mason AD, Pruitt BA Jr. Prophylactic use of high frequency percussive ventilation in patients with inhalation injury. *Ann Surg* 1991; **213**: 575–82.

52 Cioffi WG, Graves TA, McManus WF, Pruitt BA Jr. High frequency percussive ventilation in patients with inhalation injury. *J Trauma* 1989; **29**: 350–4.

53 Levine BA, Petroff PA, Slade CL, Pruitt BA Jr. Prospective trials of dexamethasone and aerosolised gentamicin in the treatment of the inhalation injury in the burned patient. *J Trauma* 1978; **18**: 188–93.

54 Robinson NB, Hudson LD, Riem M, *et al.* Steroid therapy following isolated smoke inhalation injury. *J Trauma* 1982; **22**: 876–9.

55 Welch GW, Lull RJ, Petroff PA, Hander EW, McLeod CG, Clayton WH. The use of steroids in inhalation injury. *Surg Gynaecol Obstet* 1977; **145**: 539–44.

56 Tredget EE, Yu YM. The metabolic effects of thermal injury. *World J Surg* 1992; **16**: 68–79.

57 Janzekovic Z. A new concept in the early excision and immediate grafting of burns. *J Trauma* 1970; **10**: 1103–8.

58 Heimbach DM, Engrav LH. Excision of major burns. In: *Surgical management of the burn wound*. New York: Raven, 1984: 36–49.

59 Heimbach DM. Early burn excision and grafting. *Surg Clin North Am* 1987; **67**: 93–107.

60 Tandon SM, Sutherland AB. Some problems following tangential excision and skin grafting in dermal burns. *Burns Incl Therm Inj* 1976; **3**: 96–9.

61 Engrav LH, Heimbach DM, Reus JL, Harnar TL, Marvin JA. Early excision and grafting vs. non-operative treatment of burns of indeterminate depth: a randomised prospective study. *J Trauma* 1983; **23**: 1001–4.

62 Curreri PW, Luterman A, Braun DW, Shires GT. Analysis of survival and hospitalisation time for 937 patients. *Ann Surg* 1980; **192**: 472–8.

63 Monafo WW, Bessey PQ. Benefits and limitations of burn wound excision. *World J Surg* 1992; **16**: 37–42.

64 Pruitt BA Jr. The Burn Patient: II. Later care and complications of thermal injury. *Current Problems in Surgery*, Chicago, Year Book Medical Publishers, May 1979; **16(5)**: 1–95.

16
Crush asphyxia and management of "unannounced" major incidents, with experiences from Hillsborough

JIM WARDROPE

Crush asphyxia

Definition

Crush asphyxia is the term used to describe the condition caused by a slowly applied, sustained crush to the chest and abdomen resulting in an inability to ventilate the lungs. It most commonly occurs in a crowd where large numbers of people are confined with a large weight of people pressing from behind. There are some similarities to traumatic asphyxia, where there is a sudden violent crush, but there are enough significant differences to allow distinction between the syndromes.[1]

Major incidents due to this problem are not uncommon and since crush asphyxia usually occurs in large crowds there is potential for a large number of critical casualties. These may present to the emergency services within a short period of time.

History

> The fatal event has shown how very easily a mass of human beings, driven into a corner, may asphyxiate themselves.

This quotation does not describe any of the recent crowd disasters but an incident in 1883 at the Victoria Theatre in Sunderland in which almost 200 children died.[2] They had been leaving a children's entertainment down a flight of stairs but the doors at the bottom of the staircase were barred.

There have been a number of such incidents in the recent past: Bolton (1946), Ibrox (1971), Heysel, and, most recently Hillsborough (1989). All of these have involved crowds at soccer stadia. Soccer is the commonest reason for large crowds in United Kingdom and therefore carries the greatest risk of crush asphyxia incidents. Furthermore, football grounds often have steeply sloping areas, where gravity assists the mass of bodies in crushing the victims.

After each disaster, various recommendations are made and legislation may reduce the likelihood of recurrence. However, large crowds seem to behave almost like a fluid, and if the flow of the crowd is diverted into a confined space with insufficient outlets then injury due to crush asphyxia will occur.

The most recent of these disasters occurred at the Hillsborough football stadium in Sheffield, England, in 1989.[3] Teams from Liverpool and Nottingham were using this ground as a neutral venue for a semifinal of the Football Association (FA) Cup.

Before the match large numbers of fans were still outside the ground, and in their anxiety to gain access to the ground a crush developed in front of the entry turnstiles (figure 16.1). The police, fearful that serious injury might occur, requested the opening of one of the large EXIT gates (gate C, figure 16.1). This led to an uncontrolled entry of some 2000 people within 5 minutes. This crowd flowed down a tunnel leading to the "terraces" in front of the goal area, a position favoured by football spectators. However, this area was already full.

The crowd at the front of pens 3 and 4 became slowly crushed as the new arrivals piled into the back of this confined area. There was no way of escape, due to the high fence designed to prevent hooligans invading the pitch (figure 16.2) Within 20 minutes 95 people lost their lives and over 600 were injured.[1]

Pathophysiology

Ventilation of the lungs requires that the chest or abdomen must expand to suck air into the lungs. If external pressure prevents this movement then no air will flow and the victim will asphyxiate. In the crush of a large crowd, the slow sustained pressure results in gradual loss of consciousness "like drifting off to sleep". If the victims can be extricated at this stage then full recovery is likely. However, progressive hypoxia leads to increasing cerebral damage and eventually to hypoxic cardiac arrest.

The most severely affected patients show cyanosis of the head and upper

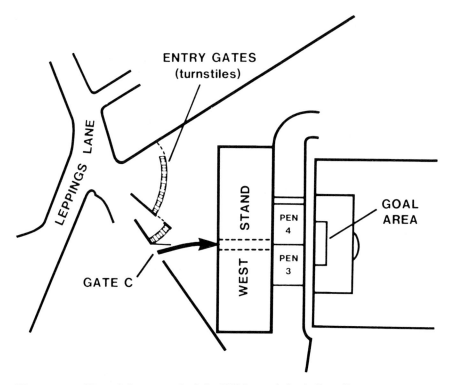

Figure 16.1—Plan of the west end of the Hillsborough football stadium.

limbs, profuse sweating, dilated pupils, and varying degrees of coma. The typical findings of traumatic asphyxia such as petechiae and subconjunctival haemorrhages are rare in crush asphyxia.[4,5]

In many of these disasters crush asphyxia is the only pathology, with a surprising lack of associated injury. In the 95 deaths at Hillsborough, crush asphyxia was the sole cause of death in 86 cases. The mode of death is hypoxic cardiac arrest, usually in asystole.

Nervous system injury

The most important organ injury is hypoxic brain damage. The main clinical signs are dilated pupils, confusion, irritability, and fits. In the early stages of a major incident there may be concern that such signs are due to direct trauma to the skull and brain. In the Hillsborough disaster there were no deaths due to intracranial bleeding.

One phenomenon observed in the survivors of Hillsborough was that of *delayed deterioration* of central nervous system (CNS) function. Some of the cases admitted for observation suddenly became confused, rapidly

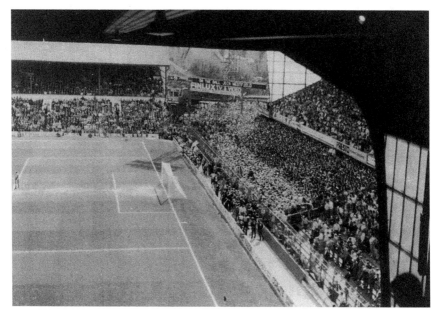

Figure 16.2—The Hillsborough disaster: the high security fence prevented escape from crushing.

progressing to grand mal convulsions. Loss of vision due to cortical disturbance was a further delayed problem in one patient. The cause of this delayed deterioration is not clear. The deterioration did not have the features of other post-anoxic syndromes.[3]

Peripheral nervous system injury: compression of the peripheral nerves resulted in neuropraxia in six patients, in three of whom the brachial plexus was affected. These nerve injuries were caused by prolonged pressure against fixed structures such as crush barriers.

Chest injury

In the 93 deaths at the ground and in the 159 patients admitted to hospital, significant chest injury was surprisingly rare. There were five pneumothoraces in the admitted patients, 17 patients had rib fractures, and one patient died from a rupture of the aorta.

Seven patients had evidence of aspiration of gastric contents on initial radiographs.

Nine patients had evidence of right heart strain diagnosed by electrocardiography (ECG) or by echocardiography. One victim who did not present to hospital on the day of the disaster was subsequently shown to have a ruptured mitral valve.[6]

Peripheral injury

Bruising and soft tissue injuries were very common but there were only five long bone fractures, one fractured femur, three fractures of the forearm, and one fracture around the ankle.

Clinical management

Pre-hospital

The response to any major incident must be flexible. The major variables affecting the efficiency of the response are the resources available, the severity of the injuries, and the rate at which the casualties present to the emergency services. In a major train or plane crash it may take may hours to free trapped casualties. In crush asphyxia it is often only a matter of lifting the victims from a pile of bodies.

Triage decisions will be difficult. Often the emergency services are on the scene before the incident occurs, due to statutory obligations to provide medical care automatically at large events.

In unconscious patients and those with respiratory arrest, basic airway care and ventilation will revive many victims. If there are large numbers of cardiac arrests much time may be wasted in prolonged cardiopulmonary resuscitation attempts. For those patients in cardiac arrest the outlook is not good. Two patients initially resuscitated in hospital from cardiac arrest following Hillsborough subsequently died, one being pronounced brain dead at 3 days after injury.

Patients who are confused or convulsing should be given priority, since this group is at most risk of long term brain injury. They should be given oxygen, the airway should be protected, and, if possible, fits should be controlled.

In the accident and emergency department

Triage

Large numbers may present within a short time span and it may be necessary to have two or more triage officers.

- Patients in cardiac arrest are unlikely to survive and should be pronounced dead unless there are adequate resources to deal with all other priority patients at the same time

- Patients who are unconscious, having fits, or markedly confused should all receive emergency resuscitation room care

- Patients with a history of loss of consciousness should be admitted

239

- Patients with difficulty breathing or with signs of shock require emergency resuscitation room assessment.

There are likely to be large numbers of "walking wounded", the upset and frightened. These patients should be seen and documented to allow formal social and psychological follow up.

Resuscitation

Normal assessment and treatment routines are carried out as laid out in the advanced trauma life support (ATLS) system. Hypoxia is the main cause of neurological problems and this should be treated aggressively.

Once life threatening problems are excluded then attention is given to the neurological state. Fits are very difficult to control with conventional anticonvulsants such as diazepam. All unconscious patients and those with fits should be intubated and ventilated. Confused patients should be fully assessed and if their conscious levels are deteriorating they should also be ventilated.

Patients requiring intubation should be given an induction agent such as thiopentone and a muscle relaxant to aid intubation and to prevent any further increase in intracranial pressure. Continuing care would be as for any brain injury, aiming to maintain the arterial oxygen tension between 15 and 20 kPa and the carbon dioxide between 3.5 and 4 kPa.

There will always be anxiety in the minds of the attending staff regarding the cause of the neurological signs. In disasters, doctors often think "head injuries" is the only cause of CNS deterioration. Urgent computed tomography (CT) is not indicated unless there is good external evidence of scalp or skull injury.

Due to the significant incidence of pneumothorax and aspiration of gastric contents, chest radiographs are required as a routine.

Crush asphyxia is likely to be the sole injury requiring resuscitation; however, other problems that may present are:

- Airway obstruction due to fractures around the larynx (probably due to the patient being stood on)

- Breathing problems due to a pneumothorax

- Hypovolaemia due to aortic rupture or abdominal injury.

Ongoing care of patients

Those patients requiring intubation receive the standard intensive care provided for any severe head injury. Ventilation and fluid balance are closely monitored. Fits may be very difficult to control and a continuous thiopentone infusion may be required. Aspiration of gastric contents is common and the use of prophylactic antibiotics seems to lessen the problems of chest infection.[3] Dexamethasone in a high dosage for 2 days was given in those severely injured at Hillsborough. Although there is little evidence that it improves the outcome in hypoxic brain injury, there were no adverse effects.[3]

The duration of ventilation will depend on the severity of the brain injury. Most of those requiring ventilation are likely to recover within 24 hours, but reduced conscious level and continuing fits are the main reasons for prolonged intensive care.

Electrocardiography should be performed and, when time allows, echocardiography is carried out. Right heart strain and pericardial effusion, although known to be associated with crush asphyxia, are not likely to cause any haemodynamic upset in an otherwise fit young person. Significant valvular damage needs to be excluded.[6]

Myoblobin levels will be raised, but there were no instances of renal failure in the Hillsborough victims.

In the management of the less severely injured *those with a history of loss of consciousness should be admitted as they have suffered a significant degree of hypoxia*. Late deterioration in neurological signs may occur. The patient may become increasingly confused and then have a grand mal convulsion. Late sudden loss of vision may also occur. These patients should also have a detailed examination, with emphasis on neurological and psychometric testing. Chest *x* ray, ECG, and echocardiography should be performed prior to discharge Few will require any treatment apart from adequate pain relief. If possible, all should receive an initial psychological assessment and a definitive plan for further follow up should be made in order to reduce the effects of post-traumatic stress disorder.

Outcome

Detailed follow up of all the patients injured in Hillsborough was not possible since many did not present to hospital on the day of the disaster and almost all lived away from Sheffield (in and around Liverpool). However, 22 patients who were seriously injured have been followed up.

Two patients who were initially resuscitated from cardiac arrest at admission subsequently died. One died after 2 hours and the other was pronounced brain dead after 3 days.

Five other patients were unconscious on admission (Glasgow coma scale less than 8). Two of these patients remained in a persistent vegetative state at 6 months after the disaster. There has been extensive publicity over the legal issue regarding the right to die of one of these patients. He died 4 years after the incident, soon after clarification of the legal position. The remaining three patients have very significant disabilities, mainly of higher cognitive function and memory.

Of the 15 other patients requiring intensive care (all but one requiring ventilation), 14 have recovered with only one having significant memory disturbance.

Crush asphyxia—summary

- All crowd events carry the risk of crush asphyxia. Such incidents may generate large numbers of casualties requiring immediate care

- Cerebral hypoxia is the major cause of neurological disability

- Priority treatment should be given to those who are unconscious but not in cardiac arrest, those who are having fits, and the markedly confused

- Intubation, controlled ventilation and control of fits are the most important interventions

- Prognosis is related to the degree of coma at initial presentation; regrettably, prolonged neurological disability is not uncommon

---

Managing "unannounced" major incidents

Introduction

The first indication of a major incident may be the arrival of large numbers of casualties at the hospital. This happened after the Bradford Stadium fire.[2] Similarly, the Sheffield hospitals involved in caring for the casualties of the Hillsborough disaster were not appropriately alerted before patients suddenly appeared in the accident departments. Communications are often cited as the most important problem in major incidents.[7,8] It is probably inevitable that there will be some failures of communication, and major incident planning should be flexible enough to plan for such eventualities.

Planning for the unexpected

The accident and emergency department will be the main portal of entry for the victims of a major incident. Therefore there should be clear planning arrangements to allow the following:

- The accident and emergency department must be able to activate the hospital major incident plan

- The responsibility for this decision should rest with a senior permanent member of staff, most probably the senior nurse on duty

- These staff must be given adequate training in this role and understand fully the mechanisms that are used to implement the major incident plan

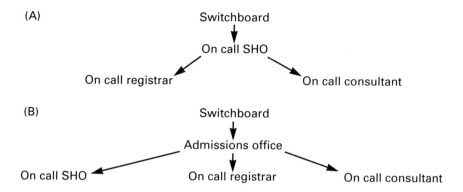

(A)

Switchboard

On call SHO

On call registrar   On call consultant

(B)

Switchboard

Admissions office

On call SHO   On call registrar   On call consultant

Figure 16.3—Call out systems. In system A the doctors may not be able to complete the call out sequence if there are large numbers of seriously ill. In system B the task of medical call out is delegated to clerical staff.

- There should be opportunities to test this part of planning. It should be made clear to staff that even if there is a "false alarm" there will be no penalty for implementing the plan: there is much more to be lost by delaying implementation in a true disaster than by being embarrassed by a wrong call out

- The structure of the hospital plan call out system should not rely on the "front line" doctors who are available in the hospital. If the disaster is unannounced then it is likely that these doctors will quickly become engaged in treating the seriously ill. The call out of senior staff from home should be delegated to the clerical/medical records/admissions staff, not telephonists (figure 16.3).

The arrival of large numbers of patients requiring urgent resuscitation is an unusual event, even in major disasters. Following Hillsborough, 28 patients requiring resuscitation arrived within 30 minutes. Four of these patients were triaged as dead on arrival, but in a further nine patients resuscitation was attempted, and in two patients cardiac output was restored. More selective triage—that is, making an early decision *not* to resuscitate—would have greatly relieved the pressure on the emergency resuscitation room.

Even with the most rigorous triage, 15 patients would have required urgent resuscitation. Most accident and emergency departments should be able to cope with such numbers. The emergency resuscitation room and adjacent areas should be able to provide at least 10 bed spaces with wall oxygen and suction. These can be converted into resuscitation points by

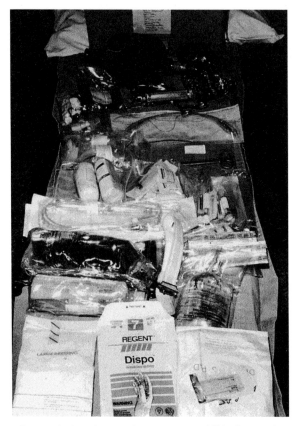

Figure 16.4—Pre-packed equipment for treatment of life threatening emergencies.

the use of pre-packed boxes containing all the equipment required for the treatment of life threatening emergencies (figure 16.4). Maintenance of this type of equipment requires regular attention and is essential to the management of such major emergencies.

Triage

Many accident and emergency departments aim to increase senior cover "out of hours", but at present it is likely that the initial triage may be carried out by junior staff who are not fully conversant with the full details of the hosptal major incident plan. Action cards are essential and should be readily available, easily read and easily understood (figure 16.5). Triage decisions may be difficult. Patients may be accompanied by friends and relatives who will place further demands on the triage officer. If possible there should be at least two triage officers.

244

ACTION CARD — TRIAGE OFFICER

— PUT ON THE TRIAGE OFFICER IDENTIFICATION
   TABARD
   (In grey cupboard marked "B")

— GO TO THE AMBULANCE DOOR

— ENSURE MEDICAL RECORDS OFFICERS HAVE
   ARRIVED
   (Call if not)

— AS PATIENTS ARRIVE CHECK FOR OUT OF
   HOSPITAL TRIAGE LABELS

— IF NO LABELS ARE PRESENT TRIAGE INTO:
   (See over for help on how to categorise)

CATEGORY	DESTINATION
Urgent	Resuscitation area, A & E
Moderate	Ward 61
Mild	Physiotherapy
Dead	Mortuary (plaster room)

(Front of action card)

TRIAGE CRITERIA

DEAD –
Victims of blunt violence with in cardiac arrest
Elderly in cardiac arrest
(not necessarily dead—penetrating trauma, hypothermia
triage decision will depend on resources available)

URGENT
Unconscious—Glasgow coma scale <12
Airway/respiratory problem:
Major facial injury   Noisy breathing
Dyspnoea   Resp. rate <12, >29.
Shocked
Obvious major bleeding   fractured pelvis
Clinical cervical spine injury

MODERATE
Stable patients with obvious injury that will require
admission
Stable patients with significant head/chest/
abdominal injury requiring full examination

NON-URGENT
Peripheral injury, e.g. Colles fracture, minor cuts
The upset

USEFUL TELEPHONE NUMBERS
Ambulance liaison ....   Mobile phone ....
Hospital control ....   A & E control ....

(Back of action card)

Figure 16.5—Action card for the accident and emergency department's officers.

Uncontrolled situation

The aim of management of a major incident is to try and maintain continuity of care, especially for the seriously injured. The ideal is for at least one doctor and one nurse (or "assistant") to provide the care for each patient requiring resuscitation. However, if the rate of arrival of the seriously injured outnumbers the available staff, then there may not be enough medical staff to allow for such individual care.

There should be a "fall back" plan put into operation until adequate help arrives. The senior doctor in the resuscitation area may have to perform a secondary triage role and assign the staff with the highest level of skills to the most needy. He should try to maintain a managerial role and should not become personally involved in practical tasks. It may be necessary to move doctors between patients to perform life saving procedures. If possible, at least one member of staff (nurse, student "assistant") should remain with the patient all the time, allowing continuity to be maintained.

Control regained

As more doctors arrive it will become easier to provide optimal care. At this point the situation should be reviewed and any problems encountered in the initial phase should be reassesed. Note keeping will have been minimal or non-existent in the early stages. As the clinical situation is stabilised, essential notes should be completed. After Hillsborough it was found that patients pronounced dead had *no* entries at all made in their major incident folders.

When more staff arrive, those involved in the early stages should be "stood down" from clinical care as quickly as possible. However, they should not be allowed to go home until there has been an opportunity for adequate debriefing.

Debriefing

Operational debriefing

Following any major incident there will be a need to compile a report. The best time to record a factual account of the event is immediately after staff are relieved from operational responsibility. Each member of staff should be individually interviewed. Notes are made concentrating on facts, timings of incidents, communications, and patients treated. Patients' records should be completed in detail. It is important that records of such debriefings are kept, preferably in typed form for ease of future reference.

Psychological debriefing

Staff involved in major incidents require support and help. There is an even greater requirement for this to be offered in the context of an "unannounced" major incident. Those staff present during the initial stages may have been subject to severe stress. These feelings may be made more acute if there has been a period where strict clinical control has been lost.

All such staff should have the opportunity to talk in confidence to a suitable counsellor. This counsellor should preferably not have been involved in the clinical management of the incident and should not be a member of the accident and emergency department staff. This should be the first part of a longer term support programme for the nursing and medical staff, which may need to be intensive over the first week. It is during this time that the external pressures from colleagues, friends and the media are likely to be greatest, with some of the reaction often being hostile to the hospital staff and emergency services.

Managing "unannounced" major incidents—summary

- All efforts should be directed to ensuring that hospitals have as much warning as possible of a major incident

- However, all plans must take into account the possibility of an "unannounced" disaster

- Action cards are an essential part of the major incident plan—they give immediate guidance to staff who may not be fully familiar with the plan

- Pre-planning and knowledge of potential problems enable an uncontrolled situation to become a controlled situation within the minimum period of time

- Psychological debriefing should be available to staff after the incident

---

1 Taylor R. *The Hillsborough stadium disaster. Interim report.* London: HMSO; 1989.
2 Lambert WO. The Sunderland catastrophe. *BMJ* 23 June 1883.
3 Wardrope J, Ryan F, Clark G, Venables G, Crosby CC, Redgrave P. The Hillsborough tragedy. *BMJ* 1991; **303**: 1381–5.
4 Sklar DP, Baack B, McFeeley P, Osler T, Marder E, Demarest G. Traumatic asphyxia in New Mexico. *Am J Emerg Med* 1988; **6**: 219–23.
5 Landercasper J, Coghill T. Long term follow up after traumatic asphyxia. *J Trauma* 1985; **25**: 838–41.
6 Gretch ED, Bellamy CM, Epstein EJ, Ramsdale DR. The Hillsborough Tragedy [letter]. *BMJ* 1992; **304**: 573–4.
7 Sharpe DT, Roberts AHN, Barclay TL, *et al.* Treatment of burn casualties after the fire at Bradford City football ground. *BMJ* 1985; **291**: 945–8.
8 Staff of the Accident and Emergency Departments for Derbyshire Royal Infirmary, Leicester Royal Infirmary, Queen's Medical Centre, Nottingham. Coping with the early stages of the M1 disaster: at the scene and on arrival in hospital. *BMJ* 1989; **298**: 651–4.

17
Dealing with chemical and radioactive decontamination in major disasters

ANDREW F DOVE

Introduction

This chapter describes the arrangements in the United Kingdom to care for casualties contaminated in an accident. It concentrates on organisational rather than clinical aspects. The principles will be the same in every country, but detailed arrangements for assistance and legal controls will vary.

Accidents resulting in the contamination of casualties are rare. When they occur, it is usually during the transport of toxic chemicals or radioactive materials. They will, however, cause disproportionate problems due to disruption of the normal functioning of the receiving hospital department. For this reason, it is imperative that pre-planning is undertaken.

The comparative rarity of such incidents means that little has been published relating to first hand experience. As is often the case, preparation for chemical contamination has been refined from war conditions[1] although some limited experience has been described from more normal civil practice.[2]

It is a tribute to the effectiveness of the regulation of the nuclear industry that few doctors have experience of the treatment of radioactively contaminated patients. Much of the reported first hand practical experience has come from Chernobyl,[3] while theoretical principles are used by a number of physicians who are involved in hospital emergency planning and the provision of care for nuclear facilities.[4]

In the United Kingdom, factories and other areas using dangerous materials are regulated by the Control in Major Accident Hazard Regulations (CIMAH) (1984). Similarly, there are effective regulations in place for the control of radioactive materials. In other countries, control is less rigid and major catastrophes have occurred—for example, at Chernobyl in Russia and Bhopal in India.

Principles of treatment

The principles of treatment are the same whether the casualty is contaminated with toxic chemicals or with radioactive materials:

- The physical condition of the casualty takes priority over decontamination procedures

- The number of staff involved in caring for the patient is kept to a minimum

- The facilities used are isolated until the patient has been decontaminated.

Where is advice available from?

One of the biggest difficulties experienced by those faced with a major contamination is obtaining information. In the majority of incidents which have occurred, as highlighted by the Bhopal tragedy, there was no accurate information available about the chemicals involved. Over 70 000 chemicals are in regular use, and it is not surprising that accurate toxicological information is often not available even when the chemical can be identified. Further research into the effects of individual incidents is likely to validate and increase present knowledge.[3,5]

Chemical contamination

In the United Kingdom, most lorries or railway carriages carrying hazardous chemicals are clearly labelled with the manufacturer's name, address, and telephone number on a HAZCHEM board. In addition, an appropriate symbol will be secured to the side (figure 17.1). The sign includes an emergency action code: in the example shown it is 3PE. The first number informs the fire and rescue service about the agent that should be used to fight the fire: 1 is water jet, 2 is water fog, 3 is foam, and 4 is a dry agent. The first letter gives information about the explosive risk, method of disposal, and protective apparatus to be used. The letter "E" appended to the number and letter means that evacuation of the surrounding area should be considered. The United Nations (UN) identification code, is an internationally recognised coding system for all chemicals; full listings of all codes used can be obtained from a regularly updated publication.[6]

Lorries carrying mixed loads in sealed drums are not required to carry

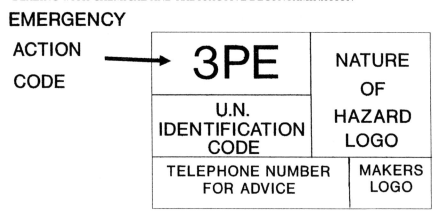

Figure 17.1—The layout of a HAZCHEM label.

any identification except for a single plain orange square on the front and the rear of the vehicle.

Hazardous loads being carried across national borders are labelled according to an agreement concerning the International Carriage of Dangerous Goods by Road (ADR). This label consists of only two numbers: the upper gives information about the nature of the hazard (toxic, radioactive, etc.) and the lower number is the UN identification code.

In the cab of any vehicle carrying toxic loads there will be a copy of the transport emergency card (Tremcard) issued by the European Council of Chemical Manufacturers Federation. This contains information about the cargo (including the nature of the hazard), protective devices to be used if handling the substance, emergency action, and any additional information provided by the manufacturer. The card must be available in the languages of the countries of dispatch, destination, and transit.

If further information is required, it may be obtained from the National Chemical Emergency Centre at Harwell.

Radioactive contamination

A multi-stage response is available. The system is laid out in HC(76)52, *National Arrangements for Incidents Involving Radioactivity and Arrangements for dealing with Contaminated and Radioactive Casualties* (NAIR).

All containers of radioactive material are prominently labelled with the black and yellow radiation symbol. If this is seen, the advisory system will be activated by the police. The first level of advice will come from radiation physicists at selected hospitals. This assistance consists of advising the police and fire and rescue services of potential hazards and the actions necessary to minimise and contain the danger.

If the scale of the incident exceeds the capacity of the initial response, further assistance will be sought through the second stage. This mobilises health physicists with industrial experience from organisations such as British Nuclear Fuels and the United Kingdom Atomic Energy Authority. The decision to invoke this level of assistance will be made by the hospital radiation physicists who made the first response.

The prime responsibility of the hospital physicist who is contacted under the NAIR arrangements is to provide advice to the police and fire and rescue service at the scene of the incident. This may mean that no advice is immediately available to the receiving accident and emergency department. This makes it especially important that some pre-planning has been undertaken to allow the situation to be controlled in hospital until help arrives.

Action at the scene

Security at the scene will be established by the police working in conjunction with the fire and rescue service. Medical services may be involved in siting a casualty clearing post and will need to take account of the prevailing winds and other relevant factors. In the M1 plane crash, kerosene was lying on the road and caused some difficulty in siting the medical facilities.

Health professionals are unlikely to be involved in evacuating casualties, as the use of breathing apparatus by untrained personnel is not recommended.

Decontamination facilities on site are likely to be provided by the fire and rescue service. Decisions about the evacuation of surrounding areas will be made by the police, fire and rescue service, and, if appropriate and possible, the medical services. Provision of temporary accommodation for evacuees is the responsibility of the emergency planning department of the local authority.

Action at the hospital

The most important factor in containing the situation in the accident and emergency department is to minimise the area affected by contamination.

If possible, casualties should be de-contaminated before entering the hospital. This may be difficult if a large number of people are involved. If the contamination is chemical, expendiency may demand that fire hoses are used in a nearby open area. Use of large quantities of water will ensure that the chemical is sufficiently diluted by the time it reaches the sewers not to cause problems. Discharge should be into a foul water sewer, however, and pre-planning for this eventuality should include identification of a suitable area. It may be possible to identify a local facility, such as swimming baths, to undertake this function but, irrespective of the well laid plans, it is still likely that the hospital will be involved.

Disposal of radioactive contamination is controlled by legislation. The consent of the Department of Environment senior radiochemical inspector should be obtained before any flushing is undertaken. If this is impossible because of the urgency of the situation, large amounts of flushing water should be used and the inspector should be notified as soon as possible. Contaminated clothes and surface material, such as soil, may only be disposed of with the consent of the inspector.

For smaller numbers of casualties, more specific arrangements may be made. Ideally, accident and emergency departments should have a decontamination room at the entrance to the unit. It should have external access and be capable of accepting ambulance and hospital stretcher trolleys. It should be tiled and the wall and floor coverings should be acid resistant. The ventilation and drainage should be self contained. Although these are official recommendations, few, if any, departments have such facilities, and makeshift arrangements are the norm.

Immediate expertise and equipment for decontamination is available from the fire and rescue service. They have mobile facilities that may be deployed to either the scene of the accident or the hospital. Careful decontamination is a time consuming affair, and it is unlikely that a mobile facility will be able to clean more than 10–12 casualties per hour.

Action within the accident and emergency department

Because of the major disruption likely to occur to the functioning of the accident and emergency department and the hospital, some elements of the major incident procedure should be activated on notification of a contamination incident with casualties. These would specifically include the communication arrangements between the hospital and the scene, the security of the department, and arrangements for dealing with press enquiries. Arrangements for making available large numbers of beds may not be necessary. Major incident plans should allow for such selective implementation.

To prepare for arrival of the casualties, an area should be identified close to the entrance of the accident and emergency department, with facilities for undertaking any necessary treatment. The number of entrances and exits should be kept to a minimum. The area should be isolated with warning signs and the boundaries marked with brightly coloured tape. The floor should be covered with plastic sheets and these sheets should be sealed at the edges with sticky tape. Clearly identified rubbish bins should be positioned for the disposal of contaminated waste. An area must also be identified for ambulance and any other non-hospital personnel to await decontamination and any necessary screening.

Key personnel should be identified who will treat the patient(s) within the contaminated area. The number of staff necessary will depend on the number of casualties and the extent of their injuries, but the staff should be as senior as possible and their number should be kept to a minimum. These doctors and nurses will wear surgical gowns, masks, hoods, double gloves, and shoe protection. If the contamination is chemical, a full length plastic gown and perspex face mask should be worn to protect against droplets. If the contamination is with radioactive material, all personnel in direct contact with the casualty should wear monitoring badges. Although with sensible precautions the risks of contamination of the treating staff is minimal, they should be aware that there is a slight risk. Pregnant women should be excluded from the area. All other personnel on duty must clearly understand their responsibilities and the importance of ensuring the isolation of the treatment area.

A member of the security staff should be positioned at the entrance to the treatment area to prevent access by unauthorised personnel. He or she will have an important role in ensuring that members of the hospital staff who are not usually based in the accident and emergency department adhere to all necessary restrictions.

When the casualty arrives, an immediate assessment with regard to the urgency of treatment will be made. This may result in immediate life saving care being undertaken or, if time permits, decontamination taking priority. All clothing will be placed in a plastic bag and retained within the contaminated area.

When the patient's condition permits, he or she will be decontaminated. If the contaminant is a chemical, the decontamination should be under-taken using Fuller's earth if there is skin contamination, followed by water. The use of neutralising agents should be confined to the scene of the accident. If radioactive materials are involved, soap, water, and soft scrubbing brushes should be used. The decontamination should be under-taken gently as any abrasions will allow systemic entry of the contaminant. Hair should be shampooed and eyes irrigated with saline.

If the accident has included the spillage of radioactive material, a detailed survey of the casualty is necessary before decontamination procedures are finished. If chemical contaminants are involved, it may be wise to take swabs for later analysis.

Further treatment

Chemically contaminated casualties

Adequately equipped accident and emergency departments will already have facilities to treat patients suffering from overdoses of drugs. Treat-ment of contaminated casualties will use many of the same therapies and techniques. It is impractical to expect that all antidotes will be held in stock. Part of the planning should, however, ensure that there is access to quantities of cyanide antidote, atropine for the muscarinic effects of organophosphorus contamination, and Fuller's earth for dry decontamination. Pralidoxime, a specific anti-cholinesterase reactivator, should also be available for organophosphorus poisoning but is only held in special centres: the hospital pharmacy will be aware of arrangements with the holding centre. Chelating agents such as British Anti-Lewisite may also be helpful. As a rule, industries using toxic chemicals will be aware of the availability of specific antidotes even if they do not hold them themselves.

Radiation victims

Medical physicists will be able to make an accurate assessment of the likely radiation dose received by the casualty and to advise about the next stage of treatment. In the United Kingdom there are only three hospitals that are equipped to care for patients who have received massive radiation doses: the Royal Marsden, the Hammersmith and the Middlesex hospitals, all in London. If necessary, admission to one of these specialised units should be arranged. Prior to transfer, blood should be taken for baseline measurements and consideration should be given to administering blocking agents if radioactive materials have been ingested.

Tidying up

Ensuring that the area used is free from contamination will be time consuming. Personnel who have been involved should use the boundary between the contaminated treatment area and the rest of the department as a changing area, and all protective clothing should be bagged and left in the contaminated area for later disposal. Disposal of radioactive material will be undertaken by the medical physicist in consultation with the Department of the Environment inspectorate. Disposal of toxic chemicals may need to await consultation with the manufacturers.

It is important to remember that dealing with seriously injured casualties is always stressful for the medical and nursing staff involved. Combining the usual stress with the limitation of the number of people involved and worries about their own safety may create an especially difficult situation for some people. Counselling may be necessary.

Conclusions

Care of contaminated casualties is difficult because of the concomitant disruption to normal hospital routines. Pre-planning and preparatory discussion with other agencies involved will make the situation manageable.

1 Shapira Y, Bar Y, Berkenstadt H, Atsmon J, Danon YL. Outline of hospital organisation for a chemical warfare attack. *Israel J Med Sci* 1991; **27**: 616–22.
2 Lavoie FW, Coomes T, Cisek JE, Fulkerson L. Emergency department external decontamination for hazardous chemical exposure. *Vet Hum Toxicol* 1992; **34**: 61–4.
3 Young RW. Chernobyl in retrospect. *Pharmacol Ther* 1988; **39**: 27–32.
4 Linneman RE. Medical experience and preparedness for handling radiation injuries. *J Med Assoc Georgia* 1989; **78**: 95–100.
5 Lorin HG, Kulling PEJ. The Bhopal tragedy—What has Swedish disaster medicine planning learned from it? *J Emerg Med* 1986; **4**: 311–16.
6 Waight DC, ed. *Dangerous substances*. Updated 1993. London: Croner.

18
Minimising injuries to occupants in aircraft accidents

DAVID J ANTON

EDITORS' INTRODUCTION

Although this book is devoted to the management of disasters and their aftermath the editors felt that the reader would be interested in the current steps being taken to improve aircraft safety particularly for impact type accidents. We are grateful to Dr Anton for reviewing the present situation and highlighting the safety measures which are being adopted currently to improve aircraft safety.

Introduction

As a form of transport, commercial scheduled aviation must be regarded as extremely safe. Wilson[1] analysed, for a variety of activities, the risks estimated to increase the chance of death in any year by 0.000001 (1 part in one million): these are given in the box.

Activities increasing the chance of death in any year by 0.000001

Activity	Cause of death
Travelling 10 miles by bicycle	Accident
Travelling 150 miles by car	Accident
Travelling 1000 miles by jet	Accident
Living for 150 years within 20 miles of a nuclear plant	Cancer caused by radiation

---

The perception of safety, however, bears little relation to real risk, and flying is regarded with apprehension by many. This appears to be because of the lack of personal control over the risk and because, when accidents happen, large numbers of people may be killed at one time. *Flight International* in an editorial in 1990 (17–23 January) commented that air travel was no longer getting safer, as the accident rate appeared to have levelled off. In this review of air travel in the 1980s, based on International Civil Aviation Organisation (ICAO) and International Air Transport Association (IATA) data, figures were presented indicating that for scheduled services of commercial aircraft of 9 tonnes maximum take off weight and over, and excluding the USSR, the decade annual average for accidents was 29 in the 1970s and 20.7 in the 1980s. Annual average passenger fatalities reduced from 825 to 670 and fatal accidents per million aircraft departures reduced from 2.9 to 1.75 (in the same decade the annual average of people killed on the roads of the United Kingdom alone was 5414). Within these figures there were wide regional difficulties in accident rates; Africa and Central and South America having a safety record between 10 and 12 times worse than North America and Europe.

Safety in commercial aviation is achieved by great attention to detail and a very high level of training and checking for its participants. Safety improvements result from improved designs and operating procedures and these in turn result, in large measure, from analysis of incidents and accidents.

The first systematic analysis of aircraft accident injuries was conducted in 1945 by De Haven in North America.[2] He concluded that:

- In accidents in which structure was distorted but remained substantially intact, the majority of serious and fatal injuries were caused by dangerous cabin installations

- Crash force, sufficient to cause partial collapse of the cabin structure, was often survived without serious injury

- The head was the first and often the only vital part of the body exposed to injury

- Fundamental causes of head injury were the presence of heavy instruments, solid instrument panels, and seat backs, and unsafe design of control wheels.

- The probability of severe injuries of the head, extremities, and chest was increased by failure of safety belt assemblies or anchorages

- Failure of the 454 kg (1000 lb) (breaking strain) safety belt occurred in 94 cases among 260 survivors of these crashes. Only seven survivors showed evidence of injury to the abdominal viscera; two of these injuries were classified as serious

257

- The tolerance to crash forces by the human body had been grossly underestimated

- If spin-stall dangers were lessened and safer cabin installations used, fatal or serious injuries should be rare in the types of aircraft studied except in extreme accidents.

In 1959, Eiband[3] summarised the literature on human tolerance to impact. He indicated that adequate torso and extremity restraint was the principle variable in establishing tolerance limits. Survival of impact forces increased with increased distribution of force to the entire skeleton, for all impacts, from all directions.

The general principles for improving impact survibability may be summarised thus:

- A protective shell, free of intrusion, must be maintained around the periphery of the occupant flail envelope

- The seat and its attachments should be as strong as the airframe to which it is attached

- The occupant should be restrained to his seat in such a way as to minimise flail

- Aircraft structures should be designed to crush and yield in such a way as to limit the load applied to the occupant.

The protective shell

Maintenance of a protective shell around the occupant requires consideration of both airframe integrity and of the integrity of items of mass which may injure occupants within the airframe. The integrity of the structure on impact is dictated by the circumstances of the crash. Unlike passenger cars and some military helicopters, passenger aircraft are not specifically designed to be crashworthy. Items of cabin furnishing and internal structure are designed for a static rather than a dynamic loading situation and only the seats require to be dynamically tested. The consequence is that structural deformation leading to changes in planned load paths can cause structural failures in otherwise minor impacts. Floor deformation or failure leads, in turn, to seat failure, which may then expose the occupant to the fatal effects of secondary impact and crushing.

A high proportion of survivable accidents occur on or in the immediate vicinity of airfields, where there is often a considerable distance (in impact terms) for the aircraft to be brought to rest. Where fuselage breaks occur these tend to be forward or aft of the centre section, where there are abrupt changes in the ultimate strength and stiffness of the airframe as well as differences in the inertia of the structure. Fuselage breaks are frequently associated with injury. This can be due to direct trauma as a result of the disruption and also to the effects of secondary failures in overhead bins and furnishings occurring as a consequence of the failure. Both these mechanisms were evident in the M1 Kegworth aircrash.

Passenger seats and restraints

In 1983 the Federal Aviation Authority (FAA) published the results of a review of crash injury protection in survivable US civil air transport accidents between 1970 and 1978. The purpose of the review was to (a) compile a database on passenger seat and restraint system performance in survivable accidents, and (b) determine if a correlation existed between occupant, seat and restraint system performance, airframe and floor deformation, and passenger injuries and fatalities. The report indicated that

Although injuries and fatalities seem to be decreasing in the more recent survivable crashes, seat performance continues to be a factor in these crashes. Failures ranging from seat pan collapse to complete breakaway of the seat assembly from the floor are reported. Floor or cabin deformation is frequently a cause of seat failure. Flailing injuries, due either to bending over the restraint system or secondary impact with the aircraft interior appear to be common.

The US study listed 327 fatalities and 294 serious injuries to passengers involved in accidents with US carriers where seats could have been a contributing factor. Four areas were indicated that had to be addressed to improve occupant protection.

- The survivable crash environment required definition so that crash loads and displacements could be established

- An understanding of structural component and whole aircraft response to the crash environment was required

- Validated analytical modelling and test engineering methods required development

- Human factors and injury mechanisms for occupants of transport aircraft required definition.

As a result of the study the FAA announced its intention to introduce new seat and restraint standards for new type certificate passenger aircraft. The then existing requirements provided that seats and safety belts should sustain the load factors given in the box. A safety factor of 1.33 was applied to the above loads. Seat manufacturers were allowed to demonstrate compliance with the load and safety factors by static testing for these "9 G" seats. The standards also applied to the supporting structure of each item of mass that could injure an occupant if it came loose in a minor crash landing.

The new FAA standards took effect in June 1988 (see box).

Federal Aviation Authority standards for static load factors assuming a minimum seat occupant weight of 77.18 kg (170 lb)

	Pre-1988	1988 standard
Forwards	$-9.0\,G_x$	$-9.0\,G_x$
Rearwards	—	$+1.5\,G_x$ (no previous requirement)
Sidewards	$\pm1.5\,G_y$	$\pm3.0\,G_y$ airframe, 4.0 G seats and attachments
Downwards	$+4.5\,G_z$	$+6.0\,G_z$
Upwards	$-2.0\,G_z$	$-3.0\,G_z$

Additionally two dynamic tests were defined, using instrumented 50th percentile 49 CFR part 572 anthropomorphic test dummies to simulate seat occupants. Test 1 approximates to a near vertical impact, with some forward speed, applying a minimum of 14 G deceleration from a minimum velocity of 10.67 m/s, canted aft 30° from the vertical axis of the seat. Test 2 approximates a horizontal impact with some yaw, applying a minimum 16 G deceleration from a minimum of 13.41 m/s, the seat yawed 10° from the direction of deceleration; thus these seats are commonly called 16 G seats. To simulate the effects of cabin floor deformation, the parallel floor rails or fittings in test 2 are misaligned by at least 10° in pitch, and 10° in roll before the dynamic test. The tests require that the seat remains attached, although it may yield to a limited extent. The tests also include a requirement limiting the pelvic load to 6.7 kN (1500 lbf), head deceleration to a head injury criterion (HIC) of $\leqslant 1000$ and axial femoral load to 10.0 kN (2250 lb). Of these two tests, test 2 is considered the more stringent. The peak deceleration (16 G) and the velocity change (13.41 m/s) were chosen as the result of a study of crash dynamics recorded from accidents, and the levels were also considered to be compatible with existing floor strengths in the current fleet of transport aircraft.

Subsequent to the promulgation of these rules the FAA issued a notice of proposed rule making (NPRM) to cover the installation of the upgraded seats in new aircraft of current type and within the existing fleet; all transport category aircraft would be required to have seats meeting these new criteria by June 1995.

The scope for reducing trauma related casualties might appear low. The FAA estimates that as a result of overall improvements in fire safety, in the air traffic control system, in training of crew members, and in the aircraft, the prospective casualty rate should show a 50% reduction compared with that in the study period (1970–8). The FAA went on to estimate that it was likely that only a small percentage of passengers would be helped by the new seat standards; the estimate being a 3–15% reduction in fatalities and a 2–9% reduction in serious injuries. It must be emphasised, however, that a significant number of deaths are due to fire. The National Aeronautics and Space Administration (NASA) sponsored a study[4] of transport aircraft crashworthiness for the period 1959–79. Data on transport aircraft world-wide were reviewed. The Boeing Commercial Aircraft Comapany, which took part in the study, selected 153 impact survivable accidents out of a worldwide total of 583. Of 3791 fatalities in the 153 impact survivable accidents, Boeing reported that 1356 were known to be due to fire, 476 to trauma, 218 to other unspecified causes, and for 1741 fatalities no known reasons could be identified. Fire clearly presents the greatest hazard, although the topic is so large that it lies outside the scope of this chapter, which is concerned only with impact trauma.

Passenger seat orientation

The question of passenger seat orientation has been a matter of debate. Eiband[3] suggested that a rear facing passenger seat would offer the best protection in an impact. He cautioned that such a seat should include a lap and chest strap, a winged back with full head rest, load bearing arm rests with recessed hand holds, and provision to prevent arm and leg flail. For maximum protection in forward facing seats Eiband recommended full body restraint and a full height seat back with integral head support.

Pinkel[5] analysed the theoretical performance of forward and rearward facing seats in transport aircraft. He assumed that passenger restraint forces were applied through the seat back attachment points on the forward facing seats, and through the seat back, at a point twice the distance of the seat belt attachments to the floor, on the rear facing seats. Using these assumptions he calculated that rear facing seats would have half of the design strength of forward facing seats, if the increase in weight due to the need for a stronger seat back was ignored. Pinkel, although recognising the lack of available actual crash data for reaching a firm decision on seat orientation, discussed the relative merits of forward and rear facing seats in the following terms:

> In crashes involving fire or ditching, it is important that the passengers survive the actual crash with only minor injuries, so that they can evacuate the aeroplane. Rearward facing seats should provide better protection from injury, and appear to have an advantage under these conditions.
> In crashes which do not involve fire or ditching, rapid and unassisted evacuation of the airplane is not so critical, and a higher level of injury might be acceptable. The forward facing seat should have greater strength than a rear facing seat of equivalent weight, and thus restrain the passenger in more severe crashes. Since a passenger who is held in place by his seat generally

261

fares better than one who breaks free, a forward facing seat appears to have an advantage under these conditions.

Mason[6] reviewed practical experience with rear facing seats. He quotes one series of investigations in which 18.9% of forward facing passengers died, compared with 5.3% of rear facing occupants. In another study 11.1% of passengers in forward facing seats were killed and 84.4% uninjured. The comparable figures for rear facing seats were 1.0% killed and 98.3% uninjured.

Notwithstanding the obvious biomechanical advantages of a rear facing seat, the overwhelming number of passengers in commercial aircraft travel facing forwards, restrained only by a lap belt. There are several reasons for this.

Firstly, as Pinkel's work[5] indicates, on a material for material basis, that rear facing seats are heavier than forward facing ones if the same impact performance is required. Increased floor strength, and hence mass, is also required if the increased loads on impact, with rear facing seats, are to be built into the structure, with no risk of failure. The cost implications of mass increase were addressed by the FAA, which calculated that each 0.45 kg (1 lb) weight increase in an aircraft would require 56.8 l (15 US gal) of additional fuel per annum.

Secondly, there is a considerable reluctance on the part of the airlines to fit rear facing seats. It is claimed that passengers do not like them. This is borne out by apparent passenger preference for forward facing seats in those aircraft where both seat types are fitted. Regrettably, many rear facing seats have not been correctly designed and are uncomfortable. Experience in those aircraft fitted only with correctly designed rear facing seats has shown that passengers are frequently not aware of seat orientation.

Thirdly, there is evidence to suggest that passengers in rear facing seats are at risk from being struck in the face by objects falling from overhead bins or the bins themselves during impacts. The risk of head and facial injury is held to be less when seats face forward.

Crashworthiness

As already indicated, commercial transport aircraft are not specifically designed to be crashworthy, in contrast to some helicopters. However, this general statement does not apply to the fuselage and items of structure, such as engines and undercarriages, that *are* designed to meet heavy landing conditions and also specifically designed to fail in a planned manner on impact. Considerable differences in impact performance exist between aircraft types. Because of their greater bulk, large aircraft such as the Boeing 747 attenuate loads on occupants much more than is the case with smaller narrow body types. In the future, the advent of very large capacity airplanes capable of seating up to 800 passengers may offer even better attenuation. Whether this is achieved will depend upon where in the fuselage the occupants are seated and how the structure actually behaves dynamically.

Guidelines exist for crashworthy design; the reader should consult the US Army *Aircraft crash survival design guide*,[7] for further information, particularly for small aircraft and helicopters.

Analytical tools—computer simulation and impact testing

In 1983, the FAA recommended that validated analytical modelling and test engineering methods required development.[8] This was a re-statement for commercial jet transport aircraft of an original joint NASA/FAA observation in 1972. In the 1970s the FAA, NASA, and the aviation industry had started a cooperative effort to develop the technology for improved crashworthiness and occupant survivability in general aviation aircraft. This work lead to the development of computer programs such as KRASH, DYCAST, and ACTION. KRASH is a hybrid digital program that solves the coupled Euler equations of motion for n interconnected lumped masses. Each mass has a maximum of 6 degrees of freedom defined by inertial coordinates and eulerian angles. The concentrated masses interact through interconnecting beams which are appropriately attached and have specifiable stiffness. KRASH was used by the UK Air Accidents Investigation Branch in the analysis of the impact of the Boeing 737-400 at Kegworth with some success. There are difficulties in using the program on this scale, however, since few are experienced in its use on large aircraft structures and a degree of engineering judgment requires to be exercised. Similar conditions apply to the use of finite element programs such as DYCAST. For a fuller description of available programs and limitations in their use the reader is referred to Jones and Wierzbicki.[9]

Some test and analytical work can be conducted on impact test tracks. These, however, suffer from a number of limitations. Most survivable aircraft crashes involve considerable stopping distances from velocities of up to 100–150 knots. During the crash the aircraft will usually experience significant forces in the x and z axes and may also experience y axis and rotational forces (the tail section of the Kegworth aircraft providing an example of this). Such forces may be applied on more than one occasion during the impact. Such a crash environment can be simulated by programs such as KRASH, and the occupant response to such a crash environment can be followed with occupant response simulations such as MADYMO. Decelerator tracks, however, can only produce an approximation of one pulse from the crash, normally at a lower impact velocity and over a relatively short stopping distance. The test seat and occupant can be oriented to permit an impact in the principal vector, although the full effects of vector change cannot be reproduced.

Investigation of a large number of survivable aircraft accidents has indicated that the principal impacts can be simulated by a single triangular pulse. The pulse is specified in terms of peak G, impact velocity, and time to peak G. These parameters vary with the size and type of aircraft. Typical examples for light aircraft, rotorcraft, and public transport aircraft are utilised in the proposed and actual new FAA seat requirements.

Anthropomorphic test devices (ATDs) or "dummies" are used in impact testing to give an indication of the loads that would be experienced by a human. Most ATDs have been developed for use in the automotive industry and have response characteristics that are optimised in the x axis; even in this axis there tend to be serious deficiencies in the response of the head and neck. Anthropomorphic test devices are particularly limited in z axis behaviour, exhibiting a response that is noticeably stiffer than a human subject. This is a significant drawback for aviation research, since almost all aircraft crashes have a significant z axis component in the principal impact vector.

However, ATDs have a very valuable part to play in understanding the detailed interactions between the occupant and the seat on impact. For such work the decelerator track limitations referred to above are not a significant drawback. Any ATD used for such work requires very sophisticated and comprehensive instrumentation. Only one ATD in current manufacture (the Hybrid III) can be so equipped, and few laboratories in the world are currently able to support such work because of the cost and complexity involved.

Can survibability be improved?

Most current commercial aircraft types will be flying with "16 G" dynamically tested seats within the next 5–10 years. New type certificate aircraft shortly entering production will be similarly equipped but, at present, both new and current types will have floors and cabin furnishings and fittings designed around the older static strength requirements. For cabin furnishings and fittings this situation could be changed, as these are items that are regularly replaced within the life of the airframe. Floor design is fixed for the life of the aircraft, and any improvements in this area will depend upon research into feasibility and regulatory activity. New large aircraft (600–800 seats) may be more crashworthy because of their bulk, although this needs to be confirmed, but new type certificate narrow body aircraft will require additional efforts on the part of manufacturers and regulators if improvements in structural crashworthiness are to be achieved.

Improvements in seat design should be sought. There is little doubt that considerable research needs to be done to understand more fully the mechanisms of occupant injury in forward facing seats. There is also no doubt that passengers restrained only by lap belts are exposed to a very high risk of incapacitating injury when exposed to the 16 G standard impact, although the introduction of this standard has been of considerable benefit. It is questionable whether, in the absence of a full harness or placing the seats unacceptably close together, there is much point in attempting to better the 16 G standard as this will only further increase the risk of injury. The introduction of rear facing seats, already extensively used in US military transports, offers the only real hope for a significant reduction in the risk of impact injury. Such a move is likely to be resisted by the airline industry, particularly on the grounds that it would be unpopular with passengers. It is clearly essential that independent market research is funded to analyse this matter and that funding be devoted to a proper understanding of the required consequential changes to cabin floors and furnishings.

Finally, in any discussion of improving survivability it must be remembered that it has to be done at a price that does not deter the customer. There is little point in making a relatively very safe form of travel so expensive that the traveller moves by other means and thus exposes himself to greater risk.

1 Wilson R. Analysing the daily risks of life. *Technol Rev* 1979; **81**(4): 40–6.
2 De Haven H. *Relationship of injuries to structure in survivable aircraft accidents.* Washington D.C.: National Research Council; 1945. (Report No. 440.)
3 Eiband AM. *Human tolerance to rapidly applied accelerations: a summary of the literature.* Cleveland, Ohio: NASA Lewis Research Centre; June 1959. (NASA Memo 5-19-59E.)
4 Widmayer E Jr, Brende OB. *Commercial jet transport crashworthiness study.* Virginia: NASA Langley Research Centre, Hampton; Atlantic City: FAA Technical Centre; Apr 1982. (Report No. NASA CR 165849/FAA-CT-82-68.)
5 Pinkel II, *A proposed criterion for the selection of forward and rearward facing seats.* New York: American Society of Mechanical Engineers; Jan 1959. (Paper No. 59-AV-28.)
6 Mason JK. *Aviation accident pathology.* London: Butterworths; 1962.
7 *Aircraft Crash Survival Design Guide.* Fort Eustis, Virginia: US Army AVRADCOM; (USARTL-TR-79-22.)
8 Federal Aviation Authority. *Crash injury protection in survivable air transport accidents— US Civil Aircraft Experience from 1970–1978.* Washington D.C.: Federal Aviation Authority, Mar 1983. (FAA Report DOT/FAA/CT-82-118.)
9 Wittlin G. In: Jones N, Wierzbicki T, eds. *Structural crashworthiness.* London: Butterworth; 1983.

19
Minimising injuries to occupants of motor cars

PETER D THOMAS, MAUREEN A BRADFORD

EDITORS' INTRODUCTION

Motor car and motorway accidents provide hospitals in the UK and Europe with many multiply injured patients but only rarely do the numbers of injured approach those which can be defined as a major incident or disaster. However, because of the increasing number of motorway incidents both in the UK and in Europe, the editors have invited Mr Thomas and Ms Bradford to describe the steps which are being taken by the motor industry to reduce the risk of injury from motor car related accidents. The editors hope that this focus on prevention of injury rather than on the management of injury will be of interest to many readers.

Introduction

Each year 25 000 car occupants are killed on the roads in Europe, equivalent to the population of a small town. These fatalities represent a disaster of a different kind to those of other transport modes. Although large numbers of deaths rarely occur in a single accident the costs to the community are many times greater. Using the 1990 UK cost per fatality of £665 000 this represents a cost to the European Community (EC) of £16 625 000 000 each year. Surviving casualties add to this sum. The reduction in these numbers is seen as a priority and research is being conducted into the most appropriate means to achieve this.

Car users form 51% of all road user deaths and are the largest single group of casualties for each country in the EC.[1] This proportion, however, varies from a minimum of 34% of total casualties in Portugal to a maximum of 80% in Luxemburg. The national priorities for each country within the EC will therefore vary. There are no statistics available that describe the numbers of surviving road user casualties in a uniform manner; some countries collect them as a matter of course—for example, the UK and

Germany—others do not. The full scale of road user injuries in the EC is therefore unknown.

Research may address vehicle safety in two ways: by investigating methods of reducing the numbers of accidents occurring and by searching for means to mitigate the severity of injuries when a crash occurs. This chapter seeks to describe the progress towards the development and implementation of car occupant injury reduction, measures known as secondary safety.

History of safety legislation

The secondary safety design of cars offers the largest potential for the reduction of fatalities and injuries for all road user categories and the level of understanding about the protection for car occupants is well developed. The introduction of secondary safety performance requirements in the early 1970s means that some current developments are simply fine tuning of the safety systems. However, there are still areas where large scale savings in human life and injury can be made. Early priority was rightly given to the reduction of fatalities, but the importance of the morbidity of the survivors has increased with the recognition that for those crashes which are survivable the numbers of casualties with long term impairment may be large.

The early EC directives and the Economic Communities of Europe (ECE) regulations dealt primarily with frontal crash protection because these constitute the largest group of impacts, at 53% of the total. Research attention moved to side impact protection in 1979 with the implementation of the EC joint biomechanics programme. The development of a test procedure and anthropometric dummies continued through the 1980s, but final agreement on the legal requirements for side impact protection has still not been reached. Research has now refocused on the subject of frontal crash protection.

Frontal crash protection

The current levels of frontal crash protection required to be built into cars include a limit of intrusion in a front barrier test in which a car travelling at 50 km/h strikes a rigid barrier with full overlap. Other regulations require occupant ride-down from the steering system and from the seat belt. The use of front seat belts is generally believed to be high in much of Europe, reaching 95% in some countries, so car designers are routinely able to use the longitudinal members in the front structures to provide additional ride-down. The validity of the front barrier test is now being heavily criticised since the test conditions are in fact rare in real world crashes.[2] The front barrier test requirement also fails to take into account the improved levels of energy management that are routinely available and it does not assess the

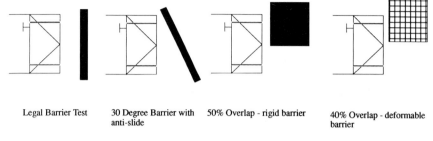

Legal Barrier Test   30 Degree Barrier with   50% Overlap - rigid barrier   40% Overlap - deformable
                 anti-slide   barrier

Figure 19.1—Types of frontal crash test.

levels of injury that the occupants might sustain. It is an easy performance requirement to achieve.

Partial overlap tests

Real-world car to car crashes more commonly involve a partial overlap of the car front. This configuration results in a concentration of the crash loads along one of the side members. There is often sufficient energy remaining to cause deformation of the vehicle interior and a reduction of the opportunity for occupant ride-down. Crash data analyses suggests that this intrusion is often associated with serious injuries which may be life threatening or may cause long term impairment.[3,4]

The development of an improved test is centring around the mitigation of the partial overlap condition.[5] Many groups are examining the 40% or 50% overlap crash[6] into a block, although a barrier set at 30° to the crash with blocks to prevent slide-off has been suggested as an alternative. Some groups are also using a deformable barrier face to simulate the characteristics of car to car crashes more accurately.[7] These crash types are illustrated in figure 19.1. An impact with a rigid barrier forces the energy absorbing side members to collapse in the designed manner. Deformable objects such as other cars are less stiff and cause the side members to collapse in a different mechanism with resulting intrusion into the passenger compartment. Intrusion is a well recognised cause of head, chest and leg injuries.

A dummy is used to measure head injury criterion, chest and pelvis acceleration, and femur loads, which reflect human tolerance to injury. A new frontal impact test will reproduce the conditions where current vehicles sustain steering wheel, fascia, and footwell intrusion. It will encourage improved car design and assess occupant loads which should be below those recognised as corresponding to severe injury.

Tests that simulate car to car crashes may not address collisions with rigid and heavy objects such as trees, lamp posts, trucks, and buses. These crashes often apply the impact loads to a localised area of the car structure, as is seen with underrun of a truck or with a collision with a cast iron lamp post. The energy management in this type of crash is much more difficult and some manufacturers are suggesting that even with full seat belt use the potential for reduction of fatalities is limited.[8] It is likely that for the forseeable future many of these crashes may not be survivable without changes to the roadside environment or to the design of trucks. Recent studies have concluded that up to 30% of fatalities resulting from underrun with a truck front could be prevented by the use of lower bumpers or other front underrun protection on the trucks themselves.[9]

Vehicle aggressivity

It is likely that a partial overlap test requirement will eventually be implemented and that car structures will become optimised for the new condition. A natural step will be for the longitudinal members at the car front to become stiffer in order to allow them to absorb more energy. This may be particularly important for small cars where crush space is more limited. These cars will have the potential to present a greater hazard if they are in collision with unmodified cars or if they strike the side of other cars and cause the struck vehicle to absorb more energy, with consequent intrusion. Many of the cars in current production that are designed for a partial overlap condition are large prestige models, they often have a relatively high mass which may tend to increase the hazard to the occupants of other cars if they collide with them in an accident.

In a similar way the use of additional side members at the top of the wings may raise the local stiffness and thus increase the hazard to pedestrians who are struck on the head or pelvic areas.

It is imperative that the development of an improved frontal crash test should be accompanied by an examination of the effects of new designs on the whole accident population. A new crash test procedure must include a systematic assessment of the aggressivity of vehicles with regard to other car occupants and pedestrians.

Side impact

The reduction of injuries in side collisions has been one of the major areas of secondary safety activity for at least the last 10 years. There is now a proposed ECE regulation describing a test using a mobile barrier and a special side impact dummy. The test aims to reproduce the essential characteristics of a car front to car side collision and will focus research into reducing head, torso, and pelvis injuries. The design of the barrier has remained largely unchanged since its description in 1985; the intervening time has been spent gaining its general acceptance. The dummy has been more difficult to develop, but the current design of the "Eurosid" dummy has recently gained the approval of the International Standards Organisation as corresponding sufficiently closely to the biological model. An EC directive requiring side impact protection is likely to be issued in 1996, probably coming into effect for cars built after 1999. The most recent delays are a consequence of the car manufacturers' wish to have the option of a computerised testing procedure as an alternative to full scale testing. Unfortunately computer simulation techniques are not yet sufficiently advanced, and the side impact proposals have been slowed up while these techniques are developed.

In contrast, the USA authorities have been able to issue an Advanced Notice of Proposed Rulemaking in 1988, the rule was issued as an amendment to FMVSS 214 in 1990 and applies to cars sold after 1995. This contrast between the European and American approaches to safety regulation raises questions over the effectiveness of the European decision making process and the coordination of the technical development of European standards.

The proposals for a side impact requirement simulate a perpendicular car front to car side collision with an approach speed of 50 km/h. Comparisons with real world crashes suggest that such a test reflects the essential characteristics of a small proportion of fatal crashes, although it simulates non-fatal crashes better.[10] In particular, 40% of all fatal side collisions are with trees or poles, which can result in a different loading to the side of the car from that caused by collisions with other cars. Also the change of velocity of fatal real world crashes is typically much higher than that seen in the test. Finally, 29% of all fatalities in side collisions are seated on the non-struck side and they sustain fatal head injuries from striking the intruding side structures in very high energy collisions. It is unlikely that any of the proposed test requirements will result in much improvement in this mechanism of injury.

The implementation of the side impact requirements will be a major piece of European secondary safety regulation, as it addresses a crash configuration that is particularly difficult to design solutions for. This difficulty has resulted in a number of design strategies; some address the profile of the intruding door face[11] while others deal with the reduction of intrusion.[12] As new cars comply with side impact protection requirements it will become essential to monitor the changes so as to facilitate identification of the most effective techniques. A "before and after" study will be of particular value in evaluating the effectiveness of the current proposals and allowing the identification of the best direction for further progress.

Whole system test

It has been suggested that the adoption of only one test in order to examine the level of protection offered by a car should be considered. This would have the advantage of reducing the cost of testing for manufacturers. However, it is not possible for a single test to examine the range of conditions that occurs in the real world. For example, a dummy might have a head contact with a part of the steering wheel during a crash test but the stiffness and hazard from the steering wheel varies—the rim is generally stiffer at the join with a spoke than between spokes. The single test will reproduce one steering wheel attitude, one contact on one part of the head, and one head attitude and velocity. Although this set of conditions might occasionally be the most severe, it is not readily controllable and will not be consistent across models of car. Items such as the steering wheel, facia, and footwell are better examined more rigorously by the use of supplementary component tests.

In addition, a single test will only examine the performance of a car at one speed, and several studies have shown that this can lead to systems that give lower protection over the whole range of crash severity.[13] Techniques are now available to optimise crash protection over the full energy spectrum.[14]

Car downsizing

International interest in environmental issues has focused intensively on the consumption of resources and pollution caused both by car manufacture and by the use of cars. One aspect has been to encourage car manufacturers to build smaller and lighter vehicles to improve fuel efficiency. The mass of a vehicle is a dominant factor in the protection offered—a heavy vehicle will experience a smaller change in velocity than a light vehicle when in collision with another vehicle. The collision between a heavy truck and a car illustrates this mass effect.

The introduction in the USA of the corporate average fuel economy standards has had the effect of encouraging the rate of reduction of car mass. In one US state the average mass decreased from 1680 kg (3700 lb) in 1984 to 1227 kg (2700 lb) in 1987. This resulted in an increased injury rate of 14% in car to car crashes, 11% in car to truck collisions and 10% in single vehicle non-rollover crashes.[15] Another study based on fatal accident data from the USA states that an increase in driver fatalities is inevitable if any car is replaced by a lighter one or if the whole population of cars is replaced by a new population of lighter but otherwise identical cars.[16] The study suggests that fuel economy and safety are intrinsically in conflict. However, the change in the numbers of fatalities resulting from pollution effects and manufacturing processes remains to be estimated. More effective use of the car mass by improved design can facilitate greater protection than is available for current cars. However, a small car can never offer greater protection than a large car fitted with the same level of technology.

Crashworthiness assessment

Safety is rapidly becoming a key selling point for many new cars. Consumers are taking account of the car makers claims for safety when choosing a new car. Folksam, a Swedish insurance company, estimates that 40% of fatalities would be prevented if every purchaser bought the safest car in the class. However, the available data evaluating safety levels are limited and this has led a number of groups in Europe to develop their own safety rating scales. These employ a variety of methods including staged collisions, real world crash studies, and vehicle inspection. Some combine the appraisal of secondary safety with primary safety effects. Each system has its own advantages and disadvantages:

- Staged collisions can test the performance in severe impacts and dummy readings can indicate the severity of injuries likely to occur but they cannot readily take account of the variety of impact types and human tolerance to injury

- Inspections rely on the protocol having a clear basis of real world crash data but, along with staged collisions, have the advantage of being effective at an early stage in the product life cycle. They address only the presence of a feature not its effectiveness, but they may take account of potential hazards to other road users. They can also include the inspection of items not subject to legal requirements—for example, the face protection offered by the steering wheel. Recent comparisons of the rank order of models inspected and featuring in real world crashes show a useful degree of consistency[17]

- Feedback from real world crashes can reflect the full variability of the crash event but requires a large data set before accurate detailed results are available for a model. They are therefore dependent on the model mix in the population under scrutiny and the size of the data collection exercise. Analysis of real world data frequently has the extra problem of insufficient exposure data

- Examinations of primary and secondary safety effects are particularly difficult to interpret in the absence of exposure data and are open to misinterpretation.

The safety rating scales in use in Europe have developed in a piecemeal fashion. There needs to be a programme to bring together techniques based on staged front and side collisions supplemented by vehicle inspections to identify the presence of safety equipment. The results would be published soon after a car was produced and the results would be supported by later feedback from crash examinations, which would supply more detailed design information. Such a programme would keep the advantages of each while avoiding many of the disadvantages and is best operated at a

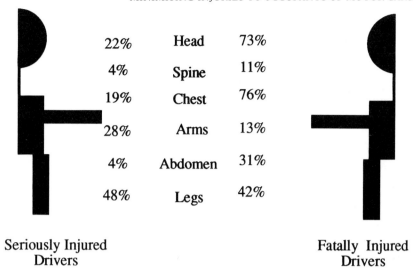

22%	Head	73%
4%	Spine	11%
19%	Chest	76%
28%	Arms	13%
4%	Abdomen	31%
48%	Legs	42%

Seriously Injured
Drivers

Fatally Injured
Drivers

Figure 19.2—Injury patterns of restrained drivers.

European level to match the European car market. Unfortunately there is no group that has the responsibility together with the resources necessary for this operation, which would undoubtedly be expensive.

Occupant injuries and contacts

The pattern of injuries sustained by restrained drivers in frontal crashes varies depending on the severity of impact and this has a consequent effect on the ensuing priorities.

When non-fatal severe injuries are examined, the legs (48%), chest (19%), and head (22%) are found to be the most commonly injured. Fatally injured occupants show a different pattern, with injuries to the chest (76%), head (73%), and abdomen (31%) being more frequent than those to the legs (42%).[18] Figure 19.2 shows these injury patterns. The issues for the survivors are therefore concerned with long term impairment, hospitalisation period, and treatment costs, particularly those resulting from leg injuries. To prevent fatalities research is now centred on the prevention of chest, head, and abdominal injuries, which would increase the chance of survival.

For this discussion "impairment" will be used to describe the physical loss of function which occurs after injury, while the use of "disability" will be avoided because of the complex relationship of "disability" to psychological factors and compensation as well as to impairment.

Seriously injured survivors have on average 1.25 body regions with an Abbreviated Injury Score (AIS) of 3 or above, while fatalities have an average of 2.58 body regions injured. This higher multiplicity of injury means that a safety measure that reduces severe injuries to just one body region may not have a large effect on the reduction of fatalities. For example, a fatality may have AIS 5 injuries to the head, chest and abdomen. Even if the AIS 5 head injury is prevented this would still leave two other AIS 5 injuries and a fatal outcome is still likely. On the other hand, a measure that prevents an AIS 3 leg injury of a survivor is likely to have a substantial benefit, since the casualty is not likely to have another injury of the same severity.

It is difficult to compare the importance of injuries to the different body regions of survivors. The normal injury severity scale used is the AIS;[19] this measures the threat to life and therefore can only be useful for assessing the priorities for fatalities. There is no equivalent scale in current use that assesses the impairment which might arise from individual injuries.

Investigations of real world frontal crashes have identified a set of typical injury-contact pairs. These include head and face lacerations from windscreen materials; facial bone fractures and minor brain injury from the steering wheel; severe head injuries from exterior objects; neck sprains following restraint use; chest bruising from seat belts; severe thoracic and abdominal injury from a combination of the steering wheel and the seat belt in higher energy crashes; and upper and lower leg fractures from the intruding fascia and footwell. Current research and development work is addressing a number of these issues. For example, improved belt systems have resulted in a reduction of slack to avoid head contact with the wheel. Equally, there are improved designs of wheel that minimise facial injury, although the supporting test methods have so far failed to be adopted as a legal requirement. Other problem areas have been only partially addressed—much frontal crash research includes the reduction of femur loads (to reduce the risk of femur fractures) but fails to address the more common and more impairing lower leg (tibia) and ankle injuries. Airbag development appears to be solely directed to a reduction of facial injuries, while any mitigation of the torso to wheel interaction is incidental. The reduction of head injuries caused by contact with external objects, a difficult task, does not seem to be addressed at all at present.

Adult restraint

Seat belts

The effectiveness of seat belts in reducing injury had been confirmed following the introduction of the mandatory use of seat belts in many countries. A number of improvements to the standard belt have been made including several types of pre-tensioner and webbing grabbers. Their use in high volume vehicles is expected to result in significant reductions of face contacts on the steering wheel and knee contacts on the fascia. Other improvements to belt systems have been suggested, including the use of 80 g maximum head deceleration, a maximum chest compression of 50 mm, and the use of a device to check lap section geometry.

Recently, belt effectiveness in protecting car occupants seated on the non-struck side in oblique side collisions has been questioned following estimates that 35% of such occupants slip out of the diagnonal section. This has been shown to result in head and face injuries from contact with the struck side of the car and also results in torso injuries induced by the belt.

Further developments in sensor technology may permit the use of intelligent restraints that use crash sensing data, occupant weight, and the position of the seat on its runners to tune the restraint performance to the needs of the crash.

Airbags

In 1984 the USA introduced a requirement for passive restraint systems that automatically protect unrestrained occupants in frontal collisions. As a result many American manufacturers have fitted airbags to the steering wheel to protect drivers. Other airbags are installed within the fascia to protect unrestrained front passengers.

The American airbags are typically set to inflate in the event of a 12 km/h frontal collision. Within 30 ms a gas generator will inflate the airbag in front of the driver. Whether restrained or unrestrained the driver will always move towards the airbag. The occupant loads force the gas out of vents or through the airbag material to provide a progressive deceleration. Figures 19.3a and 19.3b show the sequence of airbag performance.

Early estimates show that an airbag alone will reduce deaths by 18%. Use of a lap diagonal belt alone reduces deaths by 41%, while the combination with a full size airbag will provide an additional 5% reduction in deaths (that is, 46% reduction). For this reason, airbags are promoted as supplementary restraints rather than as the primary protective system.

A full size American type of driver airbag has a typical volume of 70 litres. Smaller 40 litre airbags ("Eurobags") are being installed into the steering wheels of European cars. Of injuries from the steering wheel, 72% are to the face or head while 17% are to the torso. The smaller "Eurobags" are intended to reduce the incidence of the head and face injuries, but the reduction of the torso injuries that also occur is less certain. However, head and facial injuries from the steering wheel account for only 36% of the economic cost of steering wheel injuries. Sixty per cent of the cost is attributed to the smaller numbers of torso injuries. The cost saving from injury reduction from the use of "Eurobags" may turn out to be outweighed by the costs of fitting the airbag if they do not reduce torso injuries.

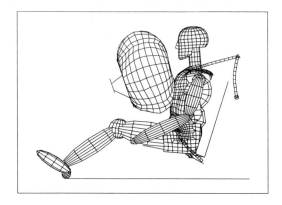

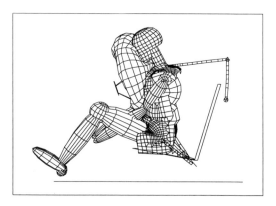

Figure 19.3—Airbag inflation sequence. Courtesy of Ove Arup and Partners.

The use of airbags in smaller European vehicles raises difficulties less frequently seen in the American market. In particular, a smaller car requires a faster trigger and inflator than a large car. Airbag development must also take account of short drivers, who sit closer to the steering wheel and may experience higher loads from contact with an inflating airbag.

A further difficulty accompanies the use of passenger side airbags together with rear facing child restraints. These airbags can be over twice the volume of a full size driver airbag. As they inflate they may impact the child restraint behind the head of the rear facing infant. In such a condition, experimental work has revealed that a child can experience very high head accelerations, double those experienced with no airbag.[20] For this reason the US National Highway Traffic Safety Administration has strongly advised that rear facing child restraints should not be placed in seat positions fitted with airbags. A similar action has been taken by the European car and restraint manufacturers.

Prototype airbag systems for side impact have been developed to provide

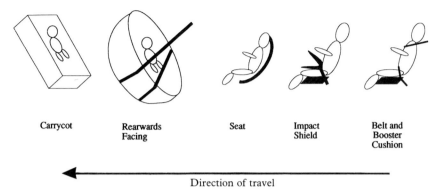

| Carrycot | Rearwards Facing | Seat | Impact Shield | Belt and Booster Cushion |

Direction of travel

Figure 19.4—Types of child restraint.

chest ride-down when deployed from an arm rest and head protection when deployed from the side header. These novel designs may provide a way of reducing head injuries from contacting exterior objects; however, there is a need for considerable development before they can be used in production vehicles.

Child restraint

Restraint types

Children have special requirements of car restraint systems. They have a lower tolerance to injury and the strong parts of their bodies are less well developed and less able to carry crash loads than is the case for adults. Infants particularly have a very different mass distribution, with a relatively large head and weak neck muscles. They may not be able to support themselves in an optimum posture. Older children may not wish to stay in one position for a long period.

A number of restraint types have been developed to address the needs of each age group; they are illustrated in figure 19.4. The very youngest children are able to use either carrycot restraints or rear facing seats. Carrycot restraints normally include an arrangement of webbing straps which encircle the carrycot and secure it in the car. The performance of the straps is specified by regulations. The performance of the carrycot, which applies the loads to the infant, is not specified. Crash tests examining these restraints have shown that the carrycot frequently provides the limiting factor. Carrycots can be designed to carry crash loads but they are frequently not. The use of these restraints may therefore give a completely false impression of security.

277

A higher degree of protection can be gained from the use of rear facing infant seats. The child faces towards the rear of the car and the loads in the most common frontal crashes are distributed through the child's back; there is no concentration of forces along the neck. Real world studies have shown that this type of restraint can provide a very high level of protection when used correctly.[21] Rear facing seats are not legal for children above 10 kg in the EC, although systems are available in Scandinavia. These are also highly effective in reducing injuries, although misuse has been found to be a compromising factor.

Forward facing child seats are frequently used for children of between 9 kg and 36 kg. They may be designed to be solely forward facing or they may also be capable of being used by infants facing rearward. Again, they have been found to be highly effective in large numbers of crashes. However, there have been a number of accident reports that have shown that cervical spine fractures can occur; these injuries are almost invariably fatal but appear to be confined to children under 2 years old. Although cervical spine fractures are extremely rare,[22] an international task force has nevertheless examined the cases available and come to the conclusion that rear facing restraints would offer greater protection, as would the use of 5- or 6-point harnesses with top tether straps on the seats.

Impact shields are restrained by a lap belt and distribute crash loads between the child's torso, pelvis, and thighs. Although there is a risk of ejection, for children below 2 years old, they can be effective for larger children. They are popular in certain countries and misuse has not been observed to be a problem. They are most appropriately used for the restraint of larger children and in seats fitted only with a lap belt.

Booster cushions raise the pelvis height of older children and ensure that crash loads are not applied to the soft parts of the abdomen. Again they are very effective in reducing injuries and encouraging seat belt use.

Child restraint misuse

The misuse of child restraints has been identified in as many as 75% of users[23] and has been observed in many countries. It has been shown by experiments to reduce the levels of protection markedly;[24] a correctly used child restraint reduces fatalities by 70%, while partial misuse reduces the risk of death by only 40%.

Misuse takes many forms. The restraint can be incorrect for the age of the child. A rear facing design might be used facing forwards. The restraint can be incorrectly strapped into the car or the child may be inadequately secured into the restraint. Most commonly the harness webbing and any adult belt may be loose, introducing excess slack and hence increasing the chance of injury.

Several groups have recommended that restraints should only be capable of being installed in one way, while new designs incorporate systems allowing harness adjustment with a single strap. A number of manufacturers are now recognising that typically 58% of rear seat occupants are children and are integrating child restraints into the rear seats of cars. Current designs feature booster cushions alone, but prototype infant restraints have also been developed.

An installation system called ISOFIX or Unifix has been developed in Sweden to avoid some of the difficulties over the installation of child restraint systems into the cars. The system uses a set of small catches on the child restraint that engage with small bars within the structure of the car seat. The positive engagement of the catches and the absence of restraining straps minimises the opportunity for incorrect installation. Through the use of electrical connectors, ISOFIX will also make it possible to provide a method of signalling the presence of a rearward facing child restraint, this signal can then be used to disengage a passenger airbag.

European accident data sources

The introduction of European Whole Vehicle Type Approval in 1994 will serve to strengthen the European car market. Decisions over vehicle design and safety performance have been made at a European level since the 1970s. This centralised activity has not been supported by an equivalent system that evaluates the problems of secondary safety in European vehicles. When any accident research is carried out, it is usually financed by individual governments or manufacturers. While the research findings and recommendations may reflect the needs of the funding group they may not be accepted by other EC countries.

There is a lack of coordinated basic information on road user casualties. For example, casualties who survive but are injured are not counted in a uniform way in the 12 member countries; European restraint use rates are unknown, nor are rates known for helmet use by motorcyclists. There are also no representative data describing the patterns and causes of European road user injuries. This makes the assessment of safety priorities difficult to establish, and there is no way in which the introduction of safety counter-measures can be monitored across Europe. There is a corresponding lack of data on the causes of accidents and the role of vehicle design.

The improvement of side impact and partial overlap protection to cars are both major safety items. There is currently no way that the effect on the complete European accident population can be adequately assessed.

This lack of a uniform European accident data set has served to delay or prevent many pieces of safety regulation. Frequently the lack of real world accident data is taken to infer that no problem exists, while in reality there are no data because there is no group that collects the data. Examples are the inordinate time taken to implement side impact countermeasures and the inability to agree on the need for a "face-friendly" steering wheel.

In contrast, the USA has an accident data system that correlates with the needs of the safety targets of the National Highways Traffic Safety Administration. The USA has a general estimates system, which uses a sample of around 46 000 accidents each year from 60 sites. These crashes represent the estimated 6 500 000 accidents nationally and supply basic data on roadway, vehicle, and road user characteristics. These data are supplemented by a greater level of detail collected for all fatal crashes within the fatal accidents reporting system and a highly detailed data set collected within the national accident sampling system which collects data on 7000 light passenger vehicles each year. The centralised consistent approach of the American accident data collection system has facilitated the early development of more demanding safety requirements and a safer vehicle population.

Summary

- The safety design of cars is changing rapidly. New types of protective systems are being introduced and new regulations are anticipated that will raise the level of protection offered to car occupants

- Improved front and side impact requirements will encourage manufacturers to tune car structures to the common crash conditions

- Improved restraints will control occupant kinematics more closely and reduce the loads experienced

- These new systems have the potential for significant reductions in injury, but the direct reductions may never be known because there is no investigation system that is able to assess the changes in the European accident population that are attributable to these systems

- The cost effectiveness of new systems may never be known because of insufficient data collection

1 European Conference of Ministers of Transport. *Statistical report on road accidents.* Department of Transport, HMSO, 1991.
2 Thomas C, Koltchakian S, Tarriere C. Inadequacy of 0 degree barrier with frontal real-world accidents. 12th International Conference on Experimental Safety Vehicles, May 29-June 1 1989, Goteborg, Sweden.
3 Mackay GM, Cheng L, Smith M, Parkin S. Restrained front seat car occupant fatalities—the nature and circumstances of their injuries. *Accident Anal Prev* 1992; 24(3): 307–315.
4 Ward E, Pattimore D, Thomas P, Bradford M. *Leg injuries in car accidents—are we doing enough?* International Conference of the Biomechanics of Impacts, September 11-13 1991, Berlin, Germany.
5 Vallet G, Cesari D, Derrien Y, Ríordán O. Test procedure comparison in frontal impact. 13th International Technical Conference on Experimental Safety Vehicles, November 4-9 1991, Paris.
6 Schmitz A, Kraemer B. Crash Tests—one element to assess passive safety of passenger cars. 13th International Technical Conference on Experimental Safety Vehicles.

7 Hobbs CA. The need for improved structural integrity in frontal car impacts. 13th International Conference on Experimental Safety Vehicles.

8 Henry C, Koltchakian S, Faverjon G, Le Coz J. Survey of "car to fixed obstacle" fatal crashes. 13th International Technical Conference on Experimental Safety Vehicles.

9 Thomas P, Clift L. *Analysis of fatal accidents involving heavy goods vehicles—front underrun accidents in 1988*. TRRL Contractor Report.

10 Thomas P, Bradford M. Side impact regulations—how do they relate to real world accidents. 12th International Technical Conference on Experimental Safety Vehicles.

11 Hobbs CA. The influence of car structures and padding on side impact injuries. 12th International Technical Conference on Experimental Safety Vehicles.

12 Deng Y. Side impact simulation and injury assessment. 12th International Technical Conference on Experimental Safety Vehicles.

13 Korner J. *A method for evaluating occupant protection by correlating accident data with laboratory test data*. Society of Automotive Engineers International Congress and Exposition, Detroit, Michigan, USA, February 27-March 3, 1989.

14 Norin H, Jernstrom C, Koch M, Ryrberg S, Svensson S. Avoiding sub-optimise occupant safety by multiple speed impact testing. 13th International Technical Conference on Experimental Safety Vehicles.

15 Klein TM, Hertz E, Borener S. A collection of recent analyses of vehicle weight and safety. 13th International Technical Conference on Experimental Safety Vehicles.

16 Evans L, Frick MC. Driver fatality risk in two-car crashes—dependence on masses of driven and striking car. 13th International Technical Conference on Experimental Safety Vehicles.

17 Krafft M, Kullgren A, Lie A, Nygren A, Tingvall C. *Car model safety rating based on real life accidents*. IRCOBI; 1991.

18 Thomas P, Bradford M, Ward E. The causes of head injuries in real-world car crashes. 13th International Technical Conference on Experimental Safety Vehicles.

19 *Abbreviated injury scale*. Association for the Advancement of Automotive Medicine, 1985, 2340 Des Plaines River Road, Des Plaines, IL60018, USA.

20 Avanessian H, Ridella S, Mani A, Krishnaswamy P. *An analytical model to study the infant seat/airbag interaction*. Analytical Modelling and Occupant Protection Technologies; Society of Automotive Engineers, February 1992. (SAE SP 906.)

21 Carlsson G, Norin H. Rearward facing child seats—the safest car restraint for children? *Accident Anal Prev* 1991; **23(2/3)**.

22 Fuchs S, Barthel N, Flannery A, Christoffel K. Cervical spine fractures sustained by young children in forward facing child seats. *Pediatrics* 1989; 2: 348–354.

23 Shelness A, Jewett J. Observed misuse of child restraints. Society of Automotive Engineers Child Injury and Restraint Conference Proceedings, October 17-18, 1983, p. 135, San Diego, California, USA.

24 Kahane C. *An evaluation of child passenger safety. The effectiveness and benefits of child safety seats*, National Highway Traffic Administration, Technical Information Service, Springfield, Virginia, USA. 1986. NHTSA Technical Report DOT HS 806889-90.

Introduction to the appendices

W ANGUS WALLACE

It is always difficult and sometimes impossible to identify an ideal emergency plan for a particular area or for a particular hospital. However, the reader will wish to study plans that have been prepared by other hospitals and regions for an indication of what might be appropriate for their particular hospital or region. The major emergency plan for the University Hospital, Queen's Medical Centre in Nottingham underwent considerable change immediately after the M1/Kegworth aircrash and as a consequence of that accident. The plan was generally simplified and streamlined. Part of the plan, including the overall major accident plan and summary relevant to the accident and emergency (A & E) department, together with the action card for the senior A & E doctor and the action card for the senior A & E nurse, are reproduced here.

A Regional Plan from the Mid-Western Health Board of the Republic of Ireland is also reproduced. This plan was devised because of the close proximity to Shannon Airport, the most westerly airport on the European continent and the one most likely to be involved in a major aircraft incident because it is the first airport reached on transatlantic flights. It must be emphasised that the plan from the Republic of Ireland does not necessarily conform to the United Kingdom standard but it does give an insight into the sort of plans that might be prepared outside the United Kingdom.

We are grateful to the Mid-Western Health Board for permission to reproduce their major emergency plans.

In addition we would refer the reader to the excellent publication *Emergency planning in Ireland*, by Patrick A O'Riordan, published in 1992 by the Institute of Public Administration (ISBN 1 872002 56 0), 57–61 Lansdowne Road, Dublin 4, Ireland. This very readable book reports on the development of emergency planning in general, reviews the literature on disasters, discusses the international situation with regard to disaster planning, and focuses on emergency planning for the Irish Republic.

Appendix A
Excerpts from the major emergency plan of the University Hospital, Queen's Medical Centre, Nottingham

ANDREW F DOVE

Introduction

When a major disaster occurs, hospitals involved will find that the medical aspects of care cause few problems; the greatest difficulties occur with the organisational requirements. It is important, therefore, that considerable pre-planning has taken place. Hospitals are complex and, for a big unit, the complete plan may run to many hundreds of pages. A central coordinating function is essential both within the hospital and between the hospital and the emergency services.

Certain general requirements for effective plans may be defined. At one level, they should be readable and not bedevilled with fine detail but, within the total plan, they should be sufficiently precise for individuals to act upon directly. Roles within the plan should be defined by position (that is, consultant orthopaedic surgeon on call) rather than name (that is, Mr Smith). Procedures and documentation used should be as close to normal routine as possible. They must provide a framework to manage any type of incident: the problems presented by a large number of patients with burns will be very different from those of caring for a large number of people with radioactive contamination. The plan must also be kept constantly under review and the responsibility for its currency at all levels clearly defined.

It is important that the plan recognises reality. It is easy to overestimate a unit's capacity and, therefore, not to anticipate requirements for assistance. Similarly, concerned relatives will ring the receiving hospital even if a police enquiry bureau is set up and publicised: failure to anticipate this may cause major disruption to the functioning of the hospital.

The plan published here was written after our experience in a major disaster and is in four parts:

(1) An overall summary of the plan is given to *all* employees.
(2) Each department (21 in all) has its own summary plan written in a common format; these are designed to fit into the back of the plan summary folder. The accident and emergency department's plan is given here.
(3) Each department has a detailed plan, which defines geography and routines.
(4) Derived from this are action cards that give a step by step guide for workers: two examples of action cards are given.

Please note that the accident and emergency department at University Hospital, Nottingham, has three consultants, one of whom would be delegated "site medical officer" at the scene and one would be "accident and emergency consultant in charge of the department."

University Hospital, Nottingham: Major Accident Plan

Introduction—scope of the plan

A *Major Accident* is an accident or emergency or combination of incidents which, because of the number and severity of live casualties, creates a demand for hospital services that requires the implementation of contingency arrangements.

This is a summary of the University Hospital Major Accident Plan and describes how the Hospital will work if it is overwhelmed with patients. Each department has its own plan and action cards and you must be familiar with the one that affects you: there is space for your *Departmental Plan* at the back of this booklet.

All departments will be involved and the contribution made by each Department will be crucial to the successful treatment of patients.

This plan describes the arrangements to:

(i)   Run the hospital and mobilise staff.
(ii) Treat patients as they arrive.
(iii) Treat patients over the medium and long term.
(iv) Care for relatives.
(v)   Care for staff.
(vi) Manage the aftermath.

Medical volunteers who do not have specific duties in the plan should report to the *Doctors Mess* (C Floor, between East Block and South Block). Volunteers from other disciplines should report to the *Volunteer Bureau* which is situated in the *Ante-Natal Waiting Room* on B Floor.

If you are off duty but are scheduled to be on duty shortly, you will be needed to relieve staff who have been working during the initial phase. Unless you are contacted by your Nurse Manager, you *should not come to the Hospital* until your scheduled start time. Staff travelling in by car should use the multi-storey and surface car parks. Keep well away from the main entrance and Accident and Emergency Department.

Accountable Managers are responsible for up-dating their plan and for ensuring that all staff are familiar with their role.

Overview

The successful management of a Major Accident requires close co-operation between all *Emergency Services*. The responsibility for the incident site and identification of fatalities rests with the *Police*. The responsibility for rescue and safety of the site rests with the *Fire and Rescue Service*. The Health Service is responsible for medical care at the scene, transport to Hospital, identification of surviving casualties and medical care of survivors.

Police Officers and an *Ambulance Liaison* Officer are stationed within the Hospital to co-ordinate activities, and may be contacted through *Hospital Control*, General Office, B Floor, East Block.

All casualties from a Major Accident will initially pass through the *Accident and Emergency Department* at the University Hospital. Decisions about disposal will be made after patients have been resuscitated. Although the *City Hospital* will not receive patients direct, specialist units there will be alerted early and some senior personnel from the City will attend the Accident and Emergency Department and assist in the initial management of casualties.

When the plan is activated, a single ward will be cleared (West F19 for adults or East D34 for children) to act as the receiving ward. All patients who are not transferred to specialist areas (i.e. ITU or Burns Unit) will initially go to the receiving ward for further treatment.

Hospital Control will also maintain contact with other Health Service agencies, including support Hospitals and District and Regional Health Authorities.

The alert

The initial warning of an accident is likely to come directly to the Accident Department from *Ambulance Control*. In the event of information arriving through other channels, the Accident and Emergency Department must be informed immediately. The decision to implement the plan will be made by the *Senior Doctor* and *Senior Nurse* in the Department in consultation, if necessary, with the on-call *General Manager*.

When the decision has been made, the *Telephone Switchboard* will be instructed to notify key personnel.

Site provision

As soon as possible, a *Site Medical Officer* and *Flying Squad* team will travel to the scene by ambulance. This will be an *Accident and Emergency Consultant*, accompanied by an *Accident and Emergency Senior House Officer* and at least *two nurses* from the Department.

The Site Medical Officer is responsible for:

(a) Providing medical advice to senior officers of other services at the scene.
(b) Co-ordinating medical care at the scene.
(c) Maintaining contact with the Hospital.

Further medical and nursing personnel and equipment will be despatched at the request of the Site Medical Officer. These may include surgical or paediatric teams.

Hospital organisation

When the plan is implemented, the *Hospital Control* is established close to the B Floor concourse and will be signposted.

The Controllers are responsible for all Hospital activities whilst the plan is in operation.

The Control Room will be staffed by:

(i) The on-call *General Manager*, with overall responsiblity for the Hospital.
(ii) The *Medical Controller (Consultant Physician on-call)*, responsible for the medical response. He will also decide which patients may be transferred and liaise with other hospitals. He is responsible for maintaining contact with the District and Regional Medical Officers.
(iii) The *Senior Nurse*, responsible for the allocation of nursing personnel, and for the co-ordination of ancillary services such as Central Sterile Supplies Department (CSSD) and Theatre Sterile Supplies Centre (TSSC).

Action cards for the controllers are held in the Control Room.

Routine activities in the *Operating Theatres, Fracture Clinic* and *Orthopaedic Clinic* will automatically cease. Normal activities will continue in other Out-Patient areas and B Floor X-Ray unless instructed otherwise by Hospital Control.

Communications

Communications are always difficult in Major Accidents. Facilities available are:

(1) *Scene to Hospital*: The Flying Squad is equipped with two Cellnet telephones— numbers are available from the Accident Department. The Ambulance radio network may also be available for communications with the scene.
(2) *Within the Hospital*: Telephones and intercoms will be available as usual but are likely to be very busy; their use is not recommended. Direct paging should be used when possible. Hospital Control will provide key personnel with two-way radios. Runners will be used.

Staff will be called in by a cascade system. The initial call will be from switchboard and thereafter further calls are the responsibility of the first person contacted. Staff should not attempt to telephone the hospital for information. Departmental plans require up-to-date lists of staff and their home telephone numbers.

Medical plan

The overall medical response will be controlled by the *Medical Controller* based in *Hospital Control*.

Direct clinical control rests with the A & E Consultant in charge of the Department and the *Clinical Controller*. The A & E Consultant, based in the Accident Department will take charge of the immediate treatment, resuscitation, diagnosis and disposal of patients as they arrive.

The *Clinical Controller* is the *Orthopaedic Consultant* on call: he will be situated on the *Receiving Ward* (F19, West Block) and will take charge of patients as they are admitted.

The anaesthetic response will be controlled by the *Consultant Anaesthetist on call*, based in the Adult Intensive Care Unit.

A senior member of medical staff will be designated by the Medical Controller to work in the operating theatres to decide priorities in conjunction with the *Clinical Controller* and the *Theatre Manager*.

On call medical staff will be called by the switchboard: *they will be told where to go*. The calling in of off duty staff will be the responsibility of the department concerned.

A Medical Volunteer Bureau will be established in the *Junior Doctors Mess* (C Floor, East Block) and run by the *General Medical Senior Registrar*. All doctors who have no specific reporting area should report there for allocation to treatment areas.

If a large number of children are involved, Ward D34 (East Block) is the designated *Receiving Ward* and the *Consultant Paediatrician on call* becomes responsible for the activities of the Paediatric Unit.

Support services

Key personnel in each Department will be contacted by the *Switchboard* or through *Hospital Control*. Each Department is responsible for calling in on a cascade system. It is the responsibility of each discipline and manager to ensure that the call out lists are kept up-to-date and are available to key personnel.

The *Medical Records* response will be controlled from the Accident and Emergency Department. Patients will be identified and documented as they leave the Accident and Emergency Department.

Any major difficulties encountered should be communicated immediately to the Hospital Control. However, all Departments will be staffed and routine requests should be directed to the Department concerned.

Liaison personnel for Pharmacy, Medical Equipment Supplies Unit (MESU) and the Mortuary will be located in the Accident and Emergency Department.

Arrangements for relatives and enquiries about patients

Relatives of casualites will be accommodated in the *Day Hospital* on A Floor. The *Hospital Chaplaincy* is responsible for this service.

Telephone enquiries about possible casualties will be directed to the *Enquiry Bureau*, organised and staffed by the *Social Work Department*, which will operate in conjunction with the *Police Casualty Bureau* at Hucknall.

No information about casualty identification will be released by anybody until the identification has been confirmed and the Hospital Controller has approved the release.

The identification of deceased patients is the responsibility of the Police in their capacity as *Coroners Officers*.

Arrangements for staff

It is important that those managing Departmental responses ensure that staff are available throughout the incident. This will probably involve a phased call out after an assessment of the likely duration has been obtained from Hospital Control.

As soon as practicable after the incident, comprehensive de-briefing will take place. All staff involved should attend de-briefing sessions. This will serve both to clarify any problems that arose and as a forum to ventilate feelings.

Formal counselling will be available for any staff who require it. Arrangements will be publicised.

Departmental Managers must be sensitive to the needs of those who were not involved. Complex emotions are generated in all those who work in a Hospital which has been involved in a Major Accident and, if these are not recognised, destructive divisions may appear.

Aftermath

Planned activity within the Hospital is likely to be disrupted for some time after the incident. *Out-patients* and *operating lists* may be cancelled. Limitations will be decided by the General Manager and arrangements made to notify patients and staff.

The media

There will be immediate interest from the press. The *General Manager* or representative is responsible for *press and media relations* and will arrange press conferences and other contacts between Hospital staff, patients and journalists. It is important that all press and media information is channelled through one person. Spontaneous remarks and comments and incautious statements can cause immense distress to patients and their relatives, as well as creating organisational difficulties for the Hospital.

Summary of the major accident plan for the Accident and Emergency Department

Role of department

The Department will provide resuscitation and immediate treatment for all patients involved in the Accident. Personnel from the Department will provide on site medical and nursing staff. Information about identity of casualties will be gathered in the Department.

Overview of plan

All patients will enter through the Walking Injured entrance, receive initial documentation and be triaged into treatment categories as they enter. Critically ill patients will go to the Emergency Room, patients on stretchers will go to the Main Department and Walking injured will be treated in Fracture Clinic. Documentation will be completed as the patient leaves the Department.

Control and reporting point

The A & E Department will be run by an A & E Consultant and Senior Nurse. They will be mobile but identifiable by means of a yellow tabard. Each treatment area will be supervised by senior personnel wearing a red tabard. All staff should report to them on arrival.

Callout procedures

The A & E Consultants will be contacted by switchboard. Further callout will be undertaken by a student nurse. Staff arriving must report to the Doctor/Nurse in Charge.

Action cards

Action cards are kept in the Sisters' Office in the Central Area.

Communications

Contact must be maintained with: the site, Hospital Control Room, the Receiving Ward, Intensive Care Unit and Theatres. This will be achieved by the Cellnet telephone, internal telephones and runners. Liaison personnel from the Mortuary, Pharmacy and TSSU will be in the Department.

Effect on normal activities

All patients arriving whilst the plan is in operation will be processed through the documentaton and triage system.

Aftermath

After standdown has been declared by the Hospital Control normal activities will resume immediately. If it is necessary to cancel follow-up Clinics, Hospital Control will be notified and undertake notification of affected patients.

Accident and Emergency Department major incident plan

Objectives within the department

To estimate the scale and nature of the incident and to remain informed of changes in the scale and nature of the incident.

To provide initial assistance at the scene.

To prepare maximum possible accommodation and equipment within a temporarily expanded A & E Department.

To utilise available staff of appropriate disciplines and competence.

To alert the Hospital switchboard and to initiate the hospital Major Incident plan.

To treat Major Incident victims requiring hospitalisation and limit their use of A & E resources to the minimum necessary for diagnosis, emergency treatment and referral for subsequent treatment.

To provide definitive treatment for Walking Injured.

To plan and implement action within the A & E Department beyond the initial response stage.

To control the response within the A & E Department and maintain it at a level which matches the changing level of the incident.

To maintain communications with Hospital Control Room, the Receiving Ward and the scene of the incident.

Reorganisation

The A & E Department will be re-organised to create:

A triage area (Reception and main waiting area)

A Walking Injured area (Fracture Clinic)

A stretcher patient/resuscitation area (Emergency Room and Main Department)

A holding area for stretcher patients awaiting a cubicle (Central Area)

An area for stretcher patients waiting for treatment and/or admission (Admissions Room—A1154)

A unique Major Incident documentation/patient identity system

A facility to identify patients as they leave the department

A "Patient Flow" system to prevent avoidable congestion in the Department

A Bed Bureau Control Centre

Normal routine patient property procedures within the Department will be suspended.

Accident and Emergency Department action cards

A & E Medical action card 1

SENIOR A & E DOCTOR 1

(1) A large number of casualties may be expected soon.

(2) Assess scale and nature of incident from information on the Major Incident Form A/E1.

(3) If the A & E Major Incident Plan only has been implemented, decide if the Hospital Major Incident Plan should be implemented and, if so, inform the Senior A & E Nurse who will advise the hospital switchboard. When alerted, the switchboard operators will contact all staff identified in the Hospital Major Incident Plan until you instruct otherwise.

(4) If there is a chemical hazard contact ambulance control for HAZCHEM information.

(5) If there is a radiation hazard, assistance is available from the Medical Physics Department. The procedure and call out list is in the radiation cupboard in the paediatric dirty utility room (A1112). A spare key is held in the adult A & E Sisters office (A1016).

(6) A yellow tabard is provided for you to wear so that you are clearly identified and you will work with the senior A & E Sister, who will also wear a yellow tabard. Neither of you should become involved with direct patient care.

(7) The A & E and other SHOs already present in the Department should be deployed in clearing patients from the Department as quickly as possible (A & E Medical Action Card 7).

(8) Your main duties include:
8.1 Promotion of smooth patient flow within and out of the A & E Department.
8.2 Assessment of information from the scene of the incident. If you conclude that the capacity of the A & E department to cope is likely to be exceeded,

inform the Medical Controller of the need to divert casualties from the scene to the supporting hospital(s).

8.3 Allocation of medical staff as they arrive. The number assigned to each area will depend on the number of patients in each triage category. The areas to be staffed are:

Triage
Resuscitation Area
Stretcher Area
Walking Injured Area
Paediatric A & E
A & E X-Ray if necessary (see para. 12 below)

(9) The doctor in charge of triage and the doctor in charge of resuscitation should be senior A & E Staff.

(10) Patients will not be sent from triage to the Walking Injured Area until you confirm to the doctor in charge of triage that there is a doctor in this area.

(11) At your discretion, A & E Theatres may be converted into an extra resuscitation area; in this case, the lower dressings cubicles may be used for minor surgery and suturing.

(12) If possible, each seriously ill patient should have a doctor and nurse allocated to them. If this is not possible, a doctor must be stationed in A & E X-Ray to ensure medical supervision of patients there.

(13) As demand subsides in an area, re-deploy the staff to other tasks (see plan of Department overleaf).

A & E Nursing action card 1

SENIOR NURSE 1

(1) A large number of casualties may be expected soon.

(2) A yellow tabard is provided for you to wear.

(3) You will take no direct part in patient care, but will work with the senior doctor and retain overall operational control of the A & E Department for the duration of the A & E Major Incident Plan.

(4) After consultation with the senior A & E Doctor immediately available inform the Hospital Switchboard that the A & E Major Incident Plan is in operation and request implementation of the Hospital Major Incident Plan.

(5) Ensure that the A & E reception, X-Ray, Paediatric A & E, Fracture Clinic and the A & E porter(s) are informed.

(6) The A & E Consultant on call will act as the Site Medical Officer: if he is prevented from reaching the Hospital by the Incident, the on call registrar will go but he *must not* leave until the Department is ready to receive casualties.

(7) Nominate, and give Action Cards to, the Sisters and Staff Nurses who will be in charge of:

Reception Area
Stretcher and Resuscitation Area
Walking Injured Area (Fracture Clinic Sister, if possible)
X-Ray Department (A & E X-Ray)—used for stretcher patients

Admissions Room

(8) Nominate a student nurse to undertake the call-out of A & E Staff (Nursing Action Card 6). She can call in Paediatric staff if necessary.

(9) Consider switching off the automatic opening devices for all the entrance doors to the Department. Bolt shut one of the stretcher entrance doors. Wedge open the A & E Reception doors. The switches are situated by the plant room at the Walking Injured entrance.

(10) Wedge open the pair of smoke doors between the reception and A & E Porters desk

(11) Arrange for existing untreated A & E patients in the waiting area to be informed of what is happening and advised to leave and seek treatment from their G.P.s.

(12) With the senior doctor, allocate nursing and medical staff as they arrive: the allocation to each area will vary according to the changing numbers of patients in each category.

(13) Issue A & E Nursing Action Card 3 to a student nurse to assist and act as runner to the nurse in charge of triage.

(14) Nominate student nurses to assist and act as runners to the nurses in charge of:
Stretcher Area and Resuscitation
Walking Injured
X-Ray
Holding Area (Admissions Room)

(15) If patients are dead on arrival at hospital, the bodies may be stored in the Clinic Area until personnel are available to transfer them to the Mortuary. If this happens, contact the Mortuary who will send a technician to take charge of property procedures.

(16) Maintain liaison with the Senior Nurse on duty for the Hospital. A member of the General Managers staff will act as liaison between the Department and the Hospital Control Room.

(17) Ensure that the nurse in charge of Resuscitation has identified an RGN who will stay by the controlled drugs (CD) cupboard and take charge of the issue of CDs and be responsible for recording their destination and the name of the doctor prescribing in the CD Register.

(18) Only people having legitimate business in the Department should be allowed in; do not hesitate to call Security or the Police to maintain order.

(19) Walking Injured patients will be X-rayed in the Orthopaedic Clinic X-Ray, all stretcher patients will be taken to A & E X-Ray.

(20) If there is a large number of children amongst the casualties, be prepared to implement the Paediatric Plan. This can be implemented by the Paediatric A & E Department. You should be prepared to lend a learner nurse to carry out their callout.

(21) Support Departments (including Pharmacy, TSSU, and Works) will send a member of staff to act as liaison officer. You should relay requirements to them.

(22) See attached plans of whole Department and Walking Injured area.

Appendix B
The major emergency plan for the Mid-Western Health Board, Republic of Ireland

J PAUL ROBINSON

Introduction

Dealing with emergencies is part of their normal work for many Health Board employees. In particular staff of the Ambulance Service and Accident and Emergency Departments are trained and experienced in coping with emergencies on a daily basis.

There are however certain rare events which, if they occur, will tend to overwhelm the normal health services. This may be due to their magnitude, duration, intensity or speed of onset. Alternatively the fact that key medical facilities and/or personnel are involved and thus rendered ineffective may be the major problem. Such events include aircraft accidents, train crashes, major fires and chemical explosions. These events are often known as Disasters and in Ireland, for planning purposes, have been designated as Major Emergencies.

Major Emergency Planning is a process whereby organisations which may have to respond to a Major Emergency prepare for such an event. The process includes an examination of the potential hazards, the preparation of Major Emergency Plans, the exercising of these plans and the co-ordination of the planning process with other potential responding organisations.

Each Garda Division, Local Authority and Health Board has an individual Major Emergency Plan [MEP] and it has been agreed that, in the event of a Major Emergency, the Plans of the three local emergency services will be activated so as to provide a co-ordinated response.

The Major Emergency Plans of the Local Authorities and the Gardai are largely based on the provision of services in the location and at the time when the Major Emergency occurs. However, in the event of a Major Emergency the Health Board will most likely be required to provide a multiplicity of services at a number of locations over a considerable period of time. This makes Emergency Planning for the Health Board quite difficult, but also extremely important.

To facilitate interservice communication the Ambulance and Communications Centre, Dooradoyle, Limerick has been designated as the contact point for the Mid-Western Health Board in the event of a Major Emergency being declared by either the Gardai or a Local Authority.

It is the intention of the Health Board that victims of any Major Emergency should be examined on the site by a medical officer, stabilised as necessary, transported to hospital (in a sequence determined by medical priorities) and treated in hospital. It is not intended that any "field hospital" type operation be established. It should also be noted that the health services do not have a rescue role in the event of a Major Emergency.

This Plan is intended to provide Health Board staff and other organisations with a guide to the general strategies which the Mid-Western Health Board intends to employ in the event of a Major Emergency. More detailed plans have been prepared for individual service units within the Board. The most important of these subplans is the Emergency Plan for the Regional Hospital Limerick, which has been designated as the main receiving hospital in the Board area in the event of a Major Emergency. At a lower level Action Cards have been prepared for many individuals specifying the actions to be taken in the event of a Major Emergency.

Copies of all of these Plans and Action Cards are maintained at the relevant locations as well as in the MEP File. The MEP File is a reference document containing:

- Detailed plans for various institutions and services

- Action Cards for individuals and

- Lists of persons and organisations which might be useful during a Major Emergency, with relevant addresses and telephone numbers

---

Copies of the MEP File are maintained at the Ambulance and Communications Centre, the Regional Hospital, and Central Office.

It is expected that all relevant staff members will acquaint themselves with this Plan as well as with the service Plan and/or Action Card applicable to their own position. It is not possible to specify every detail in a Plan such as this, but it is intended that the Plan should be exercised at regular intervals so that staff will be aware of the particulars of their own roles as well as the roles of others.

The Plan

This Plan sets out the procedures to be followed by the personnel and Services of the Mid-Western Health Board in the event of a Major Emergency being declared. In such an event this Plan will be activated as well as the corresponding Plans of the relevant Local Authority and the relevant Garda Division so as to provide a co-ordinated response.

Important

- The variations possible in the event of a Major Emergency are so numerous that no Plan can provide for all possible events which could occur

- This Plan therefore is to be regarded as flexible and must not hinder individuals in the use of initiative and common sense when dealing with situations as they arise

---

The aim of the Plan is to facilitate the Health Board in the mobilising of all necessary and available resources, both within and from outside the Board, and in the use of such resources to best advantage.

Major Emergencies

A Major Emergency is any event which causes or threatens:

- Death or injury

- Serious destruction of essential services or

- Damage to property *beyond the normal capabilities* of the Gardai, Local Authorities and Health Services

---

This definition is based on the relationship between an emergency and the available resources and may be difficult to adjudicate on in some cases. For this reason the existence of twenty serious casualties can be used as a guide in the decision to declare a Major Emergency.

Where an authorised officer of the Gardai, the Local Authority or the Health Board becomes aware that a Major Emergency has occurred or is imminent the Major Emergency Plan is to be activated. If, on the other hand, the situation is such that in the judgement of the authorised officer a Major Emergency may arise a Major Emergency Alert can be declared.

A list of the officers authorised to activate the Plan for all of the emergency agencies, together with their home and office telephone numbers, is maintained in the MEP File.

Functions of emergency services

The functions of the emergency services in a Major Emergency have been agreed and are detailed in the MEP File.

These can be summarised as:

Health Board:

- Medical Assistance at the Site

- Assessment of Casualties

- Ambulance Transport

- Hospital Treatment

- Welfare Services and Counselling

- Certification of the Dead

Local Authority:

- Extinguishing Fires
- Containment of Chemical Spills
- Rescue of Persons and Property
- Control of "Danger Areas"
- Provision of Food and Rest Facilities at the Site
- Provision of Emergency Accommodation

Gardai:

- Maintenance of Law and Order
- Securing of the Site
- Traffic and Crowd Control
- Provision of Information on Casualties
- Arrangements for the Dead

Major Emergency Alert

A Major Emergency Alert can be declared by any of the persons authorised to activate the Major Emergency Plan (see Activation of the Plan). The activating officer will immediately notify the Ambulance and Communications Centre.

All messages shall begin with the following statement:

"This is . . . . of the Mid-Western Health Board/Garda Siochana/Local Authority

There is a possibility that a Major Emergency will occur at . . . .

If necessary, the Major Emergency Plan will be put into operation

Further information will follow

Implement Alert Procedures"

Alert Procedures

The officer on duty at the Ambulance and Communications Centre will implement Emergency Alert Procedures.

These procedures are detailed on the relevant Action Cards and in the main consist of the notification of the Alert to:

- The Telephone Operator
- The different Ambulance Stations and
- Senior Ambulance Service Personnel

Activation of the Plan

The Health Board Major Emergency Plan can be activated by:

The Chief Executive Officer,
The Deputy Chief Executive Officer,
The Chief Ambulance Officer,
The Ambulance Controller,
or an officer acting in any of these posts.

The Plan will be automatically activated on notification by the Gardai or Local Authority that their Major Emergency Plans have been activated.

A Health Board Officer activating the Plan shall arrange for immediate notification to the Ambulance and Communications Centre and the relevant Garda Division

All such messages shall begin with the following statement:

"This is . . . . of the Mid-Western Health Board/Garda Siochana/Local Authority

A Major Emergency has occurred/is imminent at . . . .

The Major Emergency Plan is now in operation"

Notification of Ambulance and Communications Centre

Any Alert or Activation of the Plan must be notified immediately to the Ambulance and Communications Centre and therefore it is here that the mobilisation of the Health Board response to the emergency will begin.

If any Ambulance Centre, Hospital or other Health Service is notified of an Alert or a Major Emergency by any source other than the Ambulance and Communications Centre they must notify the Ambulance and Communications Centre immediately, if possible by transferring the call

Mobilisation

When the officer on duty at the Ambulance and Communications Centre is notified of the activation of the Plan he/she will attempt to verify that the Plan has been activated by an authorised officer and will collect as much information as possible on the location and nature of the Major Emergency.

- At this stage the action to be taken by the officer on duty will depend on the nature of the Major Emergency, but in almost all cases where there may be victims requiring medical attention the officer will implement the Ambulance Mobilisation Procedures

- As soon as possible the officer will notify the telephone operator on duty in the Ambulance and Communications Centre of the activation of the Plan and will thereafter provide updates of information to the operator as these become available

---

Ambulance Mobilisation

The ambulance mobilisation procedures are detailed on the relevant Action Card and in summary consist of:

- The dispatch of one or more ambulances to the site as necessary.

- The call up of extra ambulance personnel, including the Chief Ambulance Officer and other senior staff.

- The dispatch of an ambulance to the Regional Hospital to collect a Site Medical Team (if such is required) as soon as one is available

- The dispatch of the Mobile Control and Equipment Carrier Vehicle and further ambulances as available to the site, if required.

Site Organisation

The Major Emergency may be spread over a wide area or may be concentrated on a reasonably sized site. Communication between the site of the Major Emergency and the Ambulance and Communications Centre is vital so that information on the numbers and condition of casualties can be provided quickly and accurately to the various services within the Board. For this reason the first ambulance to arrive at the site will normally act as a communication centre for Health Board Personnel and will remain on the site until replaced by an alternative means of communication.

Where practical, the procedures for site organisation, which have been agreed between the emergency services, will be implemented. These procedures are detailed in the MEP File and on the relevant Action Cards

---

In general it has been agreed that each service will designate a Controller of Site Operations and that the three Controllers of Operations will each control, direct and co-ordinate the activities of their own service at the site and will communicate with one another so as to ensure effective co-ordination of the three services

---

The only exception to the above shall be in those situations where a "Danger Area" is deemed to exist by the Senior Fire Officer present, in which case all activities in that area will be under the control of the Senior Fire Officer.

An idealised layout of the responding services at the site of a Major Emergency is detailed in the MEP File. It has been agreed that where possible the services assembling at the site will organise themselves in accordance with this layout or, where such is not possible, an alternative layout as agreed by the three Controllers.

Arrangements for securing the perimeter of the site are the responsibility of the Gardai. Services and personnel arriving at the perimeter of the site shall be directed by the Gardai to their respective holding areas to await deployment.

Controller of Site Operations—Health Services

The Controller of Site Operations for the Mid-Western Health Board shall be the Chief Ambulance Officer or a designated alternate nominated by him.

> The functions of the Controller of Site Operations are detailed on the relevant Action Card and in brief include control, direction and co-ordination of the activities of all Health Board Services at the site, consultation and liaison with the Controllers of Site Operations of the Gardai and the Fire Authority, communication with other agencies operating at the site and the provision of secure communications with the Ambulance and Communications Centre, the Regional Hospital and other hospitals as necessary

Site Medical Team

> Where considered necessary by the Controller of Site Operations or Senior Ambulance Officer at the site a Mobile Medical Team and a Site Medical Officer will be dispatched from the Regional Hospital by ambulance to the site

The functions of the Mobile Medical Team and the Site Medical Officer are detailed on the relevant Action Cards and in brief include *the saving of life* and *the alleviation of pain, establishment of a casualty collection point, the survey of casualties, the maintenance of communication links with the Regional Hospital Medical Co-Ordinator, the allotment of casualties to designated and supporting hospitals,* in consultation with the Hospital Medical Co-Ordinator, and *the certification of the dead.*

Casualties

> The Regional Hospital Limerick has been designated as the main receiving hospital for the Mid-Western Health Board. It is not possible to be specific in relation to all possible incidents but in general it is intended that, where practical, all seriously injured victims should be transferred to that hospital

If the numbers of injured are large and/or if the incident occurs close to another hospital it may be more practical to transport less seriously injured to such other hospital, for example Ennis General, Nenagh General or St. John's Hospital.

In the event of large numbers of seriously injured victims it may be necessary to seek assistance in the form of Ambulances and staff from other Health Boards/ Hospitals or it may be considered prudent to move some victims to acute hospitals outside the Mid-Western Health Board region. In general such decisions will be taken by the Hospital Co-ordinating Group at the Regional Hospital (see Site Organisation).

In the case of incidents involving injured and dead victims priority will, of course, be given to the injured.

However as soon as possible a temporary mortuary should be designated and this mortuary will be under the control of the Gardai.

> The Health Board will provide general information only, such as the numbers being treated and the types of injuries involved (see media liaison)

It has been agreed that all information concerning individual victims will be communicated to the media, relatives and the public by the Gardai.

Regional Hospital, Limerick

(A) HOSPITAL EMERGENCY CO-ORDINATING GROUP

A Major Emergency Plan for the Regional Hosptial has been developed and copies of same are maintained at the hospital and in the MEP File. In brief this Plan envisages the mobilisation of the Hospital Emergency Co-ordinating Group, which will consist of the Hospital Medical Co-ordinator, the Senior Nursing Officer and the Senior Hospital Administrator/Deputy and will be based in the hospital control room for the duration of the emergency. The Hospital Emergency Co-ordinating Group will manage the response of the hospital to the emergency and will liaise (through the Senior Hospital Administrator) with the Crisis Management Team (see later) in relation to the need for additional resources, relations with the media etc.

(B) ACTION CARDS

A series of Action Cards has been prepared for different members of the staff including Telephone Operators, Senior Nursing Officer, Hospital Medical Co-ordinator, Senior Hospital Administrator, etc.

It is expected that all relevant members of staff will operate in accordance with the appropriate Action Cards to provide a co-ordinated response to the emergency.

(C) TRAFFIC CONTROL

It is to be expected that any Major Emergency will generate large volumes of traffic involving casualties, relatives, media personnel, volunteers and sightseers.

There is a real danger in such a situation that access to and from the hospital may be blocked or seriously impeded.

Ancillary staff at the hospital may be required to assist porters and security staff in controlling vehicular traffic at the gates of the hospital and pedestrian traffic at the entrances to the hospital itself, so as to prevent major problems in this area.

It is also expected that the Gardai will provide valuable assistance in this area and all Health Board staff are expected to co-operate fully with the Gardai.

Ennis, Nenagh and St. John's Hospitals

- Major Emergency Plans on a lesser scale have been developed for Ennis General, Nenagh General and St. John's Hospitals.
- These Plans will be activated if required by the Hospital Co-ordinating group at the Regional Hospital.
- Control of traffic and persons will also be important at these hospitals.

General Practitioners

- With hospital medical services stretched by a Major Emergency the assistance of General Practitioners is likely to be required both on the site and in hospitals. This will certainly be the case if the emergency is of long duration and staff on duty must be relieved
- General Practitioners whose services at the site of a Major Emergency are required will be contacted personally or by local radio announcement and asked to report to the Site Medical Officer/Site Medical Team for instructions and deployment
- Likewise any General Practitioner required in a hospital will be asked to report to the Hospital Medical Co-ordinator for instructions and deployment

Hazardous Substances

- The extent of transport and storage of hazardous substances in the Mid-West Area means that a major emergency may involve the release of such substances and the contamination of persons and/or surrounding areas
- All staff involved at Major Emergency Sites should be conscious of the possibility of such contamination and where any suspicion of danger exists the advice and direction of the Senior Fire Officer on duty should be sought and followed

Crisis Management Team

The Health Board Crisis Management Team is a management group which consists of the Chief Executive Officer, the Deputy C.E.O. and other senior Officers of the Board.

This team may be assembled by the C.E.O. or the Deputy C.E.O. if such is considered necessary.

The team will normally be assembled during emergencies which are of particular severity and/or which continue for an extended period of time.

When assembled the team will control, direct and co-ordinate the overall response of the Health Board to the Major Emergency. The Team will communicate with the management of the other responding services so as to achieve maximum co-ordination as well as with outside organisations such as the Department of Health.

The Crisis Management Team will meet in the Programme Manager's office at the Regional Hospital (or, should this not be suitable, in the C.E.O.'s office at Central Office).

The Crisis Management Team will collect and collate all available information, establish where extra resources are required, mobilise these resources from within the Health Board, from other Health Boards, from private concerns or from any other places where these might be available and apply these resources to the optimum effect.

The Crisis Management Team will include a media liaison officer who will be responsible for providing the media with all available, appropriate information (excluding information on individual casualties—see Casualties).

The team may also use the media to communicate to the public any information which may be relevant.

Inter-Service Co-ordination Remote from the Site

It has been argued that a Co-ordinating Group, comprising senior representatives of the Health Board, Local Authorities and Gardai, may be called together at the discretion of any of the group at any time following the activation of the Major Emergency Plan. The members of the Group are the Chief Executive of the Health Board, the County or City Manager in whose area of responsibility the emergency has occurred and the Garda Chief Superintendent or Superintendent in whose district the emergency has occurred or the designate alternates of any of these officials.

The functions of the Co-ordinating Group are detailed in full in the MEP File and in brief include the monitoring of the activity of all agencies responding to the emergency, the maintenance of liaison between these agencies, the provision of information to Government and the distribution of information to the news media and the general public.

Resources

A list of agencies and persons whose services may be useful in an Emergency, complete with telephone numbers and contact names, where applicable, is available in the MEP File.

Welfare and Support

Welfare and Support Services which are likely to be required in the event of a Major Emergency have been identified. These services include the provision of material support to relatives and victims. A Plan to mobilise such services has been prepared and can be activated by contacting the persons nominated in the Plan.

Counselling

- It is to be expected that, in the aftermath of any major disaster, many of the survivors, as well as the professionals responding to the disaster, may be traumatised by the events.

- A Plan has been developed whereby expert counsellors can be made available to provide support for those who may require it.

- These counsellors will include health professionals such as social workers, psychiatrists, psychologists, religious and members of voluntary groups.

- A copy of this Plan is also available in the MEP File and the Plan can be activated by contacting the persons so nominated in the Plan.

Voluntary Organisations

During a Major Emergency, when resources may be stretched to the limit or beyond, voluntary organisations can play a vital role in support of the statutory services.

The availability of volunteers to move existing patients from acute hospitals to other hospitals or to perform similar tasks may release Health Board services for use in the response to the emergency.

It has been agreed that, if required, the services of certain voluntary organisations, including *Order of Malta, St. John Ambulance* and *Irish Red Cross*, can be requested by the Chief Ambulance Officer. In the event of their being mobilised, voluntary ambulance crews will assemble at the Ambulance and Communications Centre and await instructions from the Chief Ambulance Officer

---

Stand Down

Since the response of the Health Board to a major emergency is likely to involve a number of different services at different locations it is likely a single stand down will not usually be appropriate. In this situation individual units will normally be stood down on the instructions of the C.E.O. or his designated alternate following consultation with other Emergency Services as appropriate.

Index